PROFESSIONAL ISSUES IN MIDWIFERY

LYNETTE A. AMENT, PhD, CNM, RN, FACNM

Associate Professor and Chair
Department of Nursing
University of New Hampshire
Durham, New Hampshire

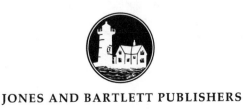

JONES AND BARTLETT PUBLISHERS
Sudbury, Massachusetts

World Headquarters

Jones and Bartlett Publishers
40 Tall Pine Drive
Sudbury, MA 01776
978-443-5000
info@jbpub.com
www.jbpub.com

Jones and Bartlett Publishers Canada
6339 Ormindale Way
Mississauga, Ontario L5V 1J2
Canada

Jones and Bartlett Publishers
International
Barb House, Barb Mews
London W6 7PA
United Kingdom

Jones and Bartlett's books and products are available through most bookstores and online booksellers. To contact Jones and Bartlett Publishers directly, call 800-832-0034, fax 978-443-8000, or visit our website www.jbpub.com.

Substantial discounts on bulk quantities of Jones and Bartlett's publications are available to corporations, professional associations, and other qualified organizations. For details and specific discount information, contact the special sales department at Jones and Bartlett via the above contact information or send an email to specialsales@jbpub.com.

The authors, editor, and publisher have made every effort to provide accurate information. However, they are not responsible for errors, omissions, or for any outcomes related to the use of the contents of this book and take no responsibility for the use of the products and procedures described. Treatments and side effects described in this book may not be applicable to all people; likewise, some people may require a dose or experience a side effect that is not described herein. Drugs and medical devices are discussed that may have limited availability controlled by the Food and Drug Administration (FDA) for use only in a research study or clinical trial. Research, clinical practice, and government regulations often change the accepted standard in this field. When consideration is being given to use of any drug in the clinical setting, the health care provider or reader is responsible for determining FDA status of the drug, reading the package insert, and reviewing prescribing information for the most up-to-date recommendations on dose, precautions, and contraindications, and determining the appropriate usage for the product. This is especially important in the case of drugs that are new or seldom used.

Production Credits
Executive Editor: Kevin Sullivan
Production Director: Amy Rose
Associate Editor: Amy Sibley
Production Editor: Carolyn F. Rogers
Associate Production Editor: Daniel Stone
Senior Marketing Manager: Emily Ekle
Cover Design: Kristin E. Ohlin
Cover Image: © Photos.com
Composition: Auburn Associates, Inc.
Printing and Binding: Malloy, Inc.
Cover Printing: Malloy, Inc.

Library of Congress Cataloging-in-Publication Data
Professional issues in midwifery / [edited by] Lynette Ament.
     p. ; cm.
     Includes bibliographical references and index.
     ISBN-13: 978-0-7637-2836-6 (pbk.)
     ISBN-10: 0-7637-2836-5 (pbk.)
        1. Midwifery—United States. 2. Childbirth—United States.
     3. Maternal health services—United States.   I. Ament, Lynette A.
     [DNLM: 1. Nurse Midwives—United States. 2. Midwifery
     —United States.   WY 157 P964 2007]
     RG950.P76 2007
     618.2—dc22
                                                                              2006012335
6048

Printed in the United States of America
10 09 08 07 06 10 9 8 7 6 5 4 3 2 1

Dedication

To my daughters, Kaitlyn, Alyssa, and Mallory, for your love, patience, and support of me in all my endeavors. You have been my light in life, and may the three of you find peace and happiness in your lives.

Contents

Chapter 13   ***Historical Perspectives on Research and the ACNM*** ***263***
LISA L. PAINE

Chapter 14   ***Professional Ethics*** ***277***
JOYCE E. THOMPSON

Chapter 15   ***Women's Health and Midwifery*** ***301***
DEBBIE JESSUP

Preface

This book is designed to focus on the distinctly unique characteristics of the profession of midwifery in the United States. It is designed as a handbook to the profession of nurse–midwifery and midwifery, the American College of Nurse–Midwives, and public health and other programs affecting the health care of women and children. This book focuses on the current issues and future directions of midwifery and is an important addition for all midwives in the United States who desire to remain current in the core issues of practice.

This book is the primary source of professional issues for student nurse–midwives, student midwives, certified nurse–midwives and certified midwives. It presents a mix of approaches to address current issues in the profession and uses case examples to illustrate the salient points. Each chapter begins with learning objectives and ends with key summary points. Several chapters include end-of-chapter exercises to practice application of the content. Many chapters include a table entitled "For Your Professional Files" that list resources available from the American College of Nurse–Midwives that midwives should gather and keep readily accessible.

The objectives of *Professional Issues in Midwifery* are to:

1. Discuss the historical relationship between midwives, nurses, and physicians.
2. Discuss the history, function, and role of the American College of Nurse–Midwives.
3. Identify key aspects of midwifery research and evidence-based practice.
4. Demonstrate an understanding of credentialing mechanisms, including licensure and privileging.
5. Evaluate the role of midwives in the delivery of care to women and children in the United States.
6. Understand the need to keep pace with the changing health system expectations.
7. Describe evolving practice patterns and staffing arrangements, including interdisciplinary teams.
8. Focus on improving quality and patient safety.
9. Analyze the regulatory and legal environment that surrounds practice.
10. Provide a basis for understanding the regulatory and professional causes of contextual issues.
11. Provide midwives with knowledge that will enhance client-centered care and the profession.

Acknowledgments

The nurse–midwives who authored these chapters contributed time, expertise, and support to this work—thank you for your invaluable contributions. Many thank yous to the people who have provided support to and acknowledgment of this work, including my midwifery colleagues in the American College of Nurse–Midwives and my colleagues at the University of New Hampshire. Thank you to Deanne Williams, Marion McCartney, and Lisa Summers for their valuable input into content and format. Amy Sibley and Katilyn Crowley from Jones and Bartlett have been of tremendous assistance and have provided patient waiting. This work would not be possible without the efforts of many.

Contributors

Diane B. Boyer, CNM, PhD, FACNM
Professor Emerita
Niehoff School of Nursing
Loyola University of Chicago
Chicago, IL

Lisa Hanson, CNM, DNSc
Associate Professor
Marquette University College of Nursing
Milwaukee, WI

**Kathryn Shisler Harrod, RN, CNM, DNSc,
    APNP, FACNM**
Associate Professor
Marquette University College of Nursing
Milwaukee, WI

Carol Howe, CNM, DNSc, FACNM
Professor and Director, Nurse–Midwifery Program
Oregon Health & Science University
School of Nursing
Portland, OR

Barbara Hughes, CNM, MS, MBA, FACNM
Director, Exempla Certified Nurse–Midwives
Exempla Saint Joseph Hospital
Denver, CO

Debbie Jessup, CNM, PhD(c), FACNM
Fairfax Station, VA

Cecilia Jevitt, CNM, PhD, ARNP
Assistant Professor
Midwifery and Nursing
University of South Florida
Tampa, FL

Nancy K. Lowe, CNM, PhD, FACNM, FAAN
Professor, Nurse–Midwifery Program
Oregon Health & Science University
School of Nursing
Portland, OR

Marion McCartney, CNM
Director, Professional Services
American College of Nurse–Midwives
Silver Spring, MD

Willliam McCool, CNM, RN, PhD, FACNM
Director and Associate Professor of Midwifery
University of Pennsylvania
Philadelphia, PA

Lisa Paine, CNM, DrPH, FACNM, FAAN
Principal & Senior Consultant
The Hutchinson Dyer Group
Cambridge, MA

Heather Reynolds, CNM, MSN, FACNM
Associate Professor
Nurse–Midwifery Program
Yale University School of Nursing
New Haven, CT

Judith P. Rooks, CNM, MPH, MS, FACNM
Past-President, ACNM
Author of *Midwifery and Childbirth in America*
Portland, OR

Joan Slager, CNM, MSN, CPC
Director, Nurse–Midwifery
Bronson Women's Services
Kalamazoo, MI

Lisa Summers, CNM, DrPH
Professional Services
American College of Nurse–Midwives
Silver Spring, MD

**Joyce Thompson, RN, CNM, DrPH, FAAN,
    FACNM**
Lacey Professor of Community Health Nursing
Bronson School of Nursing
Western Michigan University
Kalamazoo, MI

Jackie Tillett, CNM, ND
Assistant Clinical Professor
Department of Obstetrics and Gynecology
University of Wisconsin Medical School
Milwaukee Clinical Campus
Milwaukee, WI

Deanne Williams, CNM, MS, FACNM
Executive Director
American College of Nurse–Midwives
Silver Spring, MD

CHAPTER 1

Relationships Between CNMs and CMs and Other Midwives, Nurses, and Physicians

Judith P. Rooks, CNM, MPH, MS, FACNM

This chapter focuses on the interfaces and relationships between mid-wives certified under the auspices of the American College of Nurse–Midwives (ACNM) or the American Midwifery Certification Board AMCB and other professionals with whom we have overlapping identities or roles.[1] Although the emphasis is on current intra- and inter-professional relationships and issues, historic information is needed to understand the current and evolving issues, many of which have developed in important new ways during the past few years.

Learning Objectives

1. Explain the difference between a certified nurse–midwife (CNM) and a midwife who was a nurse before becoming a direct-entry midwife.
2. Identify five significant differences between CNMs and certified professional midwives (CPMs), and three significant differences between CNMs and certified midwives (CMs).
3. Identify and discuss three benefits and three disadvantages associated with nurse–midwifery's strong historical and current association with nursing.
4. Explain why procedural due process is often compromised when CNMs are disciplined by a state board of nursing.

---

[1] See Chapter 2 for information about the American College of Nurse–Midwives (ACNM). See Chapter 5 for information about the American Midwifery Certification Board (AMCB).

5. Describe four differences between obstetrician–gynecologists (Ob/Gyns) and family physicians (FPs) that affect their relationships with midwives or reflect differences in their relationships with midwives.

Relationships Between ACNM-, ACC-, or AMCB-Certified Midwives and Other Midwives

Midwifery Around the World

The word "midwife" was derived from the old English "mid," which meant "with," and "wif," which meant "wife" or "woman." The literal meaning—to be with a woman during childbirth—is the *sine qua non* of midwifery. The simplest and most widely understood definition of a midwife is a woman who assists other women during childbirth.[2]

The International Confederation of Midwives (ICM) is an international nongovernmental organization that unites 85 national midwives' associations from over 75 countries. An official international definition of "the midwife" was developed by the World Health Organization (WHO) in 1965. A revised version was adopted by ICM in 1972 and by the International Federation of Gynecologists and Obstetricians (FIGO) in 1973. The current version was adopted by ICM in 2005 (International Confederation of Midwives [ICM], 2005):

> A midwife is a person who, having been regularly admitted to a midwifery educational program, duly recognized in the country in which it is located, has successfully completed the prescribed course of studies in midwifery and has acquired the requisite qualifications to be registered and/or legally licensed to practice midwifery.
>
> The midwife must be able to give the necessary supervision, care and advice to women during pregnancy, labor and the postpartum period, to conduct deliveries on her own responsibility and to care for the newborn and the infant. This care includes preventative measures, the detection of abnormal conditions in mother and child, the procurement of medical assistance and the execution of emergency measures in the absence of medical help. She has an important task in health counseling and education, not only for the women, but also within the family and the community. The work should involve antenatal education and preparation for parenthood and extends to certain areas of gynecology, family planning and child care. She may practice in hospitals, clinics, health units, domiciliary conditions or in any other service.

A *nurse–midwife* is a graduate of a midwifery education program designed for students who have already achieved the basic knowledge and skills of a professional nurse. In the

---

[2] Although a small percentage of U.S. midwives are men, the vast majority are women, and midwifery arose from the role of women. With apology to the few wonderful men who are midwives, I will use only female pronouns in reference to midwives in this chapter.

United States, nurse–midwives have usually been referred to as "nurse–midwives" rather than "midwives," although there is a trend towards emphasizing the concept of "midwife" and "midwifery." Although most midwives in the United Kingdom (UK) and many other countries are actually *nurse*–midwives, they are usually referred to as "midwives." Their nursing background is seen mainly as an educational prerequisite.

A *direct-entry midwife* is a person who became a midwife through an experiential or formal educational process that was not predicated on the assumption that all of its students are nurses. Direct-entry midwives are usually referred to just as "midwives." Their education must lead to mastery of many skills that nurse–midwives obtain during nursing education.

Whether a country's midwives are mainly nurse–midwives or direct-entry midwives depends on the history of the development of midwifery in that country. Although the midwifery education systems in many of the countries of continental Europe produce mostly direct-entry midwives, the history of midwifery in the United States led to the development of nurse–midwifery as the predominant form of professional midwifery in this country.

Midwives in the United States

Many kinds of midwives practice in the United States. This section describes them and provides information about them and the organizations that support them. Although nurse–midwives are the largest and predominant group of midwives in this country, other chapters in this book describe the ACNM and nurse–midwifery in detail. Thus the description here is very brief. Historically, the main dichotomy in the United States has been between nurse–midwives and direct-entry midwives.

Certified nurse–midwives (CNMs) are midwives who have completed a nurse–midwifery education program accredited by the ACNM and passed the National Certification Examination administered by the ACNM from 1971 through 1991, the ACNM Certification Council (ACC) from 1992 to mid-2005, and the American Midwifery Certification Board (AMCB) since then. CNMs practice legally in every U.S. jurisdiction. Most are licensed as registered nurses (RNs), although their legal authority to practice midwifery may be based on an additional license to practice as a CNM, an advanced registered nurse practitioner (ARNP), a nurse practitioner (NP), or a nurse specialist (Reed & Roberts, 2000).

Services provided by CNMs are covered by Medicaid, Medicare, and most private healthcare insurance programs. CNMs often care for high- as well as low-risk women and provide both reproductive and primary health care to women of all ages. But most CNMs spend the majority of their time in activities related to pregnancy and primary reproductive health care (Schuiling, Sipe, & Fullerton, 2005). They practice within many settings and arrangements including employment by hospitals, health maintenance organizations, and clinics; private practices with physicians; home birth practices; and private midwifery practices with births attended in hospitals or freestanding birth centers. All practice within arrangements that provide for medical consultation and collaborative management or referral of a client to a physician, as needed.

CNMs signed the birth certificates of 7.8% of all infants who were born alive in the United States in 2002, 10.6% of live infants who were born vaginally (not delivered by cesarean section), and 96% of all infants whose birth certificates were signed by any kind of midwife during that year. Only 3% of births attended by a CNM occurred in a site other than a hospital (Martin, Hamilton, Ventura, Menacker, & Park, 2002). The proportion of United States births attended by CNMs has increased every year since 1989—the first year for which this information was available.

Direct-Entry Midwifery in the United States

Primarily black, informally trained "granny midwives" attended births in poor and/or rural communities throughout the United States, especially in the southeast, until at least the middle of the 20th century. Women generally became granny midwives in response to a need in their communities. Some were designated by other community members to fill this role; some felt they had been "called." Their primary training was through apprenticeship to older midwives, who were often family members. They were important historically, but are now almost extinct. However, informally trained direct-entry midwives still serve some small populations of women who lack access to mainstream maternity care due to race, poverty, geographic isolation, or religious or other cultural reasons that make care provided in hospitals by male physicians unacceptable. Some states make exceptions to laws that require direct-entry midwives to be licensed to allow unlicensed midwives to provide care to members of particular religious or ethnic subcultures. Examples of this would be midwives who serve members of their own religious communities in the state of Washington and midwives who are part of a cultural tradition that includes the use of indigenous midwives in Alaska. Informally trained indigenous midwives in other countries are usually referred to as *traditional birth attendants* (TBAs).

The main form of direct-entry midwifery in the United States arose from the lay-midwifery/home-birth movement that developed during the 1960s and 1970s as part of a grass roots movement by women to reclaim power over their own bodies and births and because of the criticism of male-dominated, over-medicalized, institutionalized establishment obstetrics (Davis-Floyd, 2005; Gaskin, 1975; Rooks, 1997; Schutt, personal communication, 2005). Direct-entry midwifery is also strongly associated with some religions that emphasize the sanctity of the family and home. Focusing on home births, lay midwifery developed purposefully outside of mainstream medical institutions and authority (Rooks, 1997). During the 1970s, these lay midwives and their supporters organized a variety of means to train direct-entry home-birth midwives, ranging from a formal, vocational school based on the midwifery curriculum used in the Netherlands, to programs to improve the use of apprenticeship as the main means of direct-entry midwifery education (Davis-Floyd, 2005; Rooks, 1997).

In 1982, a group of these midwives founded the Midwives Alliance of North America (MANA) as an organization open to all midwives and their supporters in Canada, the United States, and Mexico (Rooks, 1997). In 1986, MANA established an Interim Registry Board, consisting of four direct-entry midwives and one CNM to develop and administer a written test of basic, entry-level knowledge essential for responsible home-birth midwifery practice. The board also established a registry to list the names of midwives who had passed the examination (Rooks, 1997). MANA adopted its own statement of the Core Competencies for Basic Midwifery Practice in 1990 and updated it in 1994 (Midwives

Alliance of North America [MANA], 2006). The test developed by the Interim Registry Board was administered for the first time in 1991.

Also in 1991, a group of direct-entry midwifery educators founded the Midwifery Education Accreditation Council (MEAC) (http://www.meacschools.org) and charged it with developing a process for accrediting direct-entry midwifery education programs based on the core competencies and guiding principles of midwifery care established by MANA. MEAC began to accredit direct-entry midwifery education programs in 1996. Twelve programs and institutions utilizing a variety of educational models—including one-on-one apprenticeship, distance learning, and classroom-based courses—had been accredited or pre-accredited by January 2005, including schools that give degrees (Midwifery Education Accreditation Council, 2005).[3] Most current direct-entry midwifery educational programs combine a strong apprenticeship/preceptorship component with didactic classes. In 2000, MEAC received federal government recognition as an accrediting agency for direct-entry midwifery schools from the U.S. Department of Education (Davis-Floyd, 2005). Three direct-entry midwifery schools have been approved for both loans and grants through the federal Title IV student financial aid programs (Myers-Ciecko, personal communication, February 2005).

In 1994, the Interim Registry Board became incorporated as the North American Registry of Midwives (NARM). NARM, which is separate from MANA, shifted the focus from registration to certification and began to implement a process for certifying experienced direct-entry midwives in 1995. The process was expanded to include entry-level midwives in 1996.

Certified professional midwives (CPMs) are direct-entry midwives who have met all NARM standards for the professional practice of midwifery based on the Midwives Model of Care used by MANA, MEAC, and NARM,[4] and MANA's statement of the Core Competencies for Midwifery Practice, which is the knowledge and skill required to provide continuity of prenatal, intrapartum, and postpartum/neonatal care to low-risk women and their newborns in out-of-hospital settings. Criteria for certification by NARM include

---

[3] The four MEAC-accredited degree-granting institutions are the National College of Midwifery in Taos, N.M.; the Midwives College of Utah, a distance-learning institution headquartered in Orem, Utah; Bastyr University, a naturopathic university near Seattle, Wash.; and Miami-Dade Community College, in Miami, Fla. States grant authority to institutions to grant degrees.

[4] The Midwives Model of Care is based on the fact that pregnancy and birth are normal life events. The Midwives Model of Care includes:

- monitoring the physical, psychological, and social well-being of the mother throughout the childbearing cycle
- providing the mother with individualized education, counseling and prenatal care, continuous hands-on assistance during labor and delivery, and postpartum support
- minimizing technological interventions
- identifying and referring women who require obstetrical attention

The application of this model has been proven to reduce the incidence of birth injury, trauma, and cesarean section.

educational requirements; experience requirements; skills requirements; current certification in adult plus either infant or neonatal cardiopulmonary resuscitation (CPR); and verification that the applicant midwife has developed and uses appropriate practice guidelines, informed consent statements, forms and handouts describing midwifery practice, and a plan for emergency care (North American Registry of Midwives, 2004).

The education requirement can be met by: (1) successful completion of a midwifery education program accredited by MEAC, (2) certification by the ACNM or AMCB, (3) legal recognition by 1 of 12 states whose educational requirements for direct-entry midwifery licensure meet NARM's standards,[5] or (4) completion of an educational process that has been individually assessed through NARM's competency-based Portfolio Evaluation Process (the "PEP program") and judged to meet NARM standards. The midwife's educational background must include both didactic and clinical experience and cover specified content as defined by MANA's Core Competencies statement, content covered in NARM's Written Examination and Skills Assessment, and listed primary references.

The clinical component of an individually evaluated PEP program must be at least one year in duration and include at least 1,350 clinical contact hours under the supervision of a preceptor who is either a nationally certified midwife (e.g., CPM, CNM, or CM) or licensed in any North American jurisdiction as a practitioner who specializes in maternity care. The clinical experience must include prenatal, intrapartal, postpartal, and newborn care provided by the applicant midwife under the supervision of one or more preceptor(s) who were present in the room in which the care was being provided by the applicant. The applicant must have participated in at least 40 births, including 20 in which she functioned as the primary midwife; 10 of those 20 must have taken place in a home or another nonhospital setting. Minimum numbers of prenatal exams, newborn exams, and postpartum exams conducted under supervision are also specified. Candidates seeking CPM certification on the basis of ACNM or AMCB certification must have functioned as the primary midwife or primary midwife under supervision for at least 10 births in homes or other out-of-hospital settings. Candidates using the PEP process must provide three professional letters of reference and pass the NARM Skills Assessment, as judged by an evaluator qualified by NARM.

Midwives with unconventional training and experience may be individually evaluated to determine if their education is equivalent to an educational program acceptable to NARM. Examples include midwives who received most or all of their training in a country other than the United States and midwives with extensive experience who cannot document having had supervision during births. Experienced midwives must have been in primary practice for a minimum of 5 years and have attended 50 births as the primary midwife.

Most CPMs are direct-entry midwives who practice in out-of-hospital settings. The CPM is the only national credential that requires out-of-hospital birth experience. Nineteen of the 21 states that regulate direct-entry midwifery practice require either the CPM credential and/or having passed the NARM Written Examination for licensure, certification, registration, or other forms of legal sanction (MANA, 2005a). As of February 2005, more

---

[5] Alaska, Arizona, California, Colorado, Florida, Louisiana, Montana, New Mexico, Oregon, South Carolina, Texas, and Washington as of January 2005.

than one thousand CPMs have been certified, an average of about 100 per year. Fewer than five CNMs have also been certified as CPMs.

In 2001, the National Association of Certified Professional Midwives (NACPM) was founded as the professional organization for CPMs. By the end of 2004, NACPM had developed and adopted a statement of the organization's philosophy, standards, and the scope of practice of a CPM.

Although most direct-entry midwives have committed themselves to professionalizing out-of-hospital midwifery in the United States, some others oppose state regulation of out-of-hospital midwifery and do not want to be licensed. Some from this group call themselves "plain midwives"; those who are religiously oriented may call themselves "Christian midwives." As mentioned earlier, some states that require licensure make exceptions for midwives who serve particular religious or ethnic populations.

Certified Midwives (CMs)

Members of the ACNM have long debated whether it is necessary for professional midwives in the United States to also be educated and licensed as nurses (Reed & Roberts, 2000). This desire for separation was particularly strong among CNMs in New York, who were educated about this issue by Dorothea Lang, a past president of the ACNM (1975–1977) and long-time director of the Maternal and Infant Care Project of New York City. Dorothea's own birth in Japan in the 1940s was attended by professional midwives who were not nurses. Influenced by her, a committed group of New York CNMs began to envision and later lobby for a bill that would establish midwifery as an independent profession that is not regulated under the board of nursing in New York State (Davis-Floyd, 2005). Such a law was passed in 1992.

Although it does not require licensed midwives (LMs) to have completed a nursing education program, the N.Y. Midwifery Practice Act of 1992 requires applicants who are not nurses to have obtained "nursing equivalency" within their program of midwifery education. The N.Y. State Education Department Office of Comparative Education evaluates the curricula of specific non-nurse midwifery education programs to determine if they meet the state's criteria for nursing equivalency (Davis-Floyd, 2005). Applicants must also pass a written examination.

Influenced by developments in New York, ACNM members participating in the college's 1994 annual business meeting passed a motion urging the ACNM and ACC to develop processes to accredit direct-entry midwifery education programs and test and certify graduates of those programs in order to produce direct-entry midwives who are not nurses but are comparable to CNMs in all other ways. The first direct-entry midwifery education program designed to meet ACNM accreditation standards was opened by the State University of New York (SUNY) Downstate Medical Center in Brooklyn, in affiliation with the North Central Bronx Hospital, in 1996. SUNY Downstate's long-standing nurse–midwifery education program was combined with the direct-entry program as a single postbaccalaureate program with one track for nurses and one for other college graduates. Three new courses were designed to teach specified nursing and health care competencies to the direct-entry students. The two tracks are otherwise identical. A 2-year follow-up survey to the SUNY Downstate graduates and their employers elicited very positive feedback about the equivalency of CMs and CNMs (Fullerton, Shah, Schechter, & Muller, 2000). The program has graduated about five direct-entry midwives per year since 1996.

Ultimately, the state of New York contracted to use the ACC's National Certification Examination to test applicants for licensure under the 1992 law. A non-nurse applicant whose educational background is deemed equivalent to nursing education may take the examination, which was administered by the ACC until mid-2005 but is now administered by the AMCB. If she passes, she will be licensed as an LM by the state of New York and certified as a CM by the AMCB. As of January 2005, the ACC had certified 46 CMs, 29 graduates of the SUNY Downstate program, and 17 others, including midwives from other countries and graduates of programs accredited by MEAC.

The nurse–midwifery program at Baystate Medical Center in Springfield, Massachusetts, has also developed a direct-entry track, in this case designed for a physician assistant (PA). Baystate's PA track has been accredited by the ACNM, and its first and, as of 2005, only PA–midwife graduate passed the ACC exam and is now a CM. Baystate is willing to accept additional PAs, although funding is a problem. Although there is federal assistance for graduate-level nursing programs and students who are registered nurses, all federal funding for PA programs goes to basic programs, which don't include specialty education. At this time, no other ACNM-accredited nurse–midwifery education programs are known to be considering a direct-entry track.

Although the ACNM developed the CM credential to produce direct-entry midwives under the authority of the ACNM and ACC, almost 40% of all CMs certified by the ACC through the end of 2004 were not graduates of midwifery education programs accredited by the ACNM. Nevertheless, any ACC- or AMCB-certified CM is welcome to become a full-fledged voting member of the ACNM.

So far, only three states license CMs. New York gives CMs privileges equivalent to those of a CNM, including prescriptive privileges; as with CNMs, most CMs practicing in New York attend births in hospitals. New York suggests that CMs identify themselves as CNM/LMs, CM/LMs, or just as LMs, and does not require CNM/LMs to be licensed as registered nurses (RNs). New Jersey licenses CMs but does not provide prescriptive privileges, which are granted to CNMs under the New Jersey nurse practice act. As of early 2005, no CM had been given privileges by a hospital in New Jersey. Like New Jersey, Rhode Island licenses CMs, but does not provide prescriptive privileges. Students enrolled in a certified midwifery education program are eligible for federal student loans and grants but are not eligible for nurse traineeships or National Health Service Corps (NHSC) scholarships. Students enrolled in nurse–midwifery education programs that lead to a master's degree in midwifery rather than a master's degree in nursing also are not eligible for NHSC scholarships (Lichtman, personal communication, 2005).

Legal Status of Direct-Entry Midwives in the United States

Of 51 U.S. jurisdictions (50 states and Washington, D.C.), 21 require direct-entry midwives to be licensed, registered, permitted, certified, or documented in some way (MANA, 2005b). The most frequent designation is *licensed midwife*, or LM. Licensure is mandated in 20 of those 21 states, and is available—but not mandatory—for direct-entry midwives in Oregon, many of whom choose not to be licensed for a variety of reasons, including the very high cost of licensure, which is $1,500 per year. This cost is based on the state's requirement that regulation of trades and professions must be supported by licensing fees. Because relatively few direct-entry midwives have chosen to be licensed, the per-midwife fee is very high. Of 21 states that regulate direct-entry midwives, all but New York require either certification as a CPM or passing of the NARM Written Examination. Licensed or otherwise regulated direct-entry midwives in at least 12 states are permitted to administer a very limited list of drugs (Reed & Roberts, 2000). The scope of practice and prescription authority of CMs and CPMs are identical in New York.

In 22 states, out-of-hospital direct-entry midwifery practice is either not regulated but not prohibited, legal on the basis of judicial interpretation or statutory inference, or legal by statute, even though the state has not established a procedure for granting licenses. Eleven states prohibit anyone except a CNM from practicing midwifery (MANA, 2005a).

The legal status of direct-entry midwives is dynamic. Legislation to regulate direct-entry midwives was under consideration by the legislature of seven states (Illinois, Massachusetts, Missouri, Nebraska, Utah, Virginia, and Wyoming) as this chapter was being written in January 2005 (D. Pulley, personal communication, January 26–February 6, 2005).

Citizens for Midwifery is a nonprofit, volunteer grassroots organization that was founded by several women who had experienced home births with midwives and wanted to promote greater availability of this form of care. It was founded in 1996 and has close ties with MANA, NARM, and MEAC (Citizens for Midwifery, 2005).

Current Status and Number of Direct-Entry Midwives

In addition to 1,000 CPMs certified by NARM, approximately 1,000 other direct-entry midwives were practicing under state licenses as of early 2005—a total of about 2,000 direct-entry midwives with either national certification and/or licensure by a state, in addition to about 1,500 "plain" midwives who have neither state licensure nor national certification (Davis-Floyd, 2005). With few if any exceptions, direct-entry midwives other than SUNY Downstate-graduate CMs continue to attend births only in out-of-hospital settings.[6] Their services are covered by private insurance companies in most states where they are licensed, and by Medicaid in eight states. In most states, home birth attended by a direct-entry midwife is still an out-of-pocket expense. Most direct-entry midwives practice solo or in partnership with one other midwife (David-Floyd, 2005).

Out-of-Hospital Births and Who Attends Them

The United States Standard Certificate of Live Birth—a source of data regarding the numbers and percentages of births attended by midwives—did not distinguish between any kinds of midwives until the 1989 revision, which distinguishes between CNMs and other

---

[6] In states where they are licensed, a very small number of direct-entry midwives have received hospital privileges; it is very rare.

midwives. The revisions made in 2003 distinguish between midwives certified by the ACNM or AMCB—CNMs and CMs—and all other kinds of midwives.

Out-of-hospital births have accounted for less than 1% of all births in this country each year since 1989. CNMs attended fewer than 10,000 out-of-hospital births in 2002, of which the majority took place in free-standing birth centers (Martin et al., 2005). "Other midwives" attended almost 13,000 births, the majority of which were home births. Physicians attended almost 4,000 out-of-hospital births, including almost 2,000 in homes. Someone other than a midwife or physician signed the birth certificates of almost 9,000 babies born in out-of-hospital settings, including 7,500 babies born at home. Some of these were precipitous births with the baby caught by whoever was there. Some were planned home births with a family or church member attending; others were midwife-attended home births in which the father signed the birth certificate. The latter is common in states where direct-entry midwifery is unregulated or illegal (Pulley, 2005). Thus, some of those births should be attributed to "other midwives." Out-of-hospital births attended by midwives other than CNMs have consistently accounted for approximately 3 of every 1,000 births (0.3%), although the percentage varies from state to state and is much higher in some states.

Relationships Between Different Kinds of Midwives

There has been a long history of interest, antipathy, empathy, jealousy, competition, and fear between the majority of nurse–midwives, who attend births only in hospitals, and direct-entry midwives, who attend births only in out-of-hospital settings; their has also been much description and analysis of their differences (Burst, 1990; Davis-Floyd, 2005; Huntley, 1999; May & Davis-Floyd, 2005; Rooks, 1997, 1998). A small but important minority of ACNM members began as apprentice-trained midwives and value what they gained through that method of learning (Huntley, 1999). About a third of MANA members are CNMs, many of whom attend out-of-hospital births. Thus, some midwives are members of both organizations. During the mid-1990s some of these midwives, with one foot in each camp, felt the need for mutual support and a desire to increase understanding and respect among all midwives in both groups. In 1997, they formed the Bridge Club as a loosely organized group of midwives and midwifery students who wanted to build a bridge between CNMs and direct-entry midwives "from either side of the bridge" (Huntley, 1999). The Bridge Club convenes a caucus during the annual meetings of both MANA and the ACNM. It is unofficial, and its membership—usually about 100—is fluid.

During the 1998 ACNM Annual Meeting, members of the Bridge Club introduced a motion to recommend the establishment of a joint ACNM-MANA work group. The motion passed, and a formally recognized Liaison Group consisting of three members chosen by the ACNM and three by MANA was established. During its first meeting, held in June 1999, the ACNM-MANA Liaison Group developed a statement that endorsed all options of midwife certification in the United States, including the CPM. The Liaison Group statement was rejected by the ACNM Board of Directors, but was endorsed by MANA. The ACNM's budget was tight, and because the product of the group's work was inconsistent with ACNM positions, the ACNM ended its participation in the group in October 2001. In response to an outcry against this action by members attending the 2002 ACNM

Convention, the ACNM board of directors re-instituted participation in the Liaison Group with guidelines regarding topics to be addressed by the group and the understanding that ACNM representatives would be self-funded. The group meets at both the MANA and ACNM annual meetings, although more of its members are usually present at the ACNM annual meeting.

As time passes, the original dichotomy—nurse–midwives versus direct-entry midwives—is no longer straightforward. Nor is the evolved dichotomy—midwives educated and certified according to standards of the ACNM and ACC or AMCB (i.e., CNMs and CMs) versus all other midwives—since AMCB certification now extends to a small, but sure-to-grow number of midwives educated through programs accredited by MEAC. Although there is a dichotomy between midwives who attend births only in hospitals and those who attend births in homes and birth centers, nurse–midwives have led the birth center movement in the United States, and the ACNM supports home births. Perhaps we will reach a stage where we no longer feel the need to dichotomize, but we are not there yet. Possibly in time, midwives from both sides of the bridge will agree to distinguish midwives who have met national educational and certification standards defined by their professional peers—currently CNMs, CMs, and CPMs—from those who have not.

Despite deep ideological divisions between ACNM and MANA midwives about professionalism and appropriate midwifery education and scope of practice, there have been many positive relationships between CNMs/CMs and direct-entry midwives, as well as symbiosis that has benefited both groups. Former ACNM President Angela Murdaugh (1981–1983) convened a meeting that led to the founding of MANA in 1982. Former ACNM President Dorothea Lang (1975–1977) helped MANA apply for ICM membership in 1984. Virtually every ACNM president since then has made efforts toward communication and bridge building—many of which were not recognized or appreciated. In her earlier role as chair of the ACNM Division of Accreditation, ACNM President Joyce Roberts (1995–2001) explained the finer points of the ACNM's accreditation process and strategies for preserving the integrity of midwifery education in institutional settings to the direct-entry midwifery educators who went on to create MEAC (Myers-Ciecko, personal communication, 2005).

Meetings stimulated and funded by the Carnegie Foundation for the Advancement of Teaching from 1989 through 1994 brought CNMs and direct-entry midwives together to explore common ground—work that ultimately contributed to the establishment of national educational standards and NARM's certification process (Rooks, 1997). In addition, individual CNMs have supported direct-entry midwives in particular states. Current ACNM President Katherine Carr (2004–2006) has done so in her home state of Washington, where she was a founding member of the state midwives association and an early member of the faculty of the Seattle Midwifery School. CNMs are on the faculty and serve as clinical preceptors in most of the accredited direct-entry midwifery education programs; many have been both inspired and challenged by this experience (Myers-Ciecko, personal communication, 2005).

Nurse–midwives and direct-entry midwives work together in many communities—in practice partnerships providing home and/or birth center care and in collaborative relationships in which hospital-based CNMs accept referrals from direct-entry midwives when women who had planned to give birth at home or in a birth center need to go to a hospital during labor.

In the longer run, the ACNM may not be able to continue to control standards for entry into professional midwifery in the United States. ACNM Executive Director Deanne Williams has warned that the North American Free Trade Agreement (NAFTA) and other world trade agreements may eventually compel the ACNM to recognize midwife credentials that are endorsed by the United States' trade-partner countries whose educational system and standards for professional midwifery education are not equivalent to those of the ACNM (Williams, 2005).

Nurse–Midwife and ACNM Relationships with Nursing

As with relationships between different kinds of midwives, relationships between midwifery and nursing are products of their very different histories. Professional nursing in Britain and the United States arose within the context of military medicine and the terrible injuries and illnesses of war—the Crimean War, in the case of Florence Nightingale in England, and the Civil War in the United States. Midwifery, in contrast, arose within the context of women assisting and supporting other women during the normal physiologic processes and intra-psychic and social experiences of pregnancy and childbirth. Nursing developed within hospitals, whereas, until the beginning of the 20th century, most births occurred in homes. Physicians are the ultimate authority figures in hospitals, whereas pregnant women and their midwives share authority during a birth that occurs within the mother's home. As a result of these differences, the *culture* of nursing and the *culture* of midwifery have always been quite different, with the exception of public health nursing, which, like midwifery, developed outside of hospitals, with work focused on and within communities and homes.

History

The famous first nurse–midwifery service in the United States was (and still is) the Frontier *Nursing* Service (FNS), not the Frontier *Midwifery* Service. When Mary Breckinridge determined to devote herself to improving the lives of the children of poor families in the coal-mining mountains of Kentucky, she became trained as a *public health nurse.* At the end of the first World War, Breckinridge joined the Red Cross and went to France, where she created the first French Child Hygiene *Visiting Nurse* Service. Although she was impressed by the midwives she observed in France, she thought it odd that they had no background in nursing—exactly opposite from the United States, where nurses had no training in midwifery. Then she went to Britain, where she observed *nurse–midwives,* who she believed had the combination of training needed to help poor families in America. After deciding to start a nursing and midwifery service in Kentucky, she returned to England and Scotland to become trained in midwifery and recruit some British nurse–midwives to help her start the FNS. When she needed additional staff, she sent U.S. *public health nurses* to Scotland to obtain midwifery training.

In 1944, the National Organization for Public Health Nursing (NOPHN) established a section for nurse–midwives. NOPHN was dissolved in 1952 as part of a reorganization that resulted in formation of the American Nurses Association (ANA) and the National League for Nursing (NLN). Nurse–midwife Sister Theophane Shoemaker (then director of the nurse–midwifery program operated in Santa Fe, New Mexico, by members of a Roman Catholic order of missionary sisters) wrote to the presidents of the ANA and the NLN, seeking a niche for nurse–midwives within one of the new nursing organizations. Both organizations refused, based on their leaders' beliefs that nurse–midwifery is really part of medicine and thus does not belong in a nursing organization (Rooks, 1997; Tom, 1980). In 1968, the ANA reversed itself by deciding that nurse–midwifery is really a specialty within nursing (Roberts, 1995). The ACNM might never have been founded if nurse–midwifery had been acceptable to the mid-20th-century nursing leaders. In contrast to Americans, the British have always recognized that, although midwives work, and may even be educated, with both physicians and nurses, midwifery is its own profession, and not part of either medicine or nursing.

The second nurse–midwifery service was started by a New York City women's club to provide care to impoverished inner-city women and their babies (Rooks, 1997). In 1918, the City Club program became incorporated as the Maternity Center Association (MCA), a not-for-profit voluntary health agency based in Manhattan. In 1931, MCA opened the nation's first nurse–midwifery educational program in association with Columbia University's Teachers College Department of Nursing Education. The first students had to be public health nurses.

The Frontier Nursing Service was founded in 1925. Although most, perhaps all, nurse–midwifery services established during the following 35 years were paired with a nurse–midwifery education program, only a small proportion of the graduates of those programs could find employment in clinical nurse–midwifery (Rooks, 1997). As childbirth moved from homes to hospitals during the first half of the 1900s, there was a growing need for nurses to staff hospital obstetric units. Nurse–midwives were leaders in the new field of maternity nursing; often their fellow nurses did not even know that they were midwives. Nurse–midwives introduced the concept of family-centered maternity care, played a significant role in the development of childbirth education, demonstrated the radical concept of mother–baby rooming in, and urged mothers to breastfeed at a time when most hospitals were teaching them how to make formula and sterilize bottles. In 1963, the Federal Children's Bureau sponsored the first national survey of nurse–midwives in the United States (Thomas, 1965). Of 535 nurse–midwives living in the country at that time, only 34 (6%) were providing direct clinical midwifery care that included management of childbirth. Most nurse–midwifery education program graduates worked in maternity or public health nursing.

In 1954, even before the founding of the American College of Nurse–Midwifery,[7] members of the Committee on Organization drafted a document that defined a nurse–midwife as a professional who "combines the knowledge and skills of professional nursing and midwifery" (Dawley & Burst, 2005). In 1962, the ACNM approved its first definition of a nurse–midwife as "a registered nurse who by virtue of added knowledge and skill gained through an organized program of study and clinical experience has extended the limits of

---

[7] The name was changed to the American College of Nurse–Midwives in 1969 (Dawley & Burst, 2005).

her practice into the area of management of the care of mothers and babies throughout the maternity cycle." In 1978, the ACNM revised the definition to the earlier concept of a nurse–midwife as "an individual educated in the *two disciplines* of nursing and midwifery" (Dawley & Burst, 2005).

Licensure as "Advanced Practice" Nurses

Nurse-anesthetists were the first category of legally recognized nurse specialists in the United States, dating to the 1880s (Texas Association of Nurse Anesthetists, n.d.). Nurse–midwives were the second category, beginning in 1925; pediatric nurse practitioners (NPs) were the third, starting in the mid-1960s, by which time the ANA and NLN were eager to claim nurses with "expanded roles." As other categories of nurse practitioners and specialists were developed, nurse–midwives joined them in working through state nursing associations to promote legislation to legitimize and regulate CNMs and other advanced practice nurses under special subsections of state nurse practice acts (Rooks, 1997). The support of the huge nursing profession, combined with the well-documented excellent outcomes of nurse–midwifery care and the often enthusiastic support from nurse–midwifery clients, made it possible initially to pass and gradually to improve state laws that have benefited many kinds of advanced practice nurses, as well as nurse–midwives, in states throughout the country.

As of January 2000, CNMs were licensed under the state nurse practice act and regulated under the state board of nursing in 42 of the 51 U.S. jurisdictions (Reed & Roberts, 2000). In most of those states, CNMs are licensed as advanced practice nurses (APNs), advanced practice registered nurses (APRNs), nurse practitioners (NPs), or advanced registered nurse practitioners (ARNPs).

Benefits of Nurse–Midwifery's Association with Nursing

The combination of nursing and midwifery education, experience, credentials, licenses, and identities has brought many benefits to nurse–midwives and professional midwifery in the United States during the 80 years since Mary Breckinridge founded the FNS. Midwifery is a small, overworked, widely misunderstood, controversial profession, whereas nursing is huge and has a widely acknowledged and culturally accepted essential role in American health care. It has been politically necessary for nurse–midwives to align themselves with nursing at both the state and national levels in order to win fights for laws that allow them to practice legally, to administer drugs and write prescriptions, to have their services included in third-party payer programs, and to have access to professional liability insurance and government funding for nurse–midwifery education programs and scholarships for nurse–midwifery students.

It has been efficient to have students come to midwifery education with substantial health and health-care knowledge, skills, and experience. A study of factors associated with higher or lower scores on the National Certification Examination found a slight positive influence for each additional year of nursing practice prior to nurse–midwifery education, even though higher age itself (a possible confounding factor) was associated with slightly decreased scores (Fullerton & Severino, 1995). In addition, a substantially disproportionate number of nurse–midwifery clients have traditionally been low-income women with many socio-economic risks and limited access to health care (Declercq et al., 2001; Scupholme, DeJoseph, Strobino, & Paine, 1992). Many have non-pregnancy-related physical and/or mental health problems that are covered in nursing, but not midwifery education.

There are many more and a much wider variety of nursing positions than of positions in nurse–midwifery; the demand for CNMs is uneven, and the physical demands of providing midwifery care can be exhausting. CNMs who cannot find a nurse–midwifery position in a geographic area in which they prefer or need to live can usually find a position in nursing. Nursing also provides wider options for CNMs who may no longer be able to work the long hours, including nights and weekends, that clinical nurse–midwifery positions often demand. Having a wide fall-back position is often an advantage.

Disadvantages and Disagreements

There are also costs to nurse–midwifery's association with nursing, and important disagreements between nurse–midwifery and nursing regarding some critical issues. Although there are advantages to having a background in nursing, other educational backgrounds are also beneficial to individual midwives and the profession as a whole. By requiring all CNMs to be educated as nurses, nurse–midwifery loses the opportunity to enrich the profession with more midwives who have undergraduate degrees in foreign languages, sociology, anthropology, business, health education, communications, physiology, psychology, international studies, didactics, religion, nutrition, physical therapy, and other relevant courses of study. Requiring nursing as a prerequisite is costly to students in time and money and discouraging to those who complete a nursing program for the sole purpose of entering a program in midwifery. In addition, nursing education may taint pregnancy and birth with an illness orientation and requires students to override the learned nursing role in order to make independent decisions and act on them (Lichtman, personal communication, 2005). Placing nurse–midwifery education programs in schools of nursing also gives enormous power to academic nursing leaders, who may not understand midwifery or who may view it as an autonomous profession (Myers-Ciecko, personal communication, 2005).

Competency-Based Education Versus Degrees

The ACNM and organized nursing diverged on the issue of education from an early period. The ACNM was an early adopter and leader in the use of competency-based education. In contrast, the ANA and NLN educational policies have focused mainly on academic degrees to assure the quality of nursing education. Their current position is that all professional nurses should be educated through programs that lead to a bachelor of science degree in nursing (BSN), and advanced practice nurses should be educated through programs that lead to a master's degree in nursing (MSN). In 2004, the American Association of Colleges of Nursing (AACN) adopted a policy that, by 2015, all categories of advanced practice nurses, including CNMs, should be prepared in educational programs that lead to a *doctorate* in nursing practice (DNP). The rationale for this policy was based on findings from a task force that reviewed nursing curricula for advanced practice nurses (APNs) in programs across the country and found that an overwhelming majority of programs granting a master's degree to APNs had credit loads equivalent to doctoral degrees in other health professions (ACNM, 2004). The AACN represents the faculties of nursing education programs that grant baccalaureate and higher degrees in nursing.

Most nurse–midwifery educators in the late 1950s thought of midwifery as a clinical nursing specialty and believed that master's level education was desirable for nurse–midwives, in part because they hoped that the status associated with advanced university degrees would insulate nurse–midwifery from the continuing fall-out flowing from Charles Dickens's 19th-century derisive depiction of Sairey Gamp as a dirty, ugly midwife going to a birth with a bottle of gin and a pack of dirty instruments, an image that had been published in several obstetric textbooks. But only a small proportion of nurses actually had a BSN, and although three of the seven nurse–midwifery education programs operating at that time offered a master's degree in nursing, the four nondegree granting "certificate programs" included the one operated by the Frontier Nursing Service, in Hyden, Kentucky, and the one operated by the Catholic Maternity Institute, near Santa Fe, New Mexico. The need to prepare nurse–midwives for practice in poor rural areas made it necessary to continue to have some education programs that did not require a college degree for admission. Both kinds of programs were needed, and faculty from both kinds of programs worked together to develop educational standards that could be applied in various educational settings (Rooks, 1997).

Nurse–midwife educators were also concerned that the NLN system for accrediting graduate nursing education programs did not evaluate specialty practice (Sharp, 1983). In 1962, the NLN announced that it could not accredit nurse–midwifery education programs because some of them were not in graduate schools of nursing. The ACNM began to develop its own accreditation process, which was in place by 1970. By 1971, the ACNM required graduation from an ACNM-accredited nurse–midwifery education program and a passing score on the ACNM National Certification Examination for certification as a CNM. The first statement of the knowledge and skills essential for safe and effective beginning-level midwifery practice (i.e., the "core competencies" of a nurse–midwife at entrance into the profession) was approved by the ACNM Board of Directors in 1978. Since then, the ACNM core competencies statement has provided a basis for the design of nurse–midwifery education programs at every level, from nondegree certificate programs to doctoral programs; for ACNM certification of both nurse and "basic" (i.e., direct-entry) midwifery education programs; and for the National Certification Examination that is now administered by the American Midwifery Certification Board (Rooks, 1997).

In 1996, the ACNM Division of Accreditation (DOA) announced that by June 1999, all ACNM DOA accredited education programs must either require a baccalaureate degree for entrance into the program or grant no less than a baccalaureate degree at graduation from the program. Until March 2006 the ACNM had opposed all mandates for higher-level degrees, a policy that had been based in part on studies that have shown that higher academic degrees are not associated with either better performance on the National Certification Examination or greater clinical competence or success of a midwife certified by the ACNM or ACC (Rooks, Carr, & Sandvold, 1991). The similarity of outcomes regardless of degrees reflects the ability of all ACNM-accredited midwifery education programs to prepare competent beginning midwife practitioners. Other concerns about state mandates for higher degrees for licensure of CNMs included reluctance to reduce the pool of nurses who can afford to complete a midwifery education program, particularly a reluctance to reduce access to midwifery education for nurses who live in small towns and rural areas, and a desire to avoid educational mandates that increase the cost and length of midwifery education without improving the safety and effectiveness of midwifery care. Nevertheless, in March 2006 the ACNM adopted a policy that will require a graduate (master's or higher) degree for certification of CNMs and CMs who complete their midwifery education during or after 2010 (ACNM, 2006).

The most recent analysis of factors that predict performance on the National Certification Examination for nurse–midwives found that those whose highest degree was a baccalaureate degree performed slightly better than candidates with no degree or candidates with graduate degrees. Candidates who obtained their midwifery education in a certificate program performed slightly better than those whose programs led to a master's degree (Fullerton & Severino, 1995). There are some disadvantages to preparing midwives through a program that leads to an MSN degree, which, in addition to teaching the ACNM core competencies, has additional education objectives related to nursing theory, research methods, and other courses that must compete for the students' time and attention (Rooks et al., 1991).

Problems Deriving from Regulating Nurse–Midwifery Practice under State Boards of Nursing

PROBLEMS CAUSED BY NURSING'S DEMANDS FOR ACADEMIC DEGREES

Oregon was the first state to require CNMs to have a master's degree in nursing. It provides an example of some of the problems to which nurse–midwifery is vulnerable because so many states license and regulate CNMs as nurses.

Oregon CNMs are licensed and regulated by the state under the nurse practitioner (NP) part of the nurse practice act, which is administered by the board of nursing (BON). Rules requiring NPs to have academic degrees in nursing were approved in 1979, although they were not scheduled to be implemented right away. Although the new rules would not apply to NPs (including CNMs) who were already licensed to practice in Oregon, those seeking licensure in or after 1981 would be required to have at least a bachelor's degree in nursing; those applying for licensure in or after 1986 would have to have a master's degree in nursing (Howe, personal communication, 2005). The time for implementation seemed far away when the law was enacted, and the "grandmother" clause provided an escape hatch for CNMs and NPs who were living and working in Oregon when the rules were being considered. Nursing boards often use those tactics to allow time for the profession to prepare for new rules and lessen opposition to problematic proposals.

A master's degree was the highest degree for 54% of ACNM members surveyed in 2003; a baccalaureate was the highest degree for 28% (Schuiling et al., 2005). The proportion of CNMs with doctorates has varied between 3% and 5% since 1999. Of the more than 3,400 CNMs whose highest degree was at the master's level in 2003, approximately 2,800 had master's degrees in nursing. Among the more than 600 who had master's degrees in other disciplines, 263 had a master's degree in public health, 169 in a basic science, 36 in midwifery, 33 in education, and 29 in a health-related field other than nursing or midwifery. The Oregon BON does not accept a master's degree in midwifery as meeting the requirement for a master's degree in nursing (Sullivan, personal communication, 2003). This position raises questions of inconsistency in the positions of the Oregon board of nursing, which sees nurse–midwifery as a specialty of nursing but does not accept a master's degree in midwifery as equivalent to a master's degree in nursing. If nurse–midwifery is a specialty of nursing, a midwife with a master's degree in midwifery has a master's degree in nursing. If a master's degree in midwifery is not a master's degree in nursing, midwifery is not a specialty of nursing and should not be regulated by the board of nursing.

In 2003, the Oregon Board of Nursing passed a rule requiring nurse practitioners who graduate from an NP program during or after 2005 to have obtained their NP specialty education from a master's or post-master's program accredited by either the NLN or the Commission on Collegiate Nursing Education (CCNE). The Oregon Nurses Association supported adoption of this rule. Many ACNM-accredited nurse–midwifery education programs are based in graduate schools or departments of nursing and can also be accredited by one of these two nursing accreditation organizations. However, this rule would have made it impossible for graduates of any of the many ACNM-accredited education programs that are not based in schools or departments of nursing to practice midwifery in Oregon (Carol Howe, personal communication, 2005). Two CNMs with doctorates who teach at the Oregon Health and Science University in Portland were eventually able to convince the Oregon BON to accept graduates of nurse–midwifery programs accredited by either the ACNM or one of the two nursing accreditation organizations.

State BONs derive their authority from their mission of protecting the health of the public. The Oregon BON must believe that requiring CNMs to have master's degrees in nursing provides more protection, despite a lack of research-based support for that position. But despite its interest in protecting the public, the Oregon BON does not require nurse–midwives to be certified by the ACNM, ACC, or AMCB. This means that a nurse–midwifery education program graduate who fails the certification examination in nurse–midwifery/midwifery repeatedly and is never certified could be licensed in Oregon if she has an MSN. It is surprising that any state BON would not accept the ACNM/AMCB processes as adequate to protect the public, and alarming that a state BON would not require an individual nurse–midwife to have met the ACNM standards, which are nationally recognized and associated with the many positive outcomes that have been documented for nurse–midwifery practice in this country. Yet, Oregon is not alone; as of 2000, 24 US jurisdictions did not require certification by the ACNM, ACC, or AMCB (Reed & Roberts, 2000). Are some boards of nursing (despite being responsible for regulating nurse–midwifery) unaware of the ACNM/AMCB excellent quality-assurance structure? Or are these state BON decisions influenced by a desire to enhance the power of nursing and control the education and practice of nurses, combined with a lack of both understanding about and identification with midwifery?

If most CNMs continue to be licensed under state nurse practice acts and rules established by boards of nursing, it is difficult to see how nurse–midwifery will be able to adapt to current nursing leaders' visions regarding the education credentials of advanced nurse practitioners. This includes mandatory doctorates in nursing for all nurse practitioners within 10 years. In the 1950s and 1960s the ANA determined that eventually all registered nurses (RNs) should enter the profession through an educational program that grants a bachelor of science degree in nursing (BSN), and that became their policy. Yet by 1995, only about one third of all RNs actually had a BSN (U.S. Department of Labor, 2005). Nursing leaders, who have not been able to dictate the educational level of the more than 2 million employed RNs, are now trying to impose their vision of doctoral degrees for the much smaller numbers of nurse–midwives and nurse practitioners.

In addition, the ACNM now accredits midwifery education programs that do not require students to be nurses, and the AMCB now examines and certifies graduates of those programs—who are not RNs—to practice midwifery. The number of CMs is small, but the ACNM's commitment to professional direct-entry midwifery as well as nurse–midwifery is a major turning point for professional midwifery in this country. Sooner or later the ACNM and its members will have to begin the difficult work of bringing the licensure of midwives educated and certified under the authority of the ACNM, ACC, or AMCB into congruence with its mid-1990s decisions and actions leading to the education and certification of CMs.

THE IMPORTANCE OF PEER REVIEW IN THE DISCIPLINE OF CNMS

Historically, as well as in our own time and country, midwives have been subjected to unfounded accusations based on ignorance, bias, and misinformation. Although midwives are no longer burned at the stake, there is still a need to protect individual midwives against unwarranted loss of reputation and the right to practice resulting from inadequate disciplinary processes. There is also a serious responsibility to protect mothers, babies, and the public in general from incompetent or reckless unsafe midwives, and to protect the profession from the fall-out of unsafe midwifery practice.

In order to avoid erroneous discipline while preventing unsafe midwives from practicing, the processes by which a midwife could lose either her national certification or her license to practice in a particular state must embody high standards of due process. If disciplinary processes follow the fundamental principles of justice, we can rely on them to be both fair to individual midwives and effective in protecting individual women and babies and the reputation of midwifery.

More than two thousand years ago, Aristotle wrote that, "As a physician ought to be judged by the physician, so ought men to be judged by their peers" (Aristotle translated by Jowett, 1994). That concept was embodied in the British Magna Carta and carried down into the Constitution of the United States as an inherent aspect of due process, other aspects of which require that a law or regulation with the force of law be clear, fair, and have a presumption of innocence, and that accused persons have an opportunity to hear what they have been accused of, to face their accusers, and to present arguments and evidence to defend themselves, including cross-examination of those who testify against them. The law or regulation must be applied in a competent manner, and the jury must be impartial.

The due process standard should be particularly high when a person is at risk of losing her or his freedom (criminal justice), or when a professional is at risk of losing the right to practice her or his profession (professional discipline). Case law in at least one state has identified the legal processes by which a professional (a physician, in that case) risks losing his or her license to practice as "quasi criminal proceedings" that are "unavoidably punitive" (*Nguyen v. Medical Quality Assurance Commission*, 2001).

Although most CNMs practice under a state BON, it is rare for even one CNM to serve as either a member of the board or on the staff of a state BON. As of October 1998, CNMs served on the board of nursing in just 3 of the 42 states in which nurse–midwives were regulated under nursing.[8] As a result, there is often a lack of midwifery expertise and experience among key decision makers when a CNM is investigated through a disciplinary process under a BON. Physicians are disciplined by panels consisting entirely or primarily of other physicians under the authority of state boards of medicine, and nurses are disciplined by panels consisting entirely or primarily of other nurses. Few CNMs are disciplined, but those who are—including some who are guilty of incompetence or recklessness and some who are not—are at high risk of being judged by nurse practitioners or other advanced registered nurse practitioners who are not nurse–midwives and do not understand the standards for a nurse–midwife or the circumstances surrounding the events they are expected to review.

This is not just an academic consideration; several CNMs have lost their ability to practice midwifery in their home states in recent years, including a very senior, highly regarded Fellow of the American College of Nurse–Midwives (FACNM).[9] Her care in the case that stimulated the disciplinary hearing was not considered to be in error—or even questionable—in the view of the physicians involved in the situation, the quality-assurance committee of the hospital in which the care took place, several tort lawyers (who refused to bring a malpractice suit against her), and the only member of the board of nursing who was an obstetric nurse or had any experience in labor and delivery, whose recommendation that the board dismiss its charges against the CNM was not supported by the board.

NURSING CONCERN ABOUT ACNM'S DEVELOPMENT OF THE CM

Passage of the New York Midwifery Practice Act of 1992 and SUNY Downstate's development of a direct-entry track within its midwifery education program were major events in the history of the relationship between the ACNM and organized nursing. There have already been very significant adaptations on the part of the ACNM, including omission of the word "nurse" from most ACNM documents that had referred to "nurse–midwifery," and changing the title of the *Journal of Nurse–Midwifery* to the *Journal of Midwifery and Women's Health*. These changes have been seen with alarm by our colleagues in academic nursing. A 2003 paper published in *Nursing Outlook* by two advanced practice nursing leaders identified nurse–midwives (CNMs), certified registered nurse anesthetists (CRNAs), clinical nurse specialists (CNSes), and nurse practitioners (NPs) as the four distinct roles that comprise advanced practice nursing, and complained that CNMs do not re-

---

[8] The three states were Washington (Fletcher, personal communication, July 2004), Maryland, and Michigan (Reed & Roberts, 2000).

[9] Fellowship in the ACNM is an honor bestowed upon members whose professional achievements, outstanding scholarship, clinical excellence, and/or demonstrated leadership has been recognized both within and outside of the midwifery profession. Midwives elected into the ACNM Fellowship are Fellows of the ACNM and have the right to use "FACNM" after their names.

quire their specialty education to be provided through programs that lead to a master's degree in nursing (Hanson & Hamric, 2003). Nurse–midwifery's aberrancy from this otherwise unified front was described as a challenge that needs to be addressed in order to strengthen advanced practice nursing.

Nurse–midwifery is described as being in a transitional period, as compared to the other three components of advanced nursing practice, because not all midwives are nurses, and not all nurse–midwives are prepared at the master's level.

> "The current issues within nurse–midwifery are causing chasms within the APN world. The movement of the American College of Nurse Midwives to include midwives who are not nurses but who complete a certified midwifery program that is not nurse driven makes for confusion. . . . It is a professional imperative for ACNM leaders to differentiate the competencies expected of APN midwives from those expected of midwives who are not nurses or who lack graduate degrees. This differentiation is necessary to drive different certification and regulatory requirements for APN midwives versus other midwives. (Hanson & Hamric, 2003, p. 206)

The Self-Identify of the ACNM and CNMs

The ACNM is an active and leading member of the International Confederation of Midwives, which it joined in 1956 (Dawley & Burst, 2005). It is not a member of the International Council of Nurses.

In a 1990s study of how CNMs define themselves in relation to nursing, medicine, and midwifery, Scoggins found that nurse–midwives identify occupationally with midwifery, rather than nursing or medicine, even though there is some alliance with both of the other professions. The variables most strongly associated with identification with midwifery were philosophical agreement with nurse–midwifery ideologies of advocacy and the normalcy of pregnancy and birth. The tendency to differentiate themselves from both physicians and nurses was also associated with increased years of nurse–midwifery practice (Scoggin, 1996).

ACNM and CNM/CM Relationships with Medicine

Because even low-risk pregnant women may develop serious diseases and pregnancy complications, every midwife must have a functional professional relationship with one or more physicians. The primary purposes of midwifery are to educate, attend, and comfort women and their families during pregnancy, birth, and the period of family formation and reformation that follows every birth, and to maximize and protect the health of the mother and baby and the normal processes of human reproduction. The primary purposes of medicine are to prevent, diagnose, treat, control and palliate the human experience of injury and disease. Midwifery and medicine have different but complementary purposes, philosophies, and perspectives on pregnancy and birth, and different but overlapping sets of skills and bodies of knowledge (Rooks, 1999). They are separate but complementary professions. But the status and authority of physicians are much greater than that of midwives; actual working relationships depend on the circumstances of specific situations, which are more often controlled by physicians.

Early History of Medicine and Midwifery in America[10]

Midwives were among the first colonists to arrive in North America; a midwife attended three births during the *Mayflower*'s first voyage to the new world. But most of the early colonists were British, and midwifery was much slower to become professionalized in the British Isles than on the continent of Europe. A law requiring midwives to be licensed was passed in Paris in 1560. Formal, state-supported education of midwives was started. Midwives studied in the most famous obstetric hospital in France, wrote books, and developed their apprenticeship system into a full-fledged midwifery education program. By the 1800s, French midwives were teaching normal obstetrics to medical students. Midwives in the Netherlands have had to pass a rigorous examination since at least 1700. In contrast, the first law requiring British midwives to be licensed was not passed until the early 1900s—only about 100 years before publication of this book. Although midwives attended most births in the American colonies and were respected members of their communities, they did not develop schools. Some were well trained, but many were steeped in folklore. They practiced from their homes and passed their skills from one woman to another informally.

Although most of the best trained midwives came from continental Europe, they didn't speak English and stayed in their own communities. West African midwives came to America with the first boatloads of slaves. Eventually there were 4 million slaves in this country, including many black African midwives. After emancipation, they became the "Granny midwives" who took care of both black and white poor women in the South. Although midwifery was a good job for a woman, it did not develop as a profession.

Medicine was also slow to develop in America. Few colonists or immigrants came from the educated classes, so there were few university-educated physicians. Most American doctors were apprentice trained, had not attended medical school, and were in competition with homeopaths and midwives. Medicine did not become professionalized in the United States until the last half of the 1800s. When it did, it did so in a spirit of competition and the absence of a formal midwifery profession.

The 1910–1935 Campaign to Eliminate Midwives[11]

The period between 1910 and 1935 was marked by controversy about midwifery and a physician-led campaign to eliminate midwives as appropriate care for any woman who could afford a doctor. A series of events between 1910 and 1920 seem almost designed to entrench a pathology-oriented medical model of childbirth in this country. The Flexner

---

[10] This history is described in greater detail in Rooks, 1997, pp. 12–36.

[11] See Rooks, 1997, pp. 22–26, 451–452.

Report on Medical Education was published by the Carnegie Foundation for the Advancement of Teaching in 1910. After visiting every medical school in the United States and Canada, Flexner concluded that America was oversupplied with badly trained doctors and recommended that most existing medical schools be closed, leaving only the best, which should be modeled after the school at Johns Hopkins. Flexner singled out obstetrics as making the worst showing.

In 1911, Dr. J. Whitridge Williams, the leading obstetrics professor at Hopkins (and first author of *Williams Obstetrics*), conducted his own study, which confirmed Flexner's findings. The obstetric professors who responded to Williams's survey thought most women were safer with midwives than with general physicians. In 1912 Williams published his findings in the *Journal of the American Medical Association* (Williams, 1912). To improve obstetrics training, he recommended hospitalization for all deliveries and gradual abolition of midwives, who should be replaced by "obstetrical charities," which would serve as sites for training doctors.

Twilight sleep was introduced in 1914. Upper-class women eager to bring the miracle of pain relief to all women formed "twilight sleep societies." Obstetric anesthesia became a symbol of the progress possible through medicine.

In 1915, Dr. Joseph DeLee, author of the most important obstetric textbook of that time, published a paper in which he described childbirth as a pathologic process. "Obstetrics has a great pathologic dignity," he wrote. "Even natural deliveries damage both mothers and babies, often and much. If childbearing is destructive, it is pathogenic . . . if it if is pathogenic it is pathologic. . . . If the profession would realize that parturition viewed with modern eyes is no longer a normal function, but has imposing pathologic dignity, the midwife would be impossible even of mention" (DeLee, 1915, p. 134).

The first issue of the *American Journal of Obstetrics and Gynecology*, published in 1920, included an article in which DeLee proposed a sequence of interventions—including routine use of sedatives, ether, episiotomies, and forceps—designed to save women from the "evils natural to labor" (DeLee, 1920, p. 140). DeLee changed the focus from responding to problems as they arise to preventing problems through routine use of interventions to control the course of labor.

Maternal mortality and infant deaths from birth injuries increased as physicians engaged this active role. Historians analyzing data from this era associated the increases with an "orgy" of obstetrical interference in birth (Loudon, 1992). The 1925 White House Conference on Child Health and Protection concluded that "untrained midwives approach, and trained midwives surpass, the record of physicians in normal deliveries." The conference report ascribed this to "the fact that . . . many physicians . . . employ procedures which are calculated to hasten delivery, but which sometimes result harmfully to mother and child. On her part, the midwife is not permitted to and does not employ such procedures. She waits patiently and lets nature take its course" (White House Conference on Child Health and Protection, 1930).

The themes of the campaign to eliminate midwives were that midwives were untrained and incompetent, that pregnancy is a dangerous condition requiring complicated care available only from highly trained medical specialists, and that physicians needed better training in obstetrics and midwives' clients—mainly relatively poor women—were needed as "teaching material." Midwives attended approximately half of all births in 1900, but less than 15% in 1935. By the early 1930s, most practicing midwives were black or poor white granny midwives working in the rural south.

Nurse–Midwifery and Obstetrics, 1925–1970[12]

Mary Breckinridge founded the Frontier Nursing Service (FNS) in 1925, in the midst of the campaign to eliminate midwives. One of her first actions was to recruit a medical director and write protocols defining the clinical relationship between nurse–midwives and physicians.

The second nurse–midwifery service was established by the Maternity Center Association (MCA) in New York City in 1931. MCA began in 1918 as an outgrowth of a Women's City Club program to provide prenatal care and education in one zone of the city. By 1920, MCA was supervising 30 neighborhood centers in and from which public health nurses working under the direction of physicians provided prenatal care and education to pregnant women. MCA's Board of Directors soon realized that the nurses weren't adequately prepared for this work and that better homebirth care was also needed, and sought permission to open a school of nurse–midwifery. But midwifery was very controversial, and permission was hard to come by. In 1930, a group of MCA board members and others, including Mary Breckinridge, incorporated themselves as the Association for the Promotion and Standardization of Midwifery; after much work, MCA opened a nurse–midwifery service and school in Manhattan. Although the objectives specified that midwives prepared through the school would "accept responsibility for the care of normal maternity patients delegated by the obstetrician after a complete physical examination had been done" and would not be in private practice, MCA's plans drew harsh opposition, resulting in the resignations of several obstetrician members of MCA's Medical Board.

Invited into Hospitals to Help Care for the Poor[13]

The FNS was established to serve the poor in a rural area of Kentucky. MCA's nurse–midwifery service was established to serve the urban poor in Harlem, New York. The third nurse–midwifery school and service were developed to prepare nurse–midwives to meet the needs of poor black women in isolated parts of Alabama. The fourth school was a short-lived program to train black nurse–midwives in New Orleans, Louisiana. The fifth was opened by an order of Catholic sisters to serve Spanish-speaking families in a rural part of New Mexico. All of the first five schools were developed in association with midwifery services designed to meet the needs of families that lacked medical care due to geography, poverty, culture, and/or race.

Nurse–midwives did only home births until the mid-1950s, when a few midwives were invited into several of the nation's leading inner-city teaching hospitals. Obstetric leaders initiated these services to help the obstetric residents and faculty cope with the post-war

---

[12] See Rooks, 1997, pp. 36–42.

[13] See Rooks, 1997, pp. 36–45.

"baby boom" and to improve the quality of care in those hospitals. An OB department chairman speaking at a conference in the 1960s described the "shameful and humiliating circumstances" experienced by poor, black women in "our great public hospital clinics," including "attitudes of callousness" that "almost defy description," and described the competence and dedication of the nurse–midwives he had worked with during his residency and the need to introduce those attitudes into all charity-hospital obstetric services. But everyone at the meeting—including some leading nurse–midwives—agreed that nurse–midwives should be restricted to caring for the poor (Josiah Macy, Jr. Foundation, 1968).

In time, the obstetric departments of large public or charity teaching hospitals became major employers of American nurse–midwives. Nurse–midwives working in obstetric departments associated with medical schools were taught and expected to use many obstetric interventions.

What Relationship Is Required by ACNM Standards?

The 2003 version of the ACNM Standards for the Practice of Midwifery require CNMs and CMs to adhere to the following standards in regards to their relationships with physicians (ACNM, 2003). They must:

- "practice within a health care system that provides for consultation, collaborative management, or referral, as indicated by the health status of the client,"
- "demonstrate a safe mechanism for obtaining medical consultation, collaboration, and referral,"
- practice "in accord with service/practice guidelines that meet the requirements of the particular institution or practice setting," and
- develop written practice guidelines that describe "the parameters of service for independent and collaborative midwifery management and transfer of care when needed."

ACNM/ACOG Joint Statements

In 1971 the ACNM, the American College of Obstetricians and Gynecologists (ACOG), and the Nurses Association of the American College of Obstetricians and Gynecologists (now the Association of Women's Health, Obstetric and Neonatal Nurses, or AWHONN) approved a "Joint Statement on Maternity Care" which asserted that the need for quality maternity care can best be met by the cooperative efforts of physicians, nurse–midwives, obstetric nurses, and other health personnel working in teams directed by obstetrician–gynecologists. This was the first official recognition and acceptance by ACOG of the role of CNMs in the "improvement and expansion of health services" for women (Roberts, 2001). Its emphasis on the benefits of collaboration between nurse–midwives and physicians helped open the door to more private sector clinical practice positions for nurse–midwives.

In 1975, the statement was revised to expand upon and clarify "obstetrician direction of the team." The revision recognized that an obstetrician does not always need to be physically present when care is rendered, and called for representatives of each of the separate disciplines to work together to develop written agreements that specify the consultation and referral policies and "standing orders." This was the first formal agreement between the ACNM and ACOG regarding appropriate collaboration between nurse–midwives and obstetricians.

Nearly a decade later, ACOG and ACNM revised the 1975 statement as "The Joint Statement of Practice Relationships between Obstetricians and Gynecologists and Certified Nurse–midwives" (Rooks, 1997, p. 207). The 1982 statement emphasized the interdependence of obstetrician–gynecologists and CNMs working in a relationship of "mutual respect, trust and professional responsibility" and that appropriate CNM practice "includes the participation and involvement of the obstetrician/gynecologist." Although the statement urged Ob/Gyns to respond when CNMs ask for their participation, the "interdependence" between CNMs and obstetricians is not mutual and thus is not true interdependence. Physicians have support from nurses in their offices and in the hospital and can practice without collaborating with a midwife. A nurse–midwife, in contrast, cannot practice if no physician is willing to work with her. Many potential nurse–midwifery practices and birth centers have been unable to open, and others have closed because no physician in the community was willing to collaborate. Although the 1982 statement was an improvement, some people interpreted it as requiring direct physician supervision of CNMs (Roberts, 2001).

In 2001, ACOG and ACNM approved a fourth joint statement between the two organizations. The 2001 joint statement:

- Referred to CMs, as well as CNMs; every aspect of the agreement applies to all midwives certified by the ACNM or ACC
- Edited a sentence that had seemed to limit direction of a maternity care team to board-certified Ob/Gyns to also include other physicians whose hospital privileges allow them to provide complete obstetric care, such as family physicians (FPs), who work with CNMs/CMs in many rural areas
- Qualified the meaning of a supervisory relationship by placing clear responsibility for the outcomes of care with the person who directly manages the care—an important change to reduce the physician's risk of vicarious liability
- Discouraged statutory or regulatory language requiring medical supervision of CNMs/CMs
- While continuing to endorse the development of mutually agreed upon medical guidelines/protocols for CNM/CM clinical practice, used the ACNM's definitions of consultation, collaboration, and referral and referred to ACOG's *Guidelines for Implementing Collaborative Practice* in describing a pattern of collaborative care that reflects "a relationship of mutual respect, trust and professional responsibility"

One year later, a much shorter version was approved by both organizations. It consists of two simple paragraphs that should allow practices to negotiate their own clinical guidelines as appropriate for their settings:

2002 Joint Statement of Practice Relations Between Obstetrician-Gynecologists and Certified Nurse–Midwives/Certified Midwives

The American College of Obstetricians and Gynecologists (ACOG) and the American College of Nurse–Midwives (ACNM) recognize that in those circumstances in which obstetrician–gynecologists and certified nurse–midwives/certified midwives collaborate in the care of women, the quality of those practices is enhanced by a working relationship characterized by mutual respect and trust as well as professional responsibility and accountability. When obstetrician–gynecologists and certified nurse–midwives/certified midwives collaborate, they should concur on a clear mechanism for consultation, collaboration and referral based on the individual needs of each patient.

Recognizing the high level of responsibility that obstetrician–gynecologists and certified nurse–midwives/certified midwives assume when providing care to women, ACOG and ACNM affirm their commitment to promote appropriate standards for education and certification of their respective members, to support appropriate practice guidelines, and to facilitate communication and collegial relationships between obstetrician–gynecologists and certified nurse–midwives/certified midwives.

Source: American College of Nurse-Midwives, 2002a.

In 1986, Dr. Irving Cushner, a distinguished obstetrician–gynecologist and public health leader, addressed the relationship between CNMs and Ob/Gyns during a National Colloquium on Nurse–Midwifery in America (Rooks, 1997, pp. 83–84). He spoke of a developing surplus of obstetricians and the reality that nurse midwives, family practice physicians, and obstetrician–gynecologists compete to be the primary-care providers for low-risk pregnant women. Although he said that the leadership of ACOG stood behind every word of the ACOG/ACNM Joint Statement, he noted that those leaders comprised only about 50 people in an organization with approximately 25,000 members. "We cannot assume that all of the members of ACOG agree with the joint statement. Many, if not most of them, may disagree with it." At that time, approximately 8% of obstetrician–gynecologists surveyed by ACOG employed nurse–midwives in full- or part-time staff positions.

Family Physicians

Some CNMs work with family physicians, who are the only other medical specialty with an important role in primary maternity care. ACOG estimated that FPs delivered between 15% and 20% of the babies born in 1989. Although the proportion of FPs who include obstetrics in their practice is declining, their role is significant in many rural areas, especially in the West North Central region of the country (Iowa, Kansas, Minnesota, Missouri, Nebraska, North Dakota, and South Dakota), as determined by a survey conducted by the American Academy of Family Physicians (AAFP) in 1988 (Schmittling & Tsou, 1989). As of 1993, almost 40% of rural FPs provided maternal and newborn care as part of their practice.

FP practice is family-centered, and FP attitudes and beliefs about pregnancy and childbirth are, at least theoretically, relatively congruent with those of midwives. A study published in 1993 asked all midwives registered in one Canadian province and a sample of FPs and OBs working in a teaching hospital in that province about their practices, attitudes, and beliefs about childbirth (Reime et al., 2004). Cluster analysis identified three distinct clusters based on similar responses to the questions. The midwifery cluster included all of the midwives and 26% of the FPs. The OB cluster included 79% of the OBs and 16% of the FPs. The FP cluster included 58% of the FPs and 21% the OBs. Members of the OB cluster more strongly believed that women had the right to request a caesarean section without maternal/fetal indication and that increasing caesarean rates signaled improvement in obstetrics. They were also more likely to say that they would induce women as soon as possible after 41 weeks + 3 days of gestation and least likely to encourage use of birth plans. The midwifery cluster's views were opposite those of the OB cluster, while the FP cluster's views fell between those of the other two clusters. The authors concluded that obstetricians and midwives generally follow very different approaches to maternity care, while FPs' attitudes and practices are more heterogeneous; some practice more like midwives and some more like obstetricians.

Several studies have measured actual differences in care provided by FPs compared to Ob/Gyns and, in some studies, CNMs practicing in the same facilities or areas, with some mechanism to assure approximate comparability of the women cared for by each kind of clinician. Two studies conducted in Canada from the mid-1980s through the early 1990s found that family physicians were less likely than obstetrician–gynecologists to rupture the membranes, induce or augment labor, use continuous electronic fetal monitoring or forceps or vacuum, administer narcotics or provide for epidural anesthesia, cut episiotomies, or administer postpartum oxytocin (MacDonald, Voaklander, & Birtwhistle, 1993; Reid, Carroll, Ruderman, & Murray, 1989). A similar study of care provided by FPs and Ob/Gyns to women during childbirth in five sites in the United States reported that FP clients were less likely to have epidural anesthesia or episiotomies during vaginal births and had fewer cesarean sections, mainly due to less frequent diagnoses of cephalopelvic disproportion (Hueston, Applegate, Mansfield, King, & McClaflin, 1995). A study that compared maternity care provided by CNM and FP members of a co-practice in a rural hospital in Kentucky in the early 1990s found much similarity in their management of labor and delivery, except that the family physicians cut more episiotomies (Hueston & Rudy, 1993).

Nevertheless, a study of care provided to low-risk women by random samples of Ob/Gyns, FPs, and CNMs practicing in Washington State during the late 1980s found that, although CNMs were less likely than either kind of physician to use continuous electronic fetal monitoring, labor induction or augmentation, and epidural anesthesia, there was little difference between the practice patterns of obstetricians and family physicians (Rosenblatt et al., 1997). A study conducted in Michigan during the same period found that younger FPs and those affiliated with an academic family medicine department have a more family-centered approach to maternity care and use fewer intrusive practices (Smith, Green, & Carothers, 1989).

Primary maternity care in many other wealthy Western, industrialized countries is provided mainly by midwives and general practitioners—the international equivalent of North American family physicians—with a much smaller proportion provided by obstetrician-gynecologists, who practice as specialists rather than as primary care providers. A similar pattern prevails in some parts of North America. Residents in family medicine programs in the United States and Canada can choose to become trained in surgery, which is necessary if they plan to include obstetrics in their practice. A number of very successful FP/CNM practices have been described in journals of nurse–midwifery, rural health, or family medicine (Hueston & Murray, 1992; Payne & King, 1998; Reid & Galbraith, 1988; Wingeier, Bloch, & Kvale, 1988). Payne and King described a very successful CNM/FP collaboration in which a CNM joined the faculty of an academic department of family medicine that provides medical consultation and referral for a birth center sponsored by a federally funded community health center and for a CNM/family nurse-practitioner practicing in a rural area.

A later paper published by these authors—a nurse–midwife and a family physician—described the benefits for both parties of a midwifery/family medicine collaboration (Payne & King, 2001). CNMs teach management of normal childbirth to medical students and residents in most academic medical centers and are almost as likely to teach family practice residents as residents in Ob/Gyn (Harman, Summers, King, & Harman, 1998).

The American Academy of Family Physicians' Position on Nurse–Midwives

In 2003 and 2004, the American Academy of Family Physicians (AAFP) adopted policies that acknowledge the long-standing role of midwives in the provision of maternity care in the United States and encourage "cooperative and collaborative relationships among obstetricians, family physicians and nurse midwives" as "essential for provision of consistent, high-quality care to pregnant women" (AAFP, 2004). CNMs should be RNs before undergoing specific training for certification as a CNM and "only function in an integrated practice arrangement under the direction and responsible supervision of a practicing, licensed physician qualified in maternity care." AAFP "supports the concept of patient and third-party reimbursement for services of certified nurse midwives where services are provided in an integrated practice arrangement" (AAFP, 2003).

The AAFP recognizes the educational benefits of providing opportunities for family physicians to learn from and with midwives. CNMs have taught an extremely well-received workshop on nonpharmacologic methods to lessen pain and promote labor progress during the academy's annual Family-Centered Maternity Care course every year since 1997. At the same time, hundreds of CNMs have completed the AAFP program on Advanced Life Support Obstetrics (ALSO), and some have completed a course to prepare instructors for this course.

Physicians and Out-of-Hospital Birth

The movement of births from homes to hospitals was concurrent with the ascendancy of the role of physicians in childbirth. Thus, a small increase in—and much hoopla about—home births attended by lay midwives in the early 1970s was of great concern to many obstetricians, particularly because the home-birth/lay midwife phenomenon was part of a more general social and cultural upheaval that included a loud feminist critique of high-tech interventionist obstetrics, and because many of the women having midwife-attended home births were educated middle- or professional-class women (Rooks, 1997).

Although hospitalization for childbirth was almost universal by 1960, about 1% of births continued to be out-of-hospital for a variety of reasons, including geographic and financial lack of access to hospital care. The small but persisting residual of out-of-hospital births received little attention until lay-midwife home births moved into the limelight during the 1970s. Despite increasing interest in home births, the proportion of U.S. births occurring somewhere other than a hospital remained steady at between 0.9 and 1.1% until it peaked at 1.5% in 1978.[14] By 1980 it had fallen back to its usual 1%. The small, short-lived increase evoked a vituperative over-reaction by ACOG, which held press conferences in which obstetricians referred to home births as "maternal trauma" and "child abuse" and urged physicians and public safety authorities to be alert for deaths resulting from home births.

Despite no lasting increase in the proportion of out-of-hospital births, the role of physicians vis-à-vis midwives in home births did change during the 1970s. Physicians delivered about 40% of babies born in out-of-hospital settings in 1975, compared to about 30% attendance by midwives; another 30% were attributed to "other" or "unknown" birth attendants. By 1980, physicians and midwives had switched places, with midwives attending about 40% of out-of-hospital births, compared to 30% for physicians. The proportion attributed to other or unknown attendants has remained at about 30% over many decades. The role of physicians in out-of-hospital births has dropped continuously since 1975, while the role of midwives has increased. By 2002 (the most recent year with published data), physicians accounted for only 11% of out-of-hospital births, compared to 63% for midwives. Data to distinguish between CNMs and "other midwives" were not available until a change in the US Standard Certificate of Live Birth was implemented in 1989. CNMs accounted for 20% of out-of-hospital births in 1989, other midwives accounted for 26%, and physicians accounted for 27%. By 2002, CNMs' share had increased to 27%, other midwives' share had increased to 36%, and the physicians' share had dropped to 11%.

Many if not most physicians are both leery and disdainful of out-of-hospital births, of which few have had any first-hand experience. Most physicians' only experience with out-of-hospital births occurs when a mother or newborn is transferred to a hospital at some point during or shortly after the birth; that is, they see only the problems and none of the successes. Difficulty arranging for reliable physician consultation, collaboration, and referral for CNM/CM attended births in homes and birth centers is a perennial problem.

Professional Liability Concerns[15]

Many physicians—as well as hospitals, physician–hospital organizations, preferred provider organizations, health maintenance organizations, and companies that sell professional liability insurance—believe that physicians who work with midwives and hospitals that give midwives privileges are exposed to any liability incurred by negligence or malpractice on the part of the midwives. This concept is referred to as vicarious liability, that is, legal liability that is based upon a relationship rather than actual conduct.

---

[14] Data on out-of-hospital births are based on National Center for Health Statistics reports of final natality statistics for 1975, 1978, 1980, 1985, 1990, and 2002.

[15] See Jenkins, 1994.

The doctrine of vicarious liability is based on the assumption of control. Although hospitals and physicians will usually be liable for damage resulting from the conduct of any person in their actual employ, if a midwife is not a direct employee—and thus not under the control of the physician or hospital—the physician or hospital should not be subject to vicarious liability.

Hospitals have a duty to retain only competent professional staff and to oversee provision of services within their walls by use of ongoing mandatory quality-assurance mechanisms and periodic review and renewal of delineated clinical privileges for all staff members. Except when a hospital has failed to exercise due diligence in credentialing or monitoring the performance of a member of its professional staff, hospitals have rarely been held liable for care provided by physicians who are not employed by the hospital. A hospital's liability for the conduct of a state-licensed, ACNM-, ACC-, or AMCB-certified midwife who is not employed by the hospital but has been granted clinical privileges as an independent practitioner is conceptually the same as it would be for an attending physician with staff privileges.

Malpractice cases are usually highly fact specific. Determination of vicarious liability also depends on the facts of each situation. Professional consultation and collaboration per se do not imply control. But *supervision* does imply at least the right—and possibly the responsibility—of one party to control the other. A physician who consults or collaborates with a midwife may share liability depending on the facts of a particular case. In 1994, ACNM staff attorney Susan Jenkins published the article on which this discussion is mainly based. In conducting research for that article—including examination of electronic legal databases—Jenkins did not find a single case anywhere in the United States in which a physician had been held vicariously liable for the negligence of a CNM.

MD LIABILITY INSURANCE POLICY SURCHARGES[16]

The 1980s professional liability insurance crisis had several negative impacts on CNMs, including the imposition of liability insurance policy surcharges charged to some physicians who worked with midwives. A surcharge is an additional cost to purchase insurance coverage. This practice was based on the assumption that a physician is exposed to additional liability risk by working with a midwife. A survey conducted in 14 states and the District of Columbia in 1988 found that, although some surcharges were low, some amounted to more than a 25% increase in the physician's annual insurance premium—an increase of up to $23,000 in the cost of insurance per nurse–midwife per year in at least one case. A 1992 survey conducted by ACOG found that 60% of Ob/Gyns working with CNMs were paying some kind of liability insurance surcharge. These kinds of costs, as well as the underlying assumption that working with a midwife increases a physician's risk of being sued, created a formidable barrier to physicians' openness to working with CNMs.

Nurse–midwives in Illinois and Washington, D.C., challenged the legitimacy of the surcharges in court, and the problem seemed to diminish. By 1996, less than a third of ACOG members working with CNMs reported that they had been required to pay a liability

---

[16] See the ACNM Web site page on Professional Liability Information at http://www.midwife.org/education .cfm?id=202. Part 2 (Physician Surcharge) of the Professional Liability Information Packet can be downloaded directly from http://www.midwife.org/siteFiles/about/ProfessionalLiability_RP2.pdf.

insurance surcharge. However, as malpractice liability problems have again become a problem of crisis proportions, physician insurance policy surcharges are returning as an important problem for CNMs and CMs. Some physicians refuse to work with midwives and some hospitals refuse to grant clinical privileges to midwives based on vicarious liability concerns.

Vicarious liability concerns also contribute to other barriers to cost-effective CNM practice. Some insurers and hospitals require physicians to provide stringent in-person "supervision" of midwives based on the fear of vicarious liability. This sets up a circumstance that actually increases the risk that a physician or hospital could be held accountable for problems related to the practice of the midwife, because supervision, unlike consultation, is based on the assumption of the right to exercise control.

ACOG DATA ON THE PROBLEM

Data on nurse–midwives as employees and co-defendants in liability claims are available from ACOG Professional Liability surveys conducted in 1992, 1996, 1999, and 2003. Almost 8% of Ob/Gyns who participated in the 1992 survey employed at least one CNM; by 1999, almost 18% of the respondents employed CNMs. Compared to the increase between 1992 and 1999, the increase between 1999 and 2003 was modest; more than 19% of Ob/Gyns participating in the 2003 survey employed CNMs, which is almost 1 of every 5.

CNMs were named in between 2% and 3% of malpractice claims against Ob/Gyns that were either open in 1990 or were opened during the decade of the 1990s. The 2003 survey respondents were asked to identify every category of labor and delivery care provider who had been named as a co-defendant in suits brought against the Ob/Gyn between 1999 and 2002. The most frequent co-defendants were obstetricians in the same practice as the survey respondent (27%), obstetricians not associated with the respondent's practice (11.6%), residents in training (16.3%), nurses (7.1%), anesthesiologists (5.2%), pediatricians and neonatologists (3.5%), and family physicians (3.3%), with the least involvement by nurse–midwives (2.6%). ACOG has documented that Ob/Gyns who work with CNMs experience a lower average number of malpractice claims, compared to ACOG members who do not work with CNMs (Reed & Roberts, 2000).

State Laws Regarding CNM/MD Relationships[17]

The information in this section is based on an analysis of laws regulating the practice of CNMs and CMs in all U.S. jurisdictions in 2000. At that time, CNM practice in two states (New Jersey and Pennsylvania) was under the authority of each state's board of medicine. The board of nursing and board of medicine shared responsibility for regulating nurse–midwifery in five states—Alabama, Nebraska, North Carolina, South Dakota, and Virginia.

Forty states defined the required relationship between CNMs and physicians: 28 states required "consultation, collaboration and referral," and 12 states required physicians to supervise or direct the care provided by CNMs. Four of those 40 states specified that the ratio of CNMs per consultative or supervisory physician cannot be greater than 3:1 (Alabama,

---

[17] See Reed & Roberts, 2000.

Nevada, and South Carolina) or 4:1 (South Dakota). Four other states limited the number of CNMs who can consult with a single physician in regards to prescriptions (California, Colorado, Oklahoma, and Virginia).

The laws of 11 states did not describe the inter-professional relationship between midwifery and medicine.

Cross-Pollination between Midwifery and Medicine

Although there are important differences between the philosophies and care provided by physicians as compared to midwives, there is also common ground (Rooks, 1999). The knowledge and skills of midwives, obstetricians, and family physicians overlap. Midwives read books and articles written by obstetricians and use information based on their research. Midwives do their own research and write their own articles and books, which are available to, though probably less often read by, obstetricians. Many important improvements in obstetric practice during the past 30 years have resulted from obstetricians adopting some of the beliefs and methods associated with midwifery. When a physician practices them, they become part of his or her *medical* practice. CNMs and CMs have also incorporated many aspects of the medical management of pregnancy into their practices. Unfortunately, this has led to over- (i.e., unnecessary) use of some obstetric interventions by CNMs.

Physicians participate in teaching students in many nurse–midwifery programs, and CNMs teach management of normal childbirth to medical students and residents in most academic medical centers (Harman, Summers, King, & Harman, 1998). Medical students and residents interact with CNMs in the obstetric services of many teaching hospitals. Direct experience with CNMs during medical education clinical rotations has a positive effect on medical students, including better understanding of CNMs' authority to prescribe medications and more interest in working with CNMs in the future (Hanson, Tillett, & Kirby, 1997).

The Importance of Midwives' Relationships with Physicians

During the mid-1980s, the ACNM Foundation conducted a study to identify factors associated with success or failure of a nurse–midwifery practice (Haas & Rooks, 1986). The CNMs who participated in the study identified suitable physician collaboration and a good relationship between CNMs and physicians as the most important factors for success, and opposition from physicians as one of the most important obstacles. Practices without direct physician involvement were least able to attract an adequate number of clients. In 1992, the Office of the Inspector General of the Department of Health and Human Services conducted a survey to determine what CNMs perceived to be the most significant problems impeding a successful practice. Nurse–midwives who participated in that study considered attitudes and perceptions of the medical community to be the most significant barrier. The government investigators concluded that physicians probably have an impact on most of the other barriers reported by some nurse–midwives, especially inability to prescribe medications and obtain hospital privileges.

The nature of the personal working relationships between individual midwives and individual physicians depends on many factors and experiences, including the usually private assessments and judgments that professionals make of one another. In a study reported in a state medical association journal in 1994, two physicians in Oklahoma noted that, although the outcomes of maternity care provided by obstetricians, family physicians, and nurse–midwives have not been shown to differ, the attitudes and perceptions of different kinds of physicians about midwives and each other may impact access to care (Cooper & Lawler, 2001). They mailed a survey with questions on competency, attitudes, and demographics to a randomized list of 3,000 Ob/Gyns and 3,000 FPs obtained from the American Medical Association. Although the response rate was low—suggesting the possibility of bias—the findings were interesting. Both kinds of physicians expressed high confidence in the ability of Ob/Gyns to provide obstetrical care to low-risk women. FPs were not perceived to be as competent as Ob/Gyns, although FPs who were actually providing low-risk obstetrical care were more confident than Ob/Gyns of FPs' competence in low-risk obstetrics. CNMs were generally perceived as competent by both groups of physicians, who also thought that CNMs should have access to hospital privileges.

Chapter Exercises

Many of the issues described and discussed in this chapter are controversial within the profession. The following exercises are suggested to prepare you to engage these controversies from a basis of knowledge and understanding:

1. Join the American College of Nurse–Midwives.
2. Make plans to attend the next annual meeting of the American College of Nurse–Midwives.
3. Creating educational and certification pathways for direct-entry midwives has resulted in problems, challenges, and opportunities. Divide the class into two groups, one to research and present the benefits of the CM's and the ACNM's about-face in accepting the concept of direct-entry midwifery, and one to research and present the costs and risks of that action. Each team should then present its findings and conclusions, after which there should be time for questions and discussion.
4. Nurse–midwifery's historical and current associations with nursing have resulted in both benefits and disadvantages. Divide the class into two debate teams, one of which takes the position that the ACNM should retain and seek to strengthen its associations with nursing, the other of which takes the position that the ACNM should seek to unravel nurse–midwifery's educational and legal relationships with nursing. Each team should prepare itself for a debate and then have a debate on that issue.
5. Divide the class into two debate teams, one of which takes a position of support of the American Association of Colleges of Nursing's 2004 policy that, by 2015, nurse practitioners and other advanced practice nurses, including CNMs, should be prepared in educational programs that lead to a doctorate in nursing practice (DNP), and one of which takes the op-

posite position. Each team should prepare itself for a debate and then have a debate on that issue.

References

American Academy of Family Physicians (AAFP). (2003). *Nurse midwives, certified.* Retrieved March 22, 2006, from http://www.aafp.org/x6945.xml

American Academy of Family Physicians (AAFP). (2004). *AAFP-ACOG joint statement on cooperative practice and hospital privileges.* Retrieved March 22, 2006, from http://www.aafp.org/x6949.xml

American College of Nurse–Midwives (ACNM). (2002a). *Joint statement of practice relations between obstetrician-gynecologists and certified nurse–midwives/certified midwives.* Retrieved January 30, 2006, from http://www.midwife.org/display.cfm?id=471

American College of Nurse–Midwives. (2002b). *Professional liability information packet, Part 2 (physician surcharge).* Retrieved January 30, 2006, from http://www.midwife.org/siteFiles/about/ProfessionalLiability_RP2.pdf

American College of Nurse–Midwives. (2003). *Standards for the practice of midwifery.* Retrieved March 22, 2006, from http://www.midwife.org/display.cfm?id=485

American College of Nurse–Midwives. (2004). Doctor of nursing practice: AACN adopts practice doctorate. *Quickening, 35*(7), 23.

American College of Nurse–Midwives. (2006). *Mandatory degree requirements for entry into midwifery practice.* Retrieved June 6, 2006, from http://www.acnm.org/siteFiles/position/Mandatory_Degree_Requirements_3.06.pdf

Citizens for Midwifery. (2005). *What Is Citizens for Midwifery?* Retrieved February 6, 2006, from http://www.cfmidwifery.org/whatis

Cooper, C. F., & Lawler, F. H. (2001). Physician perceptions regarding competence of obstetrical providers and attitudes about other issues in obstetrical care. *Journal of the Oklahoma State Medical Association, 12,* 554–560.

Curtin, S. C. (1999). Recent changes in birth attendant, place of birth, and the use of obstetric interventions, United States, 1989–1997. *Journal of Nurse Midwifery, 44*(4), 349–354.

Davis-Floyd, R. (1999, Spring). Some thoughts on bridging the gap between nurse- and direct-entry midwives. *Midwifery Today, 49,* 15–17.

Davis-Floyd, R. (2005). ACNM and MANA: Divergent histories and convergent trends. In R. Davis-Floyd & C. Johnson (Eds.), *Mainstreaming midwives: The politics of professionalization* (Chap. 1). New York: Routledge.

Dawley, K., & Burst, H. V. (2005). The American College of Nurse-Midwives and its antecedents: A historic time line. *Journal of Midwifery and Women's Health, 50,* 16–22.

Declercq, E. R., Williams, D. R., Koontz, A. M., Paine, L. L., Streit, E. L., & McCloskey, L. (2001). Serving women in need: Nurse–midwifery practice in the United States. *Journal of Midwifery and Women's Health, 46*(1), 11–16.

DeLee, J. B. (1915). Progress toward ideal obstetrics. *Transactions of the American Association for the Study and Prevention of Infant Mortality, 6,* 114–138.

DeLee, J. B. (1920). The prophylactic forceps operation. *American Journal of Obstetrics and Gynecology, 1,* 34–44.

Fullerton, J. T., & Severino, R. (1995). Factors that predict performance on the national certification examination for nurse–midwives. *Journal of Nurse Midwifery, 40*(1), 19–25.

Fullerton, J. T., Shah, M. A., Holmes, G., Roe, V., & Campau, N. (1998). Direct entry midwifery education: Evaluation of program innovations. *Journal of Nurse Midwifery, 43*, 102–105.

Fullerton, J. T., Shah, M. A., Schechter, S., & Muller, J. H. (2000). Integrating qualified nurses and non-nurses in midwifery education: The two-year experience of an ACNM DOA Accredited Program. *Journal of Midwifery and Women's Health, 45*(1), 45–54.

Gaskin, I. M. (1975). *Spiritual midwifery.* Summertown, TN: The Book Publishing Co.

Haas, J. E., & Rooks, J. P. (1986). National survey of factors contributing to and hindering the successful practice of nurse–midwifery. Summary of the American College of Nurse–Midwives Foundation Study. *Journal of Nurse Midwifery, 31*(5), 212–215.

Hanson, C. M., & Hamric, A. B. (2003). Reflections on the continuing evolution of advanced practice nursing. *Nursing Outlook, 51*, 203–211.

Hanson, L., Tillett, J., & Kirby, R. S. (1997). Medical students' knowledge of midwifery practice after didactic and clinical exposure. *Journal of Nurse Midwifery, 42*(4), 308–315.

Harman, P. J., Summers, L., King, T., & Harman, T. F. (1998). Interdisciplinary teaching: A survey of CNM participation in medical education in the United States. *Journal of Nurse–Midwifery, 43*, 27–37.

Hueston, W., & Murray, M. (1992). A three-tier model for the delivery of rural obstetrical care: Using a nurse–midwife and family physician co-practice. *Journal of Rural Health, 3*, 283–290.

Hueston, W. J., Applegate, J. A., Mansfield, C. J., King, D. E., & McClaflin, R. R. (1995). Practice variations between family physicians and obstetricians in the management of low-risk pregnancies. *Journal of Family Practice, 40*(4), 345–351.

Hueston, W. J., & Rudy, M. (1993). A comparison of labor and delivery management between nurse midwives and family physicians. *Journal of Family Practice, 37*(5), 449–454.

Huntley, A. (1999, Spring). Build bridges, not walls. *Midwifery Today, 49*, 12–13.

International Confederation of Midwives (ICM). (2005). *Definition of the midwife.* Retrieved February 28, 2006, from http://www.medicalknowledgeinstitute.com/files/ICM%20Definition%20of%20the%20Midwife%202005.pdf

Jenkins, S. M. (1994). The myth of vicarious liability: Impact on barriers to nurse–midwifery practice. *Journal of Nurse Midwifery, 39*, 98–106.

Josiah Macy, Jr. Foundation. (1968). *The midwife in the United States: Report of a Macy conference.* New York: Author.

Jowett, B. (1994). *Politics by Aristotle: An eight-part English translation of Aristotle's Politics.* The Internet Classics Archive. Retrieved July 25, 2004, from http://classics.mit.edu/Aristotle/politics.html

Kennedy, H. P. (2000). A model of exemplary midwifery practice: Results of a Delphi study. *Journal of Midwifery and Women's Health, 45*(1), 4–19.

Loudon, I. (1992). *Death in childbirth: An international study of maternal care and maternal mortality 1800–1950.* Oxford: Clarendon Press.

MacDonald, S. E., Voaklander, K., & Birtwhistle, R. V. (1993). A comparison of family physicians' and obstetricians' intrapartum management of low-risk pregnancies. *Family Practice, 37*(5), 457–462.

Martin, J. A., Hamilton, B. E., Ventura, S. J., Menacker, F., & Park, M. M. (2002). Births: Final data for 2000. *National Vital Statistics Reports, 50*(5). Hyattsville, MD: National Center for Health Statistics.

May, M., & Davis-Floyd, R. (2005). Idealism and pragmatism in the creation of the certified midwife: The development of midwifery in New York and the New York Midwifery Practice Act of 1992. In R. Davis-Floyd & C. Johnson (Eds.), *Mainstreaming midwives: The politics of professionalization.* New York: Routledge.

Midwifery Education Accreditation Council. (2005). *List of midwifery schools.* Retrieved Febraury 6, 2006, from http://www.meacschools.org/programs/programs.html

Midwives Alliance of North America (MANA). (2005a). *Direct-entry midwifery state-by-state legal status.* Retrieved February 6, 2006, from http://www.mana.org/statechart.html

Midwives Alliance of North America (MANA). (2005b). *Direct-entry state laws and regulations.* Retrieved February 6, 2006, from http://www.mana.org/laws.html

Midwives Alliance of North America (MANA). (2006). *MANA core competences for basic midwifery practice.* Retrieved February 7, 2006, from http://mana.org/manacore.html

Nguyen v. Medical Quality Assurance Commission. (2001). 144 Wn.2d 516, 29 P.3d 689.

North American Registry of Midwives. (2004). *Position statement: Educational requirements to become a certified professional midwife (CPM).* Retrieved February 6, 2006, from http://www.narm.org/htb.htm#edrequirements

Payne, P. A., & King, V. J. (1998). A model of nurse–midwife and family physician collaborative care in a combined academic and community setting. *American Journal of Nurse–Midwifery, 43,* 19–26.

Payne, P. A., & King, V. J. (2001). What can midwives teach family physicians? *Clinics in Family Practice, 3,* 349–364.

Reed, A., & Roberts, J. E. (2000). State regulation of midwives: Issues and options. *Journal of Midwifery & Women's Health, 45*(2), 130–149.

Reid, A., & Galbraith, J. (1988). Midwifery in a family practice: A pilot study. *Canadian Family Physician, 34,* 1887–1890.

Reid, A. J., Carroll, J. C., Ruderman, J., & Murray, M. A. (1989). Differences in intrapartum obstetric care provided to women at low risk by family physicians and obstetricians. *Canadian Medical Association Journal, 140*(6), 625–633.

Reime, B., Klein, M. C., Kelly, A., Duxbury, N., Saxell, L., Liston, R., et al. (2004). Do maternity care provider groups have different attitudes towards birth? *British Journal of Obstetrics and Gynecology, 111*(12), 1388–1393.

Roberts, J. (1995). The role of graduate education in midwifery in the USA. In T. Murphy-Black (Ed.), *Issues in midwifery* (Vol. 1, pp. 119–161). New York: Churchill Livingstone.

Roberts, J. (2001). Revised "joint statement" clarifies relationships between midwives and physician collaborators. *Journal of Midwifery & Women's Health, 46*(5), 269–271.

Rooks, J. P. (1997). *Midwifery and childbirth in America.* Philadelphia: Temple University Press.

Rooks, J. P. (1998). Unity in midwifery? Realities and alternatives. *Journal of Nurse–Midwifery, 43,* 315–319.

Rooks, J. P. (1999). The midwifery model of care. *Journal of Nurse–Midwifery, 44,* 370–374.

Rooks, J. P., Carr, K. C., & Sandvold, I. (1991). The importance of non-master's degree options in nurse–midwifery education. *Journal of Nurse–Midwifery, 36,* 124–130.

Rosenblatt, R. A., Dobie, S. A., Hart, L. G., Schneeweiss, R., Gould, D., Raine, T. R., et al. (1997). Interspecialty differences in the obstetric care of low-risk women. *American Journal of Public Health, 87*(3), 344–351.

Sakala, C. (1988). Content of care by independent midwives: Assistance with pain in labor and birth. *Society of Scientific Medicine, 26*, 1141–1158.

Sakala, C. (1993). Midwifery care and out-of-hospital birth settings: How do they reduce unnecessary cesarean section births? *Society of Scientific Medicine, 37*, 1233–1250.

Schmittling, G., & Tsou, C. (1989). Obstetric privileges for family physicians: A national study. *Journal of Family Practice, 29*(2), 179–184.

Schuiling, K. D., Sipe, T. A., & Fullerton, J. (2005). Findings from the analysis of the American College of Nurse–Midwives member surveys: 2000–2003. *Journal of Midwifery & Women's Health, 50*, 8–15.

Scoggin, J. (1996). How nurse–midwives define themselves in relation to nursing, medicine, and midwifery. *Journal of Nurse–Midwifery, 41*(1), 36–42.

Scupholme, A., DeJoseph, J., Strobino, D. M., & Paine, L. L. (1992). Nurse–midwifery care to vulnerable populations. Phase I: Demographic characteristics of the national CNM sample. *Journal of Nurse–Midwifery, 37*(5), 341–348.

Sharp, E. S. (1983). Nurse–midwifery education: Its successes, failures, and future. *Journal of Nurse–Midwifery, 28*(2), 17–23.

Smith, M. A., Green, L. A., & Caruthers, B. (1989). Family practice obstetrics: Style of practice. *Family Medicine, 21*(1), 30–34.

Smucker, D. R. (1988). Obstetrics in family practice in the State of Ohio. *Journal of Family Practice, 26*, 165–168.

Texas Association of Nurse Anesthetists. (n.d.). *History of nurse anesthetists*. Retrieved February 6, 2006, from http://www.txana.org/AboutTANA/HxofNurseAnesthetis0973.asp

Thomas, M. W. (1965). *The practice of nurse–midwifery in the United States*. Washington, DC: Children's Bureau, U.S. Department of Health, Education, and Welfare.

Tom, S. (1982, December). Nurse–midwifery: A developing profession. *Law, Medicine and Health Care*, pp. 262–282.

Tom, S. A. (1980). Agnes Shoemaker Reinders: A biographical tribute. *Journal of Nurse–Midwifery, 25*(5), 9–12.

Tom, S. A. (1982). The evolution of nurse–midwifery: 1900–1960. *Journal of Nurse–Midwifery, 27*, 4–13.

U.S. Department of Labor, Bureau of Labor Statistics. (2005). *Registered nurses*. In *Occupational Outlook Handbook, 2004–2005*. Retrieved January 27, 2005, from http://stats.bls.gov/oco/pdf

Weaver, P., & Evans, S. K. (1998). *Practical skills guide for midwifery* (3rd ed.). Chugiak, AK: Morningstar Publishing.

White House Conference on Child Health and Protection (1930: Washington, D.C.). Eugene L. Bishop White House Conference on Child Health and Protection Collection. 1929–1931. Located in: Modern Manuscripts Collection, History of Medicine Division, National Library of Medicine, Bethesda, MD; MS C 266.

Williams, D. (2005). Professional midwifery in the United States: The American College of Nurse–Midwives turns 50. *Journal of Midwifery and Women's Health, 50*(1), 1–2.

Williams, J. W. (1912). Medical education and the midwife problem in the United States. *Journal of the American Medical Association, 2*, 180–204.

Wingeier, R., Bloch, S., & Kvale, J. (1988). A description of a CM-family physician joint practice in a rural setting. *Journal of Nurse–Midwifery, 33*, 86–92.

Table 1–1: For Your Professional Files 39

Table 1–1 For Your Professional Files

Name	Abbreviation	Contact	Web
American Academy of Family Physicians	AAFP	P.O. Box 11210 Shawnee Mission, KS 66207-1210 Tel: (800) 274-2237	www.aafp.org
American College of Nurse–Midwives	ACNM	8403 Colesville Road, Suite 1550 Silver Spring, MD 20910 Tel: (240) 485-1800	info@midwife.org www.midwife.org
American College of Obstetricians and Gynecologists	ACOG	P.O. Box 96920 Washington, DC 20024-6920 Tel: (202) 638-5577	www.acog.org
American Midwifery Certification Board	AMCB	849 International Drive, Suite 205 Linthicum, MD 21090	www.amcbmidwife.org
Citizens for Midwifery	CfM	P.O. Box 82227 Athens, GA 30608-2227 Tel: (888) 236-4880	info@cfmidwifery.org www.cfmidwifery.org
International Confederation of Midwives	ICM	Eisenhowerlaan 138 2517 KN The Hague The Netherlands Tel: +31 70 3060520 Fax: +31 70 3555651	info@internationalmidwives.org www.internationalmidwives.org
Journal of Midwifery & Women's Health	*J Midwifery Women's Health*	8403 Colesville Road, Suite 1550 Silver Spring, MD 20910 Tel: (240) 485-1815	www.jmwh.org www.medscape.com/ viewpublication/870
Midwifery Education Accreditation Council	MEAC	20 E. Cherry Flagstaff, AZ 86001 Tel: (928) 214-0997	info@meacschools.org www.meacschools.org
Midwives Alliance of North America	MANA	375 Rockbridge Road Suite 172-313	info@mana.org www.mana.org

continues

Organization	Abbrev.	Address	Link
		Lilburn, GA 30047 Tel: (888) 923-6262	
National Association of Certified Professional Midwives	NACPM	243 Banning Road Putney, VT 05346 Tel: (866) 704-9844	lawcing@sover.net www.nacpm.net
National Center for Health Statistics, source of data on number of births attended by birth attendant and place of birth, United States, by year	NCHS	3311 Toledo Road Hyattsville, MD 20782 Tel: (301) 458-4000	www.cdc.gov/nchs
North American Registry of Midwives	NARM	5257 Rosestone Dr. Lilburn, GA 30047 Tel: (888) 842-4784	info@narm.org www.narm.org

Document	Link
AAFP Policy on Nurse–Midwives	www.aafp.org/x6945.xml
ACNM Standards for the Practice of Midwifery	www.midwife.org/display.cfm?id=485
Jenkins, S.M. (1994). The myth of vicarious liability: Impact on barriers to nurse-midwifery practice. *J Nurse Midwifery, 39,* 98–106.	www.midwife.org/display.cfm?id=495
ACNM Professional Liability Information Packet	www.midwife.org/siteFiles/about/Professional Liability_RP.pdf
International definition of "midwife"	www.medicalknowledgeinstitute.com/files/ICM%20 Definition%20of%20the%20Midwife%202005.pdf
MANA's Statement of the Core Competencies for Basic Midwifery Practice	www.mana.org/manacore.html
Legal status of direct-entry midwives in the US	Direct-entry laws by state: www.mana.org/laws.html Direct-entry legal status by state: www.mana.org/statechart.html

CHAPTER 2

ACNM Structure and Function

Deanne R. Williams, CNM, MS, FACNM

Learning Objectives

1. Discuss the historical roots of the ACNM.
2. Describe the ACNM organizational structure.
3. Identify the five ACNM divisions and their function.
4. Describe the mission and purpose of the ACNM Foundation.
5. Understand the function and format of the ACNM Annual Meeting.
6. Discuss the history of the *Journal of Midwifery & Women's Health*.

Historical Roots

The American College of Nurse–Midwives is the professional membership organization for certified nurse–midwives (CNMs), certified midwives (CMs), and students enrolled in the ACNM Division of Accreditation accredited education programs.

Incorporated in 1955 as the American College of Nurse–Midwifery, ACNM changed its name in 1969 after it merged with the American Association of Nurse–Midwives (established in 1929). The creation of a single national organization to represent nurse–midwives places ACNM in the position of being the oldest women's health organization in the United States. In the *Journal of Midwifery & Women's Health Special Issue: 50 Years of Nurse–Midwifery/Midwifery*, Dawley (2005) outlines the quest for a new national organization for nurse–midwifery and the history of the development of the American College of Nurse–Midwives, and King (2005) tells the story of the ACNM seal.

The leaders who envisioned this organization understood the importance of setting national standards for the education, certification, and practice of midwifery and promoting the interests of midwives. Although the organization's foremothers explored a number of options that would have kept nurse–midwives within already established nursing organizations, it was their understanding of what was needed for professional autonomy that led to the decision to establish a separate organization. From fewer than 20 original members, the organization has grown to over 7,000 members. Although membership is voluntary, a majority of midwives understand how much the organization has contributed to the professional reputation now enjoyed by CNMs and CMs. The initial vision of an autonomous profession, capable of defining the scope of practice for midwifery and striving for legal recognition in all 50 states, must have seemed quite daunting at the time. Yet 50 years later, CNMs are licensed to practice in all 50 states plus all territories and are recognized in many influential federal and state laws and regulations. Although most work as employees of hospitals, physicians, or clinics, many own their own business. The standards for the education and certification of CMs, designed to be equivalent to the CNM, were adopted by ACNM in the late 1990s. Over 50 individuals have earned this credential, and licensure that recognizes the CM is available in three states.

As of 2006, the organization has set standards for the accreditation of nurse–midwifery, and then direct-entry midwifery, education programs for 44 years. The earliest nurse–midwives were certified based upon completion of their education program; however, for the past 34 years, ACNM has supported a national certification examination that is now implemented by an autonomous organization, the American Midwifery Certification Board, Inc. (formerly the ACNM Certification Council, Inc.). Over 10,000 graduates have passed the national certification exam.

Membership

All CNMs, CMs, student nurse–midwives (SNMs), and student midwives (SMs) are eligible for membership in ACNM. The three classifications of membership are:

- Active: CNMs and CMs only; may hold office or appointments on divisions, committees, and/or chapters
- Associate: CNM/CM who is a full-time student, engaged in missionary or volunteer work, retired, disabled, or not employed
- Student: Enrolled in an accredited or pre-accredited ACNM Division of Accreditation–approved nurse–midwifery or midwifery program or a graduate who is eligible to take the certification exam

ACNM members are eligible for all services of the national office, including technical assistance and consultation. Members are eligible to participate in the ACNM-endorsed professional liability insurance program, vote in elections, pay a reduced registration fee for the Annual Meeting, and receive subscriptions to the *Journal of Midwifery & Women's Health* and *Quickening*.

Governance

The ACNM Articles of Incorporation and Bylaws define the goals, objectives, and mission of the organization, how it conducts business, and its relationship to members. The most current version of these and many other documents referenced in this chapter are available on the ACNM Web site at www.acnm.org. ACNM is governed by a 10-member Board of Directors (Executive Committee plus six regional representatives). Board members are nominated by the Nominating Committee, elected by the membership, serve 3-year terms, and may serve two consecutive terms. Elections are staggered so board of directors (BOD) members' terms expire at alternating times.

The BOD has the overall responsibility to meet the objectives of the college, set policy, manage the funds of the college, approve chairpersons of divisions and committees, and approve standards of practice. The BOD consists of the president, vice president, secretary, treasurer, and representatives from six regions. The BOD meets four times each year, and all members are welcome to observe open board meetings.

To conduct the work necessary to the college, the ACNM bylaws authorize five standing divisions (Accreditation, Education, Research, Standards and Practice, and Women's Health Policy and Leadership) and the Nominating Committee. The president, with approval of the BOD, can establish specialized committees. With the exception of the Division of Accreditation and the Nominating Committee, all divisions and committees work with direction from the BOD. Members may serve on a Division or Committee for a 3-year term, limited to two consecutive terms for the same position.

ACNM Divisions

The Division of Accreditation (DOA), which is recognized by the U.S. Department of Education as an accrediting agency for nurse–midwifery education programs and direct-entry midwifery education programs for the non-nurse, has autonomous authority to plan, implement, and evaluate accreditation processes for nurse–midwifery and midwifery education programs. The DOA has a separate Board of Governors and an Advisory Committee. Refer to Chapter 4 for further information about the DOA and midwifery education.

The purpose of the Division of Education is to contribute to the health of women and newborns and the advancement of the profession of midwifery through the support and promotion of educational endeavors for and by certified nurse–midwives, certified midwives, and students in ACNM Division of Accreditation accredited programs. The DOE sections include: Basic Competency, Continuing Competency, Preceptor Development and Support, Continuing Education, and Policy.

The purpose of the Division of Research (DOR) is to contribute to knowledge about the health of women, infants, and their families and to advance the profession of midwifery by promoting the development, conduct, and dissemination of research. The DOR sections include: Research Advisory, Research Development, Networking, International, and Data and Information Management. Refer to Chapter 13 for more information about midwifery research.

The purpose of the Division of Standards and Practice (DOSP) is to contribute to the health of women and infants and the advancement of the profession of midwifery by providing, promoting, and supporting development and communication and review of midwifery philosophy, code of ethics, and standards and practice. The DOSP sections include: Clinical Practice and Structure, Home Birth, Quality Improvement, Professional Liability, and Business.

The purpose of the Division of Women's Health Policy and Leadership (commonly known as the DOW) is to improve women's health at the community, national, and international levels through coordination of the development of public health and women's health policy initiatives. The DOW sections include: Policy Development and Evaluation, Networking Development, Leadership, Women's Health Issues and Projects, and Public Information. Refer to Chapter 15 for more information on women's health and midwifery.

ACNM Committees

The purpose of the Archives committee is to establish, maintain, and preserve material of historical significance to the college for reference by members, midwifery students, and individual researchers approved by the BOD.

The purpose of the Bylaws committee is to facilitate the work of the ACNM and maintain congruence with the bylaws of the college by review of the College Standing Rules of Procedure, Chapter Bylaws and Standing Rules of Procedure, proposed bylaw amendments, and other documents as requested by the ACNM BOD.

The purpose of the Government Affairs committee is to develop economic policies, to serve as a forum for policy coordination from the divisions, and to develop strategies to carry out the implementation of political and economic policies related to midwifery practice and women's health. In addition, the Government Affairs committee will coordinate the mobilization of grassroots efforts of the membership and implement appropriate strategies through political action.

The purpose of the Uniformed Services committee is to recruit and retain members of all active, retired, and reserve commissioned corps (Army, Navy, Air Force, and Public Health Service) to ACNM, provide representation for the needs of midwives working in federal facilities, and increase awareness among the college membership of the unique issues concerning uniformed service members.

The purpose of the International Health committee is to promote awareness and provide information on international maternal and child health-care issues for ACNM members.

The purpose of the Midwives of Color committee is to recruit and retain persons of diverse ethnic and cultural backgrounds to the profession of midwifery; provide educational preparation to the ACNM membership, which will develop respect for cultural variations; and to increase awareness and responsiveness among ACNM membership to maternal/child health-care issues affecting people of color.

The purpose of the Nominating committee is to ensure the conduct of legal and proper nominations of officers and other elective positions designated by the bylaws.

The purpose of the Program committee is to plan, help coordinate, and evaluate the educational content and business meetings for the annual meeting of the college.

The purpose of the Public Relations committee is to interpret to professionals and consumers the services provided by the college, components of maternal and child health (MCH) care, and the role of the certified nurse–midwife and certified midwife in the provision of quality MCH care.

The purpose of the Student committee is to design and implement programs that support and expand the contribution of students who are enrolled in ACNM DOA accredited education programs.

ACNM Chapters

The ACNM bylaws authorize local groups of ACNM members within the same region to establish chapters. All authorized chapters must have their bylaws reviewed for compliance with ACNM bylaws, and are assigned a chapter number by the Bylaws committee. As of 2005, 98 ACNM chapters exist in the United States. Information on local chapters is available in the ACNM Membership Directory, from regional representatives, and by contacting the national office staff.

Since 1992, the certification of CNMs and CMs has been the responsibility of a separately incorporated organization, the American Midwifery Certification Board, Inc. (formerly the ACNM Certification Council, Inc.). Refer to Chapter 5 for more information on certification and licensure.

The National Office

The national office for the ACNM carries out the day-to-day activities of the college. Organized into four departments (Finance and Administration, Member Services, Professional Services, and Global Outreach), ACNM staff provide a wide range of expertise that contributes to the achievement of the organization's objectives. In partnership with the Board of Directors, divisions, committees, and individual ACNM members, staff work in the areas of expansion of midwifery practice, policy analysis and advocacy, marketing and public relations, state and federal lobbying, international development, and implementation of professional standards.

Finance and Administration

The finance and administration department is responsible for the ACNM budget and financial services.

Member Services

Member services responsibilities include a national marketing campaign; individual, chapter, and state-wide consultation and support for practice and legislative initiatives; publication of a wide variety of professional and consumer education materials; organizing at least one national meeting each year; lobbying for initiatives that increase funding for midwifery education and practice and that improve the health status of women and their families; and collaboration with other organizations on joint initiatives.

Professional Services

The professional services department provides essential services to ACNM members. The department is responsible for all aspects of clinical practice and policies. It has produced several sentinel publications, including the *Quick Info* series and articles on credentialing and professional liability. Professional services staff speak to large volumes of midwives each year about issues that affect their clinical practice. The federal lobbyist, senior policy analyst (who addresses state policy issues), senior staff researcher, and senior technical advisor are members of the professional services department.

Global Outreach

For over 15 years, ACNM has worked on safe motherhood activities in developing countries, primarily through the Department of Global Outreach (originally the Special Projects Section). It is widely known that the majority of women in resource-poor countries receive maternity care from midwives or traditional birth attendants. Saving the lives of women requires that all health-care providers have appropriate knowledge and skills, and this is particularly true when hospitals are not available or are not capable of caring for women in labor. Hundreds of CNMs have worked as consultants in these countries, and ACNM has earned a solid reputation for providing expert consultants to establish the ACNM Life Saving Skills (LSS) program as a means to train skilled birth attendants. In 2005, ACNM introduced the Home-Based Life Saving Skills program, which is designed to complement LSS by making stronger connections and expanding the support from community organizations and leaders.

The ACNM Journal

The professional reputation of CNMs and CMs is enhanced by the publication of the peer reviewed *Journal of Midwifery & Women's Health,* which is available online and listed in the Index Medicus. Established in 1955 as the *Bulletin of the American College of Nurse–Midwifery,* the name was changed in 1973 to the *Journal of Nurse–Midwifery.* In January 2000, the name was changed again to *Journal of Midwifery & Women's Health (JMWH).* The history of the journal is well documented in the March/April 2005 issue of *JMWH.* The article by Editor Emeritus Mary Ann Shah, CNM, MSN, FACNM, includes a review of the 10-year effort that preceded the 1986 acceptance into Index Medicus; the provision of intensive home study programs by and for midwives; the movement to an independent editorial board; and a number of publication milestones that have distinguished this internationally known journal.

The ACNM Foundation

Established in 1967, the ACNM Foundation, Inc. (ACNMF) is a 501(c)(3) nonprofit organization that supports the provision of high quality maternal, newborn, and well-woman health services through the practice of midwifery. The foundation collaborates closely with and complements the goals of the ACNM. Donations to the foundation are tax deductible as allowed by law. Guided by the Board of Trustees, ACNMF engages in a broad program of activities, including provision of scholarships for basic midwifery students and research; sponsorship of research, educational, and leadership programs; and recognition of accomplished midwives. On average, the foundation gives out over $20,000 in awards and scholarships each year.

Communication

ACNM communicates with members and the community at large through a number of mechanisms. Regional representatives utilize eMidwife discussion lists to post announcements and gather information. eMidwife discussion lists have been organized around topics such as clinical management, home birth, business, international, and gynecology. Members have the opportunity to share information and seek helpful hints on common dilemmas via these electronic communication tools. Members join a list via a link on the ACNM home page at www.acnm.org.

The bimonthly newsletter, *Quickening*, and professional journal, *JMWH*, are mailed to members and friends of the college. *Quickening* is often described as a news journal. With timely information that goes into detail beyond what is typically found in a newsletter, *Quickening* includes regular columns from the president, executive director, regional representatives, director of professional services, policy staff, and the communication manager. Minutes from ACNM board meetings are published in *Quickening* along with information about new products and policies that impact women's health and the practice of midwifery. Classified ads list jobs, products, services, and meetings that are relevant to the profession. **Table 2–1** lists ACNM publications.

Since 1994, ACNM has owned the Internet domains www.midwife.org and www.acnm.org. The Web site gets over 3,000 visitors per day and has been highly praised by students, midwives, members of the press, and consumers. Over the years, content on the Web site has expanded to include a large variety of announcements, current documents, and historical facts. Individuals can submit abstracts and register for ACNM meetings, purchase publications, write letters to elected officials and the media, apply for scholarships,

---

Table 2–1 ACNM Publications

Handbooks
> *Quality Management*
> *The Midwife as First Assistant*
> *Vacuum Assisted Birth in Midwifery Practice*
> *Home Birth Practice*
> *Clinical Privileges & Credentialing*
> *Minding Your Own Business: Business Plans for Midwifery Practices*
> *Getting Paid: Billing, Coding and Payment for Nurse–Midwifery Services*
> *Marketing and Public Relations*
> *Taking Action: A State Advocacy Handbook*
> *Midwifery Today: A Summary of Nurse–Midwifery Legislation*

Marketing Materials
> *Pregnancy Calculator*
> *Today's Certified Nurse–Midwife Brochures*
> *Certified Nurse–Midwives and Your GYN Health*

Bimonthly News Journal
> *Quickening*

Journal
> *Journal of Midwifery & Women's Health*

communicate with ACNM staff members, apply for membership, and make a donation to the foundation all via the ACNM Web site.

The ACNM Annual Meeting and Exhibit, which is scheduled in the spring of every year, attracts more than 1200 midwives to five days of meetings that include continuing education sessions, business meetings, an exhibit hall, and fundraising for the ACNM Foundation. A wide variety of education sessions and workshops are offered to meet the continuing education needs of midwives. In addition, a number of official and unofficial activities are planned that facilitate interaction between members and the ACNM leadership. All divisions and committees meet during the week and the members conduct the business of the College as defined in the bylaws. This is the only time when the organization's bylaws can be changed and members can bring motions to the floor for discussion and an advisory vote by those present. The Annual Meeting is an important mechanism for communicating the state of the profession to a variety of colleagues and serves as an important opportunity for midwives to expand their knowledge, scope of support, and professional pride. Special activities, such as breakfast with the BOD and preparation of a student report to the membership, are designed to introduce midwife students to the profession. Activities such as the Heart of Midwifery, Blankets for Babies, and the closing party offer attendees a chance to go beyond the scientific boundaries to the heart of what binds the profession together **(Box 2–1)**.

ACNM also publishes a number of handbooks, guidelines, reference packets, and marketing materials designed to meet the needs of midwives that are available to purchase online. Many ACNM documents can be downloaded without charge.

MidwifeJobs.com (www.midwifejobs.com) is the only online job search site dedicated to matching midwives with employers who are seeking the services of a midwife. Members can post their resumes online and can sign up to receive notification of any new

---

Box 2–1   In the Words of a Student

Having attended the ACNM Annual Meeting 2 years in a row as a student I must say that what I have come away with both years is a greater understanding and awareness of the "culture" of the profession. I believe it is important for the organization to gather like this on a consistent basis since the density of midwives throughout the country is not very high. If we did not come together in such ways we would slowly become absorbed by the healthcare system and lose our identity in the process. There's strength in numbers as we all know, so maintaining a strong, unified organization is crucial to the advancement of any profession. You should know that each year is different, and heavily dependent upon the location where the conference is held. Last year, it was New Orleans; we stayed 2 blocks off Bourbon Street. Needless to say, it was a much different atmosphere than this year's politically focused meeting. Last year there was a palpable energy in the lobby of the hotel where we stayed, mainly due to the nightlife that everyone was enjoying. This year, the same amount of energy was present, but focused on Capitol Hill. I appreciate both types of agendas, making friends and making political progress.

Hope to see you next year!

Samantha Nardella
Kansas University Medical Center

job postings. Listings are organized geographically. Like virtually all ACNM services, the success of any one program is a direct measure of how many members chose to participate. MidwifeJobs.com receives high marks from those looking to hire a midwife!

ACNM also supports two consumer-focused Web sites: www.gotmom.org and www.myMidwife.org. GotMom provides breastfeeding information and resources to mothers and families; and myMidwife provides information on midwifery, maternity, women's health, and family-centered health care. ACNM has also published four editions of the consumer magazine, *Every Baby*. Over 250,000 copies are available for distribution by members each year.

ACNM Honors and Awards

The ACNM Fellowship program was established in 1994. Election to ACNM Fellowship is an honor that is celebrated at each ACNM Annual Meeting. Fellows earn the credential based on their professional achievement, outstanding scholarship, clinical excellence, and/or leadership. The mission of the Fellowship is to serve the ACNM in a consultative and advisory capacity.

First awarded in 1997, the Hattie Hemschemeyer Award is bestowed annually to an outstanding ACNM member who is a CNM/CM, has been certified for at least 10 years, and has demonstrated outstanding contributions or distinguished service to midwifery or maternal child heath. The award is named after the first ACNM president. The Kitty Ernst Award, affectionately named the "young whippersnapper" award, is named after the youngest ACNM president, known for her flamboyant hats and purple boa. The Kitty Ernst award honors a CNM/CM who is an active ACNM member and has been certified for less than 10 years. The award is presented annually to an individual who has demonstrated innovative, creative endeavors in midwifery and/or women's health clinical practice, education, administration, or research.

Other awards presented at the ACNM Annual Meeting include the Regional Award for Excellence, which honors one CNM/CM from each region during the regional meetings. The recipients of this award are elected by members within each individual region. The Dorothea M. Lang Pioneer Award is named after an ACNM president and visionary leader, and honors an exceptional CNM/CM who has been certified for 10 years, has not received the Hattie Hemschemeyer Award, and demonstrates vision and leadership. The With Women for a Lifetime commendation honors midwifery services, and the Midwifing Midwives for a Lifetime commendation honors midwifery education programs that have provided innovative and compassionate care to families, expanded access to women's health care to CNMs/CMs, and educated future CNMs/CMs.

Support for Students

ACNM has designed a number of programs with the student in mind. From membership dues to the annual meeting registration, deep discounts are offered to students. Students are welcome to serve on divisions and committees, speak at the business meetings, and participate in the annual preparation of a report for the membership on the needs of students.

Many ACNM publications focus on the business of midwifery because this is an area that is hard to fit into most education programs, but becomes critically important shortly after graduation. ACNM provides expert consultation for midwives who need to apply for hospital privileges and need to be credentialed by health insurance companies. Student members can post their resume on MidwifeJobs.com for free, and ACNM offers a certification exam prep course at the Annual Meeting. A student-only breakfast with the ACNM Board of Directors is scheduled during the Annual Meeting. Students are welcome to serve as interns at the ACNM national office. In addition, the ACNM Foundation awards a number of student scholarships each year.

Summary

Fifty years after its incorporation as an independent voice for the profession of nurse–midwifery, ACNM has surpassed the vision of its founders. Now representing certified nurse–midwives and certified midwives, ACNM is well-known and widely respected for the role it plays in promoting the health of women and newborns throughout the world. All CNMs and CMs, whether members or not, are well served by the role ACNM plays in a wide variety of areas. Whether it is assuring that laws, regulations, and policies that influence access to women's health care are midwife-friendly, creating a demand for midwifery care, educating members on the business of midwifery, or doing the hard work that comes with being a professional, ACNM members and staff have always been up to the task.

Table 2–2 For Your Professional Files

ACNM Articles of Incorporation
ACNM Bylaws
ACNM Mission Statement
ACNM Philosophy and Code of Ethics

References

Dawley, K. (2005). Doubling back over roads once traveled: Creating a national organization for nurse–midwifery. *Journal of Midwifery & Women's Health, 50*(2), 71–82.

King, T. (2005). The emblem of the American College of Nurse–Midwives. *Journal of Midwifery & Women's Health, 50*(2), 83–84.

Shah, M. A. (2005). The *Journal of Midwifery and Women's Health* 1995–2005: Its historic milestones and evolutionary changes. *Journal of Midwifery & Women's Health, 50*(2), 159–168.

CHAPTER 3

Public Health and Midwifery

Heather Reynolds, CNM, MSN, FACNM

Learning Objectives

1. Analyze the historical developments in health care and public policy that have contributed to present day practice in the care of women and infants.
2. Identify the history and role of the United States government in maternal–child health.
3. Discuss the role of the Maternal and Child Health Bureau and Title V in maternal–child health.
4. Discuss the role of Title X of the Public Health Service Act.
5. Identify Healthy People 2010 objectives that relate to maternal–child health.
6. Discuss the purpose and elements of a community assessment.

In 1910, U.S. President Taft noted in his support for the establishment of a Federal Children's Bureau that, "We have an agricultural Department and we are spending $14 million or $15 million a year to tell the farmers . . . how they ought to treat the cattle and the horses with a view to having . . . good cattle and good horses. . . . If out of the public treasury at Washington we can establish a department for that purpose, it does not seem to be a long step or a stretch of logic to say we have the power to spend the money on a Bureau of Research to tell how we may develop good men and women" (Bradbury & Eliot, 1956, p. 3). The responsibility for the public's social and health well-being had historically resided with the individual states and local communities (Bradbury & Eliot, 1956; Meckel, 1990; Mustard, 1945; Smilie, 1949; Soule & MacKenzie, 1940). When states encountered major problems that overwhelmed their resources, they often looked to the federal government for solutions and assistance (Mullan, 1989). When local and state authorities and everyday citizens turned to the federal government for help in addressing critical child welfare issues, the government eventually responded with the establishment of the Federal Children's Bureau in 1912 (Bradbury & Eliot, 1956). It took 9 years (1903–1912) from its conception to its authorization by the U.S. Congress. The movers and shakers who were unrelenting in their efforts to see this bureau exist grew out of the 1800s–1900s social reform movement in the U.S. Known as Progressivism, this reform movement was a response to the rapid changes occurring in American society as a result of immigration, urbanization, and industrialization.

Social Reformers

The development of maternal–child health care and public health policies in the United States is inextricably linked to the efforts of the social reformers of the late 1800s (Bradbury & Eliot, 1956; Meckel, 1990; Mullan, 1989; Smilie, 1949). A number of these reformers were educated women of high social standing who were unable to exercise their talents and skills in the broader U.S. community due to the social and gender constraints of that period. "In an age when domesticity and motherhood were considered the only proper functions of 'ladies,' young women who desired careers that would take them away from the home faced ridicule from large segments of the population" (Litoff, 1978, p. 13). These college/seminary educated, socially and economically well-heeled women took up residence in settlement houses and worked directly with the poor. Their objectives included educating and assisting immigrants to adjust to life in the United States and assuring that these immigrants would assume their civic and community responsibilities (Hull-House Residents, 1895). Though their initial goals may not be perceived as altruistic and perhaps were primarily geared toward "Americanizing" these new immigrants, their orientation towards and their perceptions of these immigrants changed once they became familiar with their circumstances. The eyes of the women working in these communities were opened to the despicable conditions in which families were living. Not only were the living spaces overcrowded, but sanitation resources were inadequate and underused by these new immigrants, thus fostering health epidemics that resulted in loss of lives (Hull-House Residents, 1895; Meckel, 1990). Between 1880 and 1900 the population in Chicago had quadrupled, with more than 75% of the population born outside of the United States (Wattenberg, n.d.). These women focused their attention on addressing the ills that plagued the poor and burgeoning immigrant populations in urban communities such as New York City and Chicago (Hull-House Residents, 1895).

Along with the social reform movement of that time, the local public health care system was also evolving as it attempted to grapple with health concerns that arose with the increasing immigrant population of the late 1800s and early 1900s. Infectious disease encouraged by poor working and living conditions dictated the need for a sound public health infrastructure (Mustard, 1945; Price, 1919; Soule & MacKenzie, 1940). This, coupled with efforts to improve the lot of women and children in the poor and immigrant populations, provided impetus for the development of federal policies and programs that would promote health in these communities.

Infant mortality rate (IMR) became the sentinel marker for the health and well-being of a community. As was noted in the Secretary of the Commonwealth of Massachusetts' annual reports (1866–1875), the IMR in Suffolk County, Massachusetts, showed consistent disparities in rates among children of native-born parents versus those whose parents were foreign-born. Differences in the IMRs between these two groups ranged from a low of 5.8 to 32.6 infant deaths per 1000 live births (Meckel, 1990). In 7 of the 10 years of this survey, infants of foreign-born parents had an IMR that was 16 points greater than that of infants of native-born parents. These findings were consistent with other communities as well (Dorey, 1999). The settlement house workers, by going door to door, were able to gather data that provided in "graphic form a few facts concerning the section" wherein the settlements were located (Hull-House Residents, 1895, p. 7). Some of the data compiled in this way were gleaned from governmental agencies interested in the conditions in these slums. Municipalities as well as a broader audience were thus informed of the tenuous conditions of these slum dwellers and could reasonably assess the nature and depth of social and health problems in these communities (Hull-House Residents, 1895).

The early advocacy for a national focus on maternal and child health issues came from women working in settlement houses in cities like New York and Chicago (Bradbury & Eliot, 1956; Meckel, 1990; Rosen, 2003). These settlement houses were modeled after the university settlement movement in England that was spearheaded by those seeking social reform there (Addams, 1910; Gorst, 1895). On returning from a visit to England, Jane Addams and Ellen Starr established the Hull House settlement in 1889 in Chicago, Illinois; though not the first of its kind in the United States, it was one of the most successful and well known (Brown, 1999). Subsequently, in 1895, Lillian Wald, a nurse and social worker (though not formally trained as a social worker, early public health nurses by virtue of their work were often called nurse-social workers) founded the Henry Street Settlement house in New York City. Social reformers went on to wage campaigns against child labor, sweatshops, abuse of women laborers, and other social ills that beset the poor. Living and working with the poor in these settlement houses afforded the incubating and avid reformers first-hand experiences with the human destruction and loss resulting from poverty, lack of education, and crowded living conditions (Hull-House Residents, 1895).

In addition to her work at Henry Street Settlement, Lillian Wald is credited with introducing a resolution that would allow the education of nurses in midwifery and the concept of nursing in public health (Bradbury & Eliot, 1956). Additionally, Wald is noted as being the first person to suggest, in 1903, the need to develop a Federal Children's Bureau. Lillian Wald first introduced the bureau concept to Florence Kelley of the National Consumer's League, and this link proved fateful in getting the ear of then-President Teddy Roosevelt (Bradbury & Eliot, 1956; Meckel, 1990). Both Wald and Kelley were strong advocates for social reform and were connected to organizations that were prominent in the early 1900s for advocacy and lobbying the government on social and health-related issues. The National Consumer's League, whose first executive secretary was Florence Kelley, was an ardent advocate for a fair marketplace for workers and product safety for consumers, and was pivotal in the passage of the federal Fair Labor Standards Act of 1938.

Child Welfare

These women were connected on many levels and in many varied circumstances. Ms. Kelley had spent time at Hull House and supervised a federally sanctioned survey of the community in which Hull House was located (Hull-House Residents, 1895). As part of the Progressive Movement, they collaborated on a number of initiatives such as child labor, child welfare, and other social welfare issues. Social activists who led the charge to transform the practice of child labor worked through the National Child Labor Committee, which was formed in 1904. While working on the issue of child labor, these reformers embraced other welfare and health issues related to children and forged alliances to enact changes in the status quo. For example, practices such as child labor had always been an integral part of the fabric of the United States agrarian system, and this practice easily transitioned into factory and textile jobs generated by the Industrial Revolution. It was generally accepted that children beginning at age 10 years were suitable for employment to augment their families' incomes (Bradbury & Eliot, 1956; Brown, 1999; Meckel, 1990; Trattner, 1970). Many state-level organizations worked tirelessly to enact laws that would change child labor practices in their respective communities.

The Children's Bureau studies on child labor resulted in the Child Labor Law of 1917, which was administered by the bureau. Although it was declared unconstitutional 9 months after its enactment, it laid the foundation for later activities in this area (Addams, 1935; Bradbury & Eliot, 1990). After the Great Depression and the implementation of the National Industry Recovery Act's subsequent Fair Labor Standards Act in 1938, strict guidelines for child labor were developed at the federal level. Other efforts for child welfare bore fruit before that year at the local level.

Many members of these organizations, and especially the National Child Labor Committee and the National Consumer's League, were instrumental in making the Federal Children's Bureau a reality. At its December 1905 meeting in Washington D.C., the National Child Labor Committee drafted legislation to create a Federal Children's Bureau. This draft served as the basis for the 11 unsuccessful bills submitted in the United States Congress through 1911 as well as the bill that launched the establishment of the Children's Bureau (Bradbury & Eliot, 1956; Meckel, 1990).

The year 1909 was a pivotal one for promoting the idea of a Federal Children's Bureau. Two important meetings that year energized and solidified the need and support for this bureau. The first White House Conference on the Care of Dependent Children and the American Academy of Medicine (AAM) meeting in New Haven, Connecticut, which saw the establishment of the American Association for the Study and Prevention of Infant Mortality (AASPIM), both laid the foundation for the bureau's development.

The first White House Conference on the Care of Dependent Children was called by President Theodore Roosevelt and convened in Washington, D.C., on January 25 and 26 (Bradbury & Eliot, 1956; Meckel, 1990; Roosevelt, 1909). The attendees at this conference included social workers, educators, juvenile court judges, labor leaders, and social reformers. Both men and women concerned with the welfare of children attended. This conference formally recommended that a Federal Children's Bureau be established that would collect and disseminate information affecting the welfare of children. Echoing his support for this recommendation, President Roosevelt exhorted Congress to act on this bill, though his efforts were initially unsuccessful.

Helen Putnam, a practicing physician from Rhode Island and the President of AAM, had proposed and successfully got AAM to commit to designing a conference on infant mortality. The AAM committee that formed to tackle infant mortality enlisted a multi-disciplinary advisory group, and together they planned and convened the infant mortality conference in New Haven, Connecticut, in 1909. At this conference, a number of organizations were represented and contributed to the discussions around the causes and methods for the prevention of infant mortality. A number of social reformers were either on the advisory committee for this meeting (Jane Addams of Hull House) or were in attendance (Florence Kelley, Lillian Wald, Julia Lathrop, and Dr. Alice Tallant, who was Professor of Obstetrics at Women's Medical College of Pennsylvania) (American Association for the Study and Prevention of Infant Mortality [AASPIM], 1912; Meckel, 1990). The American Association for the Study and Prevention of Infant Mortality (AASPIM) was formed at this meeting and its members included a number of individuals in support of a Federal Children's Bureau (Meckel, 1990). In fact, one of the five AASPIM objectives stated that "by arousing public sentiment and lobbying legislatures and government officials, it would work for the establishment of municipal, state and federal infant and child health bureaus" (Meckel, 1990, p. 110). On the other hand, this new organization served as a forum to address the issues related to the practice of midwifery. During AASPIM's second annual meeting held in Chicago, Illinois, on November 16–18, 1911, the Committee on Midwifery, chaired by Dr. Mary Sherwood of Baltimore, Md., had six commissioned papers presented. The topics of these papers were:

- "The Midwife Problem and Medical Education in the United States" by Dr. J. Whitridge Williams, Professor of Obstetrics, Johns Hopkins University
- "Has the Trained and Supervised Midwife Made Good?" by Drs. Arthur Brewster Emmons, II, and James Lincoln Huntington, both from Boston, Massachusetts
- "Obstetric Care in the Congested Districts of our Large American Cities" by Dr. Arthur Brewster Emmons, II
- "The Problem of Midwifery from the Standpoint of Administration," by Dr. Marshall Langton Price, Baltimore, Maryland
- "Registration and Practice of Midwifery," by Dr. Fredrick V. Beitler, Baltimore, Maryland
- "School for Midwives," by Dr. S. Josephine Baker, Director of Child Hygiene, Department of Health, New York City.

The "Midwife Problem"

Dr. J. Whitridge Williams's address to the AASPIM body regarding the "midwife problem" and the state of medical education in the United States reflected the prevailing attitude in a portion of the medical and nursing professions (Meckel, 1990). His comments, which were subsequently published in 1912 (Williams, 1912), characterized most of the physicians who were practicing obstetrics as being incompetent and perhaps causing more harm to women and children than the midwives. In his survey of medical school professors, Williams found that "more than three-quarters of the professors of obstetrics in all parts of the country, in reply to my questionnaire, state that incompetent doctors kill more women each year by improperly performed operations than the ignorant midwife does by neglect of aseptic precaution" (AASPIM, 1912, p. 180). Although the majority of the professors whom he surveyed felt that the midwife problem could be solved by education and regulation of midwives (AASPIM, 1912), Williams was less enthusiastic, feeling "very dubious concerning the possibility of developing satisfactory midwives by any method of instruction (AASPIM, 1912, p. 192). Rather than support efforts to license and regulate the midwives, he advocated their abolishment. "Reform is urgently needed, and can be accomplished more speedily by radical improvement in medical education than by attempting the most impossible task of improving midwives" (Williams, 1912, p. 6). Williams chose to support improving the training and caliber of practicing obstetricians, noting that the institutionalization of midwifery would result in competition for physicians and lower fees for physician services (Litoff, 1978; Meckel, 1990).

On the other hand, Dr. S. Josephine Baker, the director of the New York City Bureau of Child Hygiene and a strong advocate of training and regulation of midwives, presented a more supportive perspective on midwives than Dr. Williams, based on her research at the same AASPIM meeting in 1911. When she first assumed her position as director of this bureau, Dr. Baker experienced success in reducing infections in children by educating their mothers. She next turned her attention towards the midwives as another avenue to further reduce infant and child mortality and morbidity. Though she regarded the immigrant midwives as "densely ignorant, and therefore filthy, superstitious, hidebound, everything a good midwife should not be" (Baker, 1939, p. 112), Baker recognized that the immigrant women were culturally and traditionally wedded to midwifery care. Her research findings supported the use and efficacy of trained midwives. With this as a backdrop, Baker went about the business of installing an efficient licensing system for midwives. She was able to receive new, strict licensing laws from the New York State Legislature for New York City. Midwives came in droves to receive their licenses once the law was instituted, almost four-thousand strong (Baker, 1939). Over time, the "unfit" midwives were weeded out and subsequent to the initial licensing, new applicants had to demonstrate that they graduated from either the Bellevue Hospital Midwifery School or a comparable European school. Her testament to midwifery care speaks volumes about her respect for midwives: "If I had a daughter who was going to have a baby, I would rather see her in the hands of one of those competent Scandinavian midwives. A well-trained midwife deserves all possible respect as a practical specialist" (Baker, 1939, p. 114). Baker had published figures that clearly demonstrated that the maternal mortality rate from infection related to childbirth was far higher in hospital-based physician-delivered women than in those delivered at home by midwives (Baker, 1939). Dr. Baker's research on European-trained midwives indicated that they were the best in the country. Furthermore, Baker supported schools for training midwives and an avenue for registering and regulating their practice (Litoff, 1978, 1986). Unfortunately, the Flexner Report, which criticized the excessive numbers of medical schools ($N = 155$) and the poor caliber of graduates from these institutions, was released in 1910. This report undoubtedly influenced the priority for the 1911 AASPIM meeting, where the emphasis was more on improving the physicians' obstetrical requirements and training, rather than on the institutionalization of midwifery practice in the United States. Given the mixed reports on midwifery at this AASPIM meeting, the committee's resolution on midwifery reflected this impasse: "That the study of local midwifery conditions is urged as a means of collecting facts with which to direct public opinion in regard to this important subject" (AASPIM, 1912, p. 164).

The "midwife problem" and the declining use of midwives had their roots in a number of circumstances, including medical innovations, and economic and social concerns

(Dawley, 2001; Litoff, 1978, 1986). The use of anesthesia and forceps in childbirth ostensibly afforded a select group of women, mostly economically well-disposed, to engage the services of male midwives, the predecessors of obstetricians (Bullough & Rosen, 1992; Dawley, 2000; Litoff, 1978, 1986). Poor women, including minorities and immigrants, continued to use the services of midwives in the early 1900s (Dawley, 2000; Litoff, 1978, 1986). Despite the relatively better outcomes with midwives versus obstetricians in the early 1900s, the midwives were blamed for the high maternal and infant mortality rate. Given the midwives' economic status and in many instances illiteracy, they were an easy target for denunciation and blame. The more affluent physicians encouraged social reformers such as Elizabeth Lowell Putnam, who at one time was the president of AASPIM, to advocate for the elimination of midwives.

The Children's Bureau

It took until 1912 for the Children's Bureau to be legislated by Congress. The authorized responsibility of the Children's Bureau was "to investigate and report upon all matters pertaining to the welfare of children and child life among all classes of people" (Bradbury & Eliot, 1956, p. 87). This marked the first time the federal government had ventured into social welfare as related to common citizens. Prior to this, the responsibility for the health and welfare of citizens was solely under the auspices of the states. Since there was no specific delegation of authority provided to the federal government by the Constitution, the prevailing attitude was that the states held the responsibilities for the health and welfare of its citizens. The federal government's legitimacy in assuming the responsibility for and a role in health care delivery and policy development hinged on the constitutional obligation to provide for the welfare of the people (Bradbury & Eliot, 1956; Meckel, 1990; Mullan, 1989).

After President Taft signed the new legislation for the Children's Bureau in 1912, he selected Julia Lathrop to be the director. Lathrop, a social reformer, emerged from the settlement house experience to lead the way in articulating the social and health concerns of children in the United States. Prior to leading the Children's Bureau, Ms. Lathrop worked at Hull House, and along with its co-founders, Jane Addams and Ellen Starr, had been educated at the Rockford Female Seminary. Lathrop, a lawyer, was trained by her father, William Lathrop, who was an attorney as well as a U.S. congressman (Hull House, 2002). With her background, she had the experience and expertise to assume the leadership of this new bureau. Lathrop undertook the data gathering priority of the Children's Bureau with zeal: "We did not know accurately how many babies were born each year, how many die or why they die" (Bradbury & Eliot, 1956, p. 6). Statistics of birth and mortality were needed to assess the scope of the problem and to address the issues appropriately.

The early years of the Children's Bureau were occupied with investigating and reporting on the social, health, and employment issues of children. Additionally, the bureau collected and analyzed data on both maternal and infant mortality and morbidity. The data generated by the efforts of the bureau clearly demonstrated that improved economic conditions, maternal availability to and breastfeeding of a child through its first year, and good sanitation were linked to an improved chance of survival of children in the first year of life (Bradbury & Eliot, 1956). Lathrop presented information on preventive strategies that improved outcomes in countries such as New Zealand, and used this information to articulate the bureau's function of finding solutions to, rather than just reporting on, the problems (Meckel, 1990). In her 1914 report on New Zealand's Baby Saving work, Lathrop highlighted successful strategies used there, including establishing maternity hospitals for treatment of problem cases and training of nurses, state registration and training of midwives, compulsory registration of births, national educational endeavors through prenatal care centers, well baby clinics, and a visiting nurse program.

The Children's Bureau embraced efforts to disseminate health information, including publication of pamphlets for parents on issues such as prenatal care (published in 1913) and on infant care. Grace Miegs, the director of the Children's Bureau's Division of Child Hygiene, authored the 1916 report for the bureau on the importance of maternal mortality and its profound impact on infant mortality (Meckel, 1990). Miegs's report appeared to move the bureau from its original mandate of child welfare into the arena of maternity care. Miegs was able to reconcile this move into maternity care by noting that "In the progress of work for the prevention of infant mortality . . . It must be plain, then, to what a degree the sickness and death of the mother lessens the chances of the baby for life and health" (Meigs, 1917, p. 9). Furthermore, the bureau acknowledged that maternal mortality in the United States was related to "ignorance of the dangers connected with childbirth," plus the need for prenatal care and good hygiene (Meckel, 1990, p. 203). In her 1917 report to Congress, Julia Lathrop made recommendations that they produce legislation that would provide matching grants to states to establish maternal and child health centers and expand the visiting nurse services, particularly in rural areas where health services were either not accessible or not available.

Following Julia Lathrop's recommendations in her 1917 report, many congressional bills were proposed to enact her recommendations. Each year following her report, bills were introduced and defeated until finally one was passed in 1921. This 1921 bill was an iteration of a bill introduced by Representative Jeanette Rankin in 1918 and was introduced in 1919 by Senator Morris Sheppard from Texas, a Democrat, and Representative Horace Towner from Iowa, a Republican. So much publicity was generated by various citizen groups in support of this bill that Congress relented and passed the bill commonly referred to as the Sheppard-Towner Act or the Maternity and Infant Act (Meckel, 1990).

The Sheppard-Towner Act

The Sheppard-Towner Act passed in 1921 and was authorized to focus on the health and well-being of women and children. Although this act was repealed in 1929, it was the first time the federal government allocated monies to states for health services (Meckel, 1990). During its early years, the Children's Bureau argued for programs that would include the use of public health nurses (PHN) to instruct pregnant women on how to care for themselves and their babies, as well as programs to support the granny midwives who provided care to these women (Hogan, 1975). Under the Sheppard-Towner Act, a number of southern states established programs where PHNs were involved in educating and supervising granny midwives. Furthermore, in their studies on maternity care in rural communities, the Children's Bureau included data on the granny midwives who attended the vast majority of births in these communities (Litoff, 1978). Most of these grannies were illiterate and lacked training in infection prevention and hygiene related to childbirth practices. However, despite their shortcomings, most of these grannies welcomed the opportunity to learn and improve their capacity to care for these childbearing women (Rooks, 1997; Thomas, 1942).

To place these developments of midwifery in context, it is important to note that in the early 20th century, roughly 40–50% of all births in the United States were attended by mid-wives (Dawley, 2000, 2003; Litoff, 1978, 1986; Rooks, 1997; Van Blarcom, 1914). In some communities, more than of 90% of births were attended by granny midwives (Dawley, 2000; Litoff, 1978; Raisler & Kennedy, 2005; Rooks, 1997). The immigrant mid-wives came with the influx of immigrants in the late 1800s to 1900s. Anna E. Rude's study for the Children's Bureau revealed that in 31 states there were 26,627 midwives who had legal sanction to practice and over 17,000 others who were practicing without legal au-thority (Bullough & Rosen, 1992; Meckel, 1990; Rosen, 1975; Thomas, 1942). Over the years, the Children's Bureau, through its surveys, has played a role in highlighting the jour-ney of nurse–midwifery practice in the United States. Its survey in 1963 (Thomas, 1965) captured the under-utilization of nurse–midwives in providing direct clinical services, when only 6.4% of midwives were engaged in such practice. In the late 1960s and early 1970s, the Children's Bureau's funds were used to develop nurse–midwifery programs in Indian Health services across the country. Up until its change in focus after a reorganization in the federal agencies in 1968, the Children's Bureau was instrumental in funding a number of nurse–midwifery educational programs. After 1968, the newly constituted Maternal and Child Health Bureau (MCHB), housed in the Health Resources and Services Administration (HRSA), took up the baton to continue supporting selected programs in nurse–midwifery education. Along with another HRSA program, the Division of Nursing, the MCHB has been one of the major sources of financing of nurse–midwifery education in the United States at the federal level.

Although in the early years of the Children's Bureau there was some support and advo-cacy for legislating, licensing, and regulating midwives, other forces were at work to elim-inate this as a viable option both at the federal level and in some local municipalities. Notably, some social reformers who supported child welfare and child health improvements looked askance at the equal rights movement for women and midwifery care for women. Prominent socialite and reformer Elizabeth Lowell Putnam, though supportive of the Children's Bureau during Julia Lathrop's tenure, began to denounce the activities of the bu-reau, particularly regarding implementation of the Sheppard-Towner Act (Rosen, 2003). Putnam's views generated high visibility in the MCH community, particularly with her dis-tinction as the 1918 elected president of AASPIM and her 5-year study demonstrating the efficacy of prenatal care in decreasing maternal and infant mortality (Rosen, 1975). As an ardent anti-suffragist, as well as a proponent for prenatal care and safety for mothers and infants, she campaigned against the Sheppard-Towner Act as implemented by the Children's Bureau. Putnam felt that health-related issues should be housed under the U.S. Pubic Health Service (USPHS) and physician authority rather than in the Children's Bureau. Whereas the Children's Bureau director, Grace Abbott, encouraged states to de-velop programs for the training and licensing of midwives, Putnam criticized this view as ignorant and lacking regard for the lives of women (Rosen, 1975). She took the position of organized medicine that midwifery was "second class care" (Rosen, 1975). Organized medicine, along with these social reformers, successfully lobbied to repeal the Sheppard-Towner Act, because they viewed it as a harbinger of socialized medicine and thus felt it did not reflect the democratic intent of our forefathers and could ultimately be an impediment to independent/private medical practice.

Title V

Putnam viewed maternal and infant mortality as a medical problem that had little to do with social events (Putnam, 1925). Putnam lobbied at both the state and federal levels to successfully defeat a 1924 bill that was introduced in the Massachusetts Legislature to legalize and license the practice of midwifery (Rosen, 2003). After the loss of the Sheppard-Towner Act, it took until after the Great Depression in 1929 for Congress, under much pressure from President F.D. Roosevelt and their constituents, to enact social and economic reforms and programs to address the needs and dislocation that resulted from the Depression. Title V in the Social Security Act of 1935, one of the social reform programs, brought back the practice of the federal government providing grants to states for maternal–child health programs. The Sheppard-Towner Act served as the template for the Title V program instituted under the Social Security Act of 1935.

Title V legislation provides block grants (funds given to states by the federal government to run programs within defined guidelines) for states to use to address deficits and/or needs in local health delivery systems for women and children. By allotting monies to states, the federal government allows states to develop strategies specific to the needs of their local communities, which during its early years allowed for the training and deployment of nurse–midwives to communities with limited or no resources (Rooks, 1997; Thomas, 1942). Even with this mixed history, midwifery and midwives have been and continue to be a force in the articulation of programs within the Federal Maternal and Child Health Programs. The Tuskegee School of Nurse–Midwifery, the first nurse–midwifery program at a historically black college and the third school of nurse–midwifery in the United States, opened in 1943 with funds provided by the Children's Bureau, the Maternity Center Association (MCA), and others (Maternity Center Association, 1943).

Maternal and Child Health Bureau

Administration of Title V remained under the auspices of the Children's Bureau until 1968, when the then Secretary of Health, Education, and Welfare, John W. Gardner, reorganized the bureau and the Maternal and Child Health Bureau (MCHB) was formed. The Children's Bureau continued its work in child welfare, focusing on issues such as adoption, foster care, and children with special needs. The Children's Bureau currently operates under the auspices of the Administration for Children and Families in the Department of Health and Human Services. Currently the MCHB carries out the health-related activities that were part of the Children's Bureau. The MCHB continues to be the designated federal entity under which the majority of MCH services and programs are housed. In 1912, the Children's Bureau began with a budget of $50,000, as compared to the $1.3 million allocated to the Department of Agriculture to do research on cows. In 2004, the MCHB had an operating budget of approximately $949 million (Bradbury & Eliot, 1956; Meckel, 1990; Maternal and Child Health Bureau, 2000; Office of Budgets, 2005). The MCHB operates under Title V of the Social Security Act to assure the health of mothers and children in the United States. The MCHB is currently housed in the Department of Health and Human Services under the Health Resources and Services Administration (HRSA) (see **Figure 3–1**).

Following the Social Security Act of 1935 and Title V, a significant amount of legislation related to MCH transformed the provision of and access to health care for women and children. New sentinel legislation included Title X in 1965 for family planning services; Medicaid in 1965; the Nutrition Act of 1966 for the Women, Infants, and Children Program (WIC); and the Personal Responsibility and Work Opportunity Reconciliation Act of 1996 for welfare reform (PRWORA, Public Law 104-193).

All of these programs/legislations have increased the federal government's role in providing a wider range of health services to women and children. Throughout the history of nurse–midwifery in the United States, nurse–midwives have consistently attended births with predominantly low-income women (Raisler & Kennedy, 2005; Rooks, 1997). Some of these programs have provided avenues for nurse–midwifery practice to expand into family planning services. For example, Title X and Medicaid target poor, medically underserved populations. Since these populations have been the cornerstone market for nurse–midwives, these programs supported proliferation of jobs opportunities for nurse–midwives.

Figure 3–1 Department of Health and Human Services

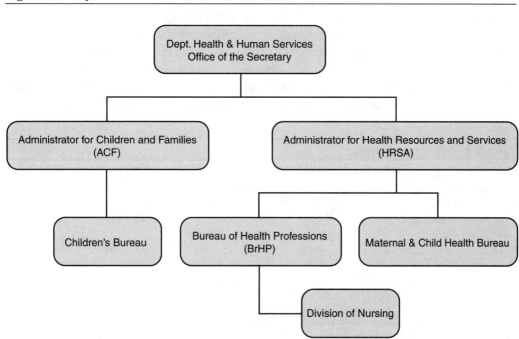

Title X

Title X legislation, providing for population research and voluntary family planning programs, was enacted in 1970 under the Public Health Service Act (Public Law 91-572). Title X is administered through the Office of Family Planning and 10 nationwide regional DHHS offices, and allocates funds through public or not-for-profit entities for family planning and selected prevention services (Office of Population Affairs, n.d.). The funding for Title X has grown from $30 million in 1970 to $288 million in Fiscal Year 2005, and is one of the primary sources of subsidized family planning services in the United States. Title X is specifically devoted to family planning and reproductive health care/preventive services to a primarily low income population. Included under the rubric of preventive health services are:

- Patient education and counseling
- Breast and pelvic exams
- Screening for cervical cancer, sexually transmitted infections (STIs), and human immunodeficiency virus (HIV)
- Pregnancy diagnoses and counseling (Gold & Sonfield, 1999)

In 1992, a collaborative effort with the Centers for Disease Control (CDC), state family planning administrators, and Title X grantees initiated the Family Planning Services Surveillance Project (FPSS) to describe the women who had received family planning services from Title X in Fiscal Year 1991. The data demonstrated that over 4 million people (both men and women) received family planning services in 1991, with oral contraceptives being the most frequently selected method for family planning. Over 64% of users of family planning services were at or below the federal poverty level (FPL). From 1991 to the most recent examination of the Title X population and other users of federal family planning subsidized programs, the demographics and utilization data of this service have been consistent, though expanding in numbers of recipients of service (see **Table 3–1**).

Subsidization of family planning services comes from several programs: Title X, Title V (MCH block grants), Title XIX (Medicare), and Title XX (Medicaid). Although Medicaid provides the lion share of subsidized funds for these services, Title X provides a

Table 3–1 Title X demographics

	1991	*2001*	*2002*	*2003*
Total population served	4,218,412	4,857,717	4,974,874	5,012,048
Females served	Not available	4,658,472	4,772,254	4,784,889
% of females served <24 yrs old	61.8	59.8	60	59
% used oral contraception for FP	69.4	45.3	Not available	48
% lived in households at or below FPL	64.6	65.4	65	67

Reference: Mosher, Martinez, Chandra, Abma, & Willson (2004); Office of Population Affairs (2005); Maternal and Child Health Bureau (2003); Centers for Disease Control and Prevention (1994).

significant service to low income women who may not be eligible for Medicaid, including the working poor (Alan Guttmacher Institute, 2002). Again, the private, not-for-profit, and public institutions that receive funds through Title X have historically employed large numbers of nurse practitioners and nurse–midwives. Mid-level providers such as physician assistants, nurse practitioners, and certified nurse–midwives continue to provide the bulk of services to the population served in this program (see **Table 3–2**).

The range of Title X services continues to reflect the original intent of the legislation for health promotion and disease prevention services beyond the family planning emphasis (see **Table 3–3**).

The Child Nutrition Act of 1966 (Public Law 89-642, October 11, 1966) was initiated under the Johnson Administration as part of its "War on Poverty." This act authorized the provision of supplemental foods and nutrition education to pregnant, postpartum, and breastfeeding women, and infants and young children from families who, by virtue of their limited income, were at physical and mental health risk. In its current iteration, amended through Public Law 108-498 (December 23, 2004), under section 17, the Women, Infants and Children's program (WIC) provides cash grants to states so that designated state entities may provide supplemental foods and nutrition to eligible individuals. Underlying the legislative intent is that individuals in this program are linked to a health delivery system and thus the program serves as an "adjunct to good health care" (Child Nutrition Act, 1966, p. 2-21). The act specifically covers:

- Breastfeeding women up to 1 year postpartum and breastfeeding their infants
- Children ages 1 year through 5 years
- Postpartum women up to 6 months after birth
- Pregnant women who have one or more fetuses in utero
- Children under 1 year of age (Child Nutrition Act, 1966, pp. 2-21–2-22)

One of the critical elements in the WIC program's implementation is the promotion of breastfeeding, a practice that is near and dear to the heart of midwives. Since 1974, the

Table 3–2 Profile of staff of subsidized family planning services

Provider	FTEs	Total Patient Encounters
Physicians	524.93	912,035
CNMs, PAs, NPs	2,407.92	5,418,248

Reference: Alan Guttmacher Institute (2004).

Table 3–3 Services provided to women in Title X programs in 2003

Service Provided	Number of Women Served
Pap smear	2,852,438
Breast exam	2,771,671
STI screening excluding HIV	4,792,211
HIV screening	454,602

Reference: Alan Guttmacher Institute (2004).

amounts of monies expended and individuals served in this program have consistently grown (see **Tables 3–4** and **3–5**).

Welfare Reform

The Personal Responsibility and Work Opportunity Reconciliation Act (PRWORA) was enacted in 1996 to address the increasing costs for state and federal support of single parent households and the need to locate and obtain financial support from the absent, non-financially supporting parent. Based on data indicating that the number of individuals receiving Aid to Families with Dependent Children (AFDC) had more than tripled since 1965, this legislation sought to stem the tide. Furthermore, more than two thirds of AFDC recipients were children, and 85% of these lived in homes without a father. PRWORA required states to develop a data system using social security, employment, and other information sources to track and locate "deadbeat" parents. It also gave states the latitude to require genetic testing to establish paternity of individuals suspected of being the father of children receiving aid. Since the law specifically cites "deadbeat dads" as the target, it infers that the vast majority of single parent households are headed by women. The implication of nonsupport of children by noncustodial parents was that it placed a financial burden on the local and state entities to assume the costs for both medical (through Medicaid) and nonmedical (AFDC) services to such families.

U.S. Public Health Service

Parallel to the MCH activities at the federal level, the Public Health Service grew from the federally designated program of Marine Hospitals for "sick and disabled seamen" into the current structure known as the U.S. Public Health Service (USPHS) (Mullan, 1989; Mustard, 1945). Though federally legislated, the Marine Hospitals were funded by levying

Table 3–4 Average number of participants in WIC

Year	Number of Participants	Average Costs Per Month/Individual ($)
1974	88,000	15.68
2001	7.3 million	34.31
2002	7.4 million	34.82
2003	7.6 million	35.28
2004	7.9 million	37.54

Reference: U.S. Department of Agriculture, 2006.

Table 3–5 National totals of expenditure for WIC

Fiscal Year (FY)	Dollars Allocated
2004	5,150,356,692
2003	4,645,860,005
2002	4,446,913,761
2001	4,180,055,755

a 20 cents per month charge on the wages of American seamen. This charge represented the first forced health insurance program in the U.S. federal government (Mullan, 1989). Each Marine Hospital was administered by the local governments where they were located, but over time they became the USPHS, with direct administrative ties to the federal government (Mullan, 1989). The USPHS received an infusion of funds from Title VI of the SSA of 1935. Prior to Title VI allocations, the USPHS had provided counsel, assistance, and partnership with local public health officials to develop and enhance their public health infrastructures (Mullan, 1989). With the receipt of Title VI funds, the USPHS was able to continue the work it had already begun in these local and state communities.

Post-World War I, nurses became an integral part of the USPHS. Nurses staffed hospitals and clinics that operated under the aegis of the USPHS. Nurses' role in the USPHS would become more dramatic during World War II. The civilian nursing shortage wrought by the increased need and utilization of nurses by the military resulted in the passage of the Nurse Training Act of 1943. This act created the U.S. Cadet Nurse Corps, quite similar to the current National Health Services Corp Program. Sixty-five thousand women were recruited into nursing and enrolled into approved nursing programs throughout the country. The USPHS covered the costs of tuition and living of the student nurse, who, after graduation, was obligated to work for 2 years in an assigned position. In providing financial support to schools, while developing and enforcing standards for nursing education, the USPHS was instrumental in establishing schools of nursing outside of the traditional hospital domain (Mullan, 1989). The Division of Nursing, which was created in 1946, became an integral part of the federal government structure as needs for nursing personnel grew and there was acknowledgement that a national nursing focus was important for the health of the nation (U.S. Public Health Service, 1997). The Division of Nursing, which has funded a number of nurse–midwifery educational programs, is located in the Bureau of Health Professions in the Department of Health and Human Services (HHS) (see Figure 3–1).

Now operating under the Department of Health and Human Services and led by the Surgeon General, the USPHS continues to provide opportunities for nurse–midwives to work in underserved communities. Through the National Health Services Corps (NHSC) or loan repayment programs, costs for education as a nurse–midwife are paid by the government, with the nurse–midwife obligated to work in underserved communities for 2–3 years. The NHSC was born during the Vietnam War, when conscientious objectors (COs) were trying to find alternative assignments to the military in order to fulfill their draft obligations. One such CO, Dr. Lawrence Pitt, proposed the NHSC in 1969.

Healthy People 2010

The Surgeon General's role became pivotal in moving the national focus from specific high morbidity/mortality diseases to examining health goals over a prescribed period of time. The seminal work in the health goal and disease prevention model began with the work of Dr. Julius Richmond, Assistant Secretary for HHS and Surgeon General from 1976–1981. In the 1979 "The Surgeon General's Report on Health Promotion and Disease Prevention" he addressed the antecedents of high mortality rates, including smoking, alcohol use, poor diet, sedentary living, and poor safety practices (U.S. Department of

Health, Education, and Welfare, 1979). In this document, Dr. Richmond outlined goals for achieving healthier outcomes by 1990. This format has been utilized by subsequent Surgeon Generals, providing a 10-year window in which we can improve healthy behaviors and health outcomes for all segments of the U.S. population. Healthy People 2010 (HP2010) has two major goals:

- To increase the quality and years of healthy life for all individuals
- To eliminate health disparities that exists among segments of the U.S. population

There are 28 health/disease focus areas in which specific objectives are articulated for improvement. HP2010 has a wide range of objectives for women's health outside of the maternity cycle. Specifically, all of the health objectives have significant relevance for both men and women in such focus areas as arthritis, osteoporosis, cancer, environmental health, nutrition, and obesity. As providers of primary health care, nurse–midwives and certified midwives should be conversant with these objectives, which can be readily accessed at http://www.healthypeople.gov. **Tables 3–6** and **3–7** highlight objectives and goals related to family planning and MCH.

While the federal government was moving forward with its involvement in the social and health issues of the nation, local municipalities persisted in their efforts to address these same issues in their respective communities. Some of the programs and strategies devised at local levels were widely disseminated and adopted in communities across the nation. During the late 1800s and throughout the 1900s, New York City engaged in a number of initiatives focused on maternal and child health that served as a template for programs in other areas of the United States (Dorey, 1999; Litoff, 1978; Meckel, 1990). Following a survey in 1905 that showed midwives conducted 42% of the births in New York City, the Board of Health assumed responsibility for licensing and regulating midwives (Meckel, 1990). In 1908, New York City established the Bureau for Child Hygiene within its Department of Health to more specifically address the health of children. This represented the first municipal bureau in the United States focused on improving infant and child health (Van Inger, 1921). Dr. S. Josephine Baker became the first director of this bureau and served in that position for over 25 years (Litoff, 1978; Meckel, 1990). A review of the practice of midwives in New York City was favorable and encouraged the city to open the School of Midwifery at Bellevue Hospital in 1911 (Rooks, 1997). Supported by tax funds, this school operated successfully until its closing in 1935. Other cities such as Newark, New Jersey, and Philadelphia, Pennsylvania, developed programs that licensed, supervised, and improved the practices of midwives in their respective communities (Dawley, 2003; Litoff, 1978; Rooks, 1997). All of these midwives had decreases in their maternal mortality rates in the population where they provided care (Litoff, 1978). More privately funded and orchestrated efforts also were occurring at the local level. One such initiative was the Maternity Center Association (MCA).

Maternity Center Association

MCA was formed in the midst of Word War I when a few physicians and citizens met at the home of Joan Rogers, a New York City socialite, to discuss and plan for ways to address the

Table 3–6 Summary of MCH HP2010 objectives

Goal: Improve the health and well-being of women, infants, children, and families.

Fetal, Infant, Child, and Adolescent Deaths
16-1   Fetal and infant deaths
16-2   Child deaths
16-3   Adolescent and young adult deaths

Maternal Deaths and Illnesses
16-4   Maternal deaths
16-5   Maternal illness and complications due to pregnancy

Prenatal Care
16-6   Prenatal care
16-7   Childbirth classes

Obstetrical Care
16-8   Very low birth weight infants born at level III hospitals
16-9   Cesarean births

Risk Factors
16-10   Low birth weight and very low birth weight
16-11   Preterm births
16-12   Weight gain during pregnancy
16-13   Infants put to sleep on their backs

Developmental Disabilities and Neural Tube Defects
16-14   Developmental disabilities
16-15   Spina bifida and other neural tube defects
16-16   Optimum folic acid levels

Prenatal Substance Exposure
16-17   Prenatal substance exposure
16-18   Fetal alcohol syndrome

Breastfeeding, Newborn Screening, and Service Systems
16-19   Breastfeeding
16-20   Newborn bloodspot screening
16-21   Sepsis among children with sickle cell disease
16-22   Medical homes for children with special health care needs
16-23   Service systems for children with special health care needs

poor maternal health and mortality that continued to challenge their city. The MCA model was truly an interdisciplinary model that included physicians, nurses, health officials, and hospital administrators. The stated purpose of MCA was "to teach mothers and fathers the importance of safe maternity care, to teach nurses how to render better care, to stimulate doctors to improve the standard of medical care, to teach community leaders the importance of making and carrying out a plan which would provide safe care for every mother regardless of her ability to pay" (Maternity Center Association, 1943, p. 6). In its purpose, the MCA architects appreciated the complexity of the task at hand and the need to apply a multi-pronged approach. This approach extended from the individual woman/family's education to crafting a delivery system that would be accessible and available to those who needed it.

Table 3–7 HP2010 family planning objectives

Goal: Improve pregnancy planning and spacing and prevent unintended pregnancy.

Objective #	Objective Focus Area
9-1	Intended pregnancy
9-2	Birth spacing
9-3	Contraceptive use
9-4	Contraceptive failure
9-5	Emergency contraception
9-6	Male involvement in pregnancy prevention
9-7	Adolescent pregnancy
9-8	Abstinence before age 15 years
9-9	Abstinence among adolescents aged 15 to 17 years
9-10	Pregnancy prevention and sexually transmitted disease (STD) protection
9-11	Pregnancy prevention education
9-12	Problems in becoming pregnant and maintaining a pregnancy
9-13	Insurance coverage for contraceptive supplies and services

In 1915 the Health Commissioner of New York City, Dr. Hoven Emerson, appointed a committee to assess childbirth issues in Manhattan. The three committee members were Dr. Ralph W. Lobenstein, Dr. J. Clifton Edgar, and Dr. Phillip Van Inger. The committee's goals were to:

- Extend the facilities for prenatal work
- Coordinate and standardize the efforts of all agencies engaged in this work
- Improve the obstetric care at the time of delivery

The committee recommended providing maternity centers throughout the city where education and prenatal care would be provided. Sponsored by the Women's City Club, the first center opened in 1917. Eventually, 30 prenatal clinics throughout the city were operating, where public health nurses provided health education and care to pregnant women and their families.

Prior to the inception of MCA, the obstetrics practices in New York provided minimal to no care for pregnant women. Medical students would open their own obstetrics practice as physicians in the city after observing several births (Meckel, 1990). Though many hospitals had maternity service, care of the pregnant woman generally began in the seventh month unless the woman had problems that brought her into the system earlier. Once discharged from the hospital, the woman was left on her own (Maternity Center Association, 1943; Meckel, 1990).

Over the years, MCA engaged in classes for expectant mothers, outreach to families through nurses going door to door, maternity centers throughout the city for the provision of prenatal care, as well as classes on safe motherhood. When the MCA programs were in full force during 1918 to 1943, those communities served demonstrated a fall in maternal mortality rate from a high of 9.2 per 1000 births to less than 3 per 1000 live births in 1942 (Maternity Center Association, 1943). Hazel Corbin and Dr. Louis Dublin co-authored a report on improved outcomes in women who received care at these community centers.

Their extrapolation of the data, including all maternal deaths in the United States and the potential reduction with interventions as at the MCA centers, provided impetus to campaign vigorously across the country for new practices to save maternal lives. Mother's Day served as the ideal time to launch the MCA effort for more education (Maternity Center Association, 1943).

With the success of MCA, many communities across the country clamored for information on its programs. MCA developed a widely disseminated educational brochure containing 12 helpful talks. Approximately 120 million copies of this brochure were distributed (Maternity Center Association, 1943).

MCA embraced the concept of nurses trained in the art of midwifery as a way to provide safe and appropriate maternity care. The data for this position were documented via outcomes in countries where midwives were trained and regulated, and in the Frontier Nursing Services work in Hyden, Kentucky. The medical board of MCA, under the leadership of Dr. Lobenstine, recommended the establishment of a school of midwifery (Maternity Center Association, 1943; Shoemaker, 1947). It was not until after his death that the Lobenstine School of Midwifery was established, linking with the Lobenstine Midwifery Clinic that had been operating since 1931. Though this initiative resulted in the loss of several prominent obstetricians who were on its medical board, the MCA persisted in its efforts and joined the Lobenstine Midwifery Clinic and School in 1934 (Shoemaker, 1947). For more information on midwifery education refer to Chapter 4.

MCA's study and report on the antecedents of maternal deaths included inadequately trained and/or incompetent medical staff. Other communities studied the causes of infant mortality in their respective areas, with some of their findings being published and disseminated by MCA. One such community, Onondaga County of New York, focused on educating both the medical staff and the general public on the issues. As with the MCA communities, Onondaga County experienced decreased maternal and infant deaths with the implementation of advanced and specialized training in obstetrics (Maternity Center Association, 1943). Eventually, obstetric care that had previously been relegated to untrained and/or poorly trained medical students now required high standards of practice for certification by the American College of Surgeons (Maternity Center Association, 1943). Both rural and urban communities began the mission to study maternal and infant deaths and to develop ways to prevent unnecessary deaths and injuries. The New York Academy of Medicine conducted one such survey, demonstrating that two thirds of all maternal deaths were preventable and that the incompetence of the birth attendant accounted for 60% of these deaths (Hooker, 1933; Maternity Center Association, 1943).

MCA continues its tradition of extolling the needs, issues, and problems in the maternity care environment and creatively looking for ways to raise the level of care to women and children. Consistent with its advocacy work has been the support for the efficacy of midwifery care in improving outcomes in at-risk populations. MCA has been a pioneer on many fronts of maternity care, including the first demonstration project in 1975 for out of hospital births at the Childbearing Center in New York City; the first neighborhood-based birth center in the Morris Heights section of the Bronx, New York City; and the first multi-site study of outcomes of birth centers published in the New England Journal of Medicine in 1989 (Rooks et al., 1989). In 2001, MCA became the first Web site (www.maternitywise.org) to focus on evidence-based maternity care. Evidence has always been the bedrock of MCA's activities since its inception, and continues to be the platform from which its programs and initiatives are derived. The goals of MCA have remained consistent over the 87 years of its existence and continue to define its work for mothers and children.

Summary

The development of the U.S. Public Health System closely parallels and is intricately intertwined with the growth of midwifery in the United States. It was the work of social reformers, who were primarily women, that brought to our nation's forefront the issue of maternal and child health. Their work was instrumental in developing the Children's Bureau, and ultimately the Maternal and Child Health Bureau and other government programs that are designed to support the health and well-being of vulnerable populations.

Chapter Exercises

This chapter has demonstrated the importance of careful data collection when examining the health of women and children in communities and the ability to use these data when working to improve maternal–child health. As part of your learning activity for this chapter you will complete a maternal–child community assessment.

Select a community to assess. It could be your hometown or the area where you are currently in clinical practice.

1. Ascertain the demographic characteristics of the women and infants in your community. Include the following:
   a. Number and percentage of population that are women
   b. Number and percentage of population that are age 1 or less
   c. Birth rate
   d. Fertility rate
   e. Age distribution of the women
   f. Life expectancy of the women
   g. Income level of households (percentage in each income bracket)
   h. Income level of women (percentage in each income bracket)
   i. Number and percentage of single parent, female head of household
   j. Educational status of women (percentage in each educational bracket)
2. Obtain the following morbidity and mortality statistics in this population:
   a. Maternal
   b. Fetal
   c. Neonatal
   d. Perinatal
   e. Infant

3. Identify maternal–child population needs based on your analysis of the demographics and morbidity and mortality statistics.
4. Identify the services and human resources within your community that provide health care services for women and infants.
5. Evaluate if the currently available resources are sufficient in number and quality to meet the population's needs.
6. Select a Healthy People 2010 goal that is pertinent to one of the maternal–child needs you have identified in your community. Identify and discuss your plan to help your community meet that HP2010 goal. Identify obstacles that will/may make it challenging for your community to meet this goal, and then develop an evaluation plan for your selected HP2010 goal.
7. Present your community assessment to your agency or your class.

Adapted from Health Care of Women and Infants: Public Policy and Programs, Yale School of Nursing.

Box 3–1   Historical Synopsis

MCH and other health related events that evolved into key MCH policy
- 1798   Act for the relief of sick and disabled seamen is signed by President Adams.
- 1801   The first Marine (Seamen) Hospital is established in Virginia.
- 1889   Hull House Settlement is founded by Jane Addams and Ellen Starr.
- 1890   Julia Lathrop, later to become the first director of the Children s Bureau, becomes a resident of Hull House.
- 1895   Lillian Wald and Mary M. Brewster found the Henry Street Settlement House in New York City. It is the first home of the Visiting Nurses Association (VNA).
- 1899   The National Consumers League, with Florence Kelley as its executive secretary, launches a campaign against child labor and sweatshops, and works for minimum wage legislation, shorter work hours, and better and safer working conditions.
- 1902   The Marine Hospital's name is changed to Public Health and Marine Hospital Service, with six divisions.
- 1903   Lillian Wald, nurse, social worker, and founder of Henry St. Settlement, introduces the idea of a Federal Children's Bureau to Florence Kelley in the early 1900s. The National Consumers League advocated for a national commission to assess the status of children in the United Stated in seven areas:
- Infant mortality
- Birth registration
- Orphanage
- Child labor
- Desertion
- Illegitimacy
- Degeneracy

- 1903   Dr. Edward T. Devine, Sociologist at Columbia University and a trustee of the National Child Labor Committee (NCLC), contacts President Theodore Roosevelt regarding Lillian Ward's idea for a Children's Bureau.
- 1903–1905   With approval of President Theodore Roosevelt, there is a concerted effort to make the Children's Bureau a reality.
- 1904   The National Child Labor Committee is established by Lillian Wald, Florence Kelley, and others.
- 1905   Draft of legislation for the Federal Children's Bureau is presented to the annual meeting of the National Child Labor Committee.
- 1906   Bill is introduced in both houses of Congress for the Federal Children's Bureau.
- 1909   President Theodore Roosevelt calls the first White House Conference on the Care of Dependent Children. The conference concludes that a Federal Children's Bureau bill should be passed.
- 1910   President Taft endorses the proposed bill for a Federal Children's Bureau.
- 1912   Bill for the Children's Bureau, submitted by Senator William E. Borah, passes.
- April 2, 1912   The bill passes in the House.
- April 9, 1912   President Taft signs into law the bill for the Federal Children's Bureau.
- 1912   Julia C. Lathrop, formerly of the Hull House Settlement in Chicago, is appointed as the first head of the Children's Bureau.
- 1918   Maternity Center Association is formed in New York City.
- 1921   Sheppard-Towner (Maternity & Infant) Act (Public Law 67-97) is passed by the United States Congress and signed into law by President Harding. It provides matching federal funds for state-funded maternity services and child health centers.
- 1921   Grace Abbott becomes the second director of the Children's Bureau.
- 1929   The Sheppard-Towner Act is repealed, with much lobbying for its demise done by the American Medical Association (AMA).
- 1935   The Social Security Act is enacted, providing for Title V, which promoted the development of the infrastructure for MCH programs within state health agencies.
- 1939   The Reorganization Act moves the Public Health Services from the Department of the Treasury to the newly established Federal Security Agency.
- 1941   The Nurse Training Act is passed (Public Law 77-146) providing funds to develop and increase enrollment in schools of nursing.
- 1944   The Public Health Service Act is enacted (Public Law 78-40), which places all public health services under one statute.
- 1954   The Indian Health Act is enacted and transfers the operations of Indian Health Services to the Public Health Service.
- 1958   The Social Security Act (SSA) Amendment provides states with MCH grants.
- 1963   MCH and mental retardation planning amendments provides for comprehensive maternal and infant care and mental retardation prevention services.
- 1965   The Social Security Act (SSA) Amendment (Public Law 89-97) establishes health insurance for the elderly and assistance to states for the care of the poor (Medicare and Medicaid, respectively).
- 1965   The U.S. Supreme Court rules in *Griswald v the State of Connecticut* that laws prohibiting the use of birth control are unconstitutional.
- 1966   The PHS reorganizes with the Office of the Surgeon General now under the Secretary of Health Education and Welfare (HEW, the predecessor to today's HHS).
- 1966   The Child Nutrition Act (Public Law 89-642) establishes the federal program of research and support for child nutrition and the Women, Infants and Childrens' program (WIC, Sect. 17 [42 USC. 1786]).

- 1967 The Social Security Act (SSA) Amendment (Public Law 90-248) consolidates MCH authority and extends grants for family planning and dental health.
- 1970 The Family Planning Services and Population Research Act (Public Law 91-572) coordinates and expands services for family planning and research activities.
- 1970 The Emergency Health Personnel Act establishes the National Health Services Corps to recruit and engage health professionals who would practice in underserved communities.
- 1972 The Social Security Act (SSA) Amendment (Public Act 92-603) extends health insurance benefits to the disabled.
- 1973 The U.S. Supreme Court rules in the *Roe v Wade* case that a woman has a constitutional right to an abortion.
- 1976 *Toward Improving the Outcome of Pregnancy: Recommendations for Regional and Perinatal Health Services* (TIOP-1) published.
- 1981 The Omnibus Budget Reconciliation Act (OBRA) combines Title V funds with other MCH programs as a block grant to states.
- 1986 Medicaid expansion covers AFDC recipients.
- 1989 OBRA of 1989. Reporting requirements instituted for Title V grantees.
- 1991 The MCH office becomes a bureau.
- 1993 TIOP-2: The 90s and Beyond published.
- 1993 Family and Medical Leave Act requires employers to grant leave for certain family or medical reasons, including maternity leave.
- 1996 Personal Responsibility and Work Opportunity Reconciliation Act imposes time limits on receipt of welfare aid and focuses on immediate job placement.
- 1998 MCHB national performance guidelines measures required for Title V services applicants and providers.

References

Addams, J. (1910). *Twenty years at Hull-House, with autobiographical notes*. New York: MacMillan.

Addams, J. (1935). *Forty years at Hull-House*. New York: Macmillan.

Alan Guttmacher Institute. (2002). *Family planning annual report 2001*. Washington, DC: Summary Office of Populations Affairs, U.S. Department of Health and Human Services.

Alan Guttmacher Institute. (2004, August). *Family planning annual report: 2003 summary*. Washington, DC: Office of Population Affairs, U.S. Department of Health and Human Services. Retrieved February 7, 2006, from http://opa.osophs.dhhs.gov/titlex/2003-fpar-part1.pdf

American Association for the Study and Prevention of Infant Mortality. (1912). *Transactions of the 2nd annual meeting of the Association for the Study and Prevention of Infant Mortality* (pp. 232–243, November 16–18, 1911, Chicago, IL). Baltimore, MD: Franklin Printing Company.

Baker, S. J. (1912). Schools for midwives. In *Transactions of the 2nd annual meeting of the Association for the Study and Prevention of Infant Mortality* (pp. 232–243, November 16–18, 1911, Chicago, IL). Baltimore, MD: Franklin Printing Company.

Baker, S. J. (1939). *Fighting for life*. New York: MacMillan.

Bradbury, D. E., & Eliot, M. M. (1956). *Four decades of action for children: A short history of the Children's Bureau, U.S. Department of Health, Education, and Welfare, Social Security Administration, Children's Bureau.* Washington, DC: U.S. Government Printing Office.

Brown, V. B. (1999). *Twenty years at Hull-House, with biographical notes by Jane Addams.* (The Bedford Series in History and Culture). New York: Bedford/St. Martin's.

Bullough, B., & Rosen, G. (1992). *Preventive medicine in the United States 1900–1990: Trends and interpretations.* Canton, MA: Science History Publications.

Centers for Disease Control and Prevention. (1994). Characteristics of women receiving family planning services at Title X clinics—United States 1991. *Morbidity and Mortality Weekly Reports, 43*(2), 31–34.

Child Nutrition Act, 42 U.S.C. § 1786 *et seq.* (1966).

Dawley, K. (2000). The campaign to eliminate the midwife. *American Journal of Nursing, 100*(10), 50–56.

Dawley, K. (2001). Ideology and self-interest. Nursing, medicine, and the elimination of the midwife. *Nursing History Review, 9,* 99–126.

Dawley, K. (2003). Origins of nurse–midwifery in the United States and its expansion in the 1940s. *Journal of Midwifery and Women's Health, 48*(2), 86–95.

Dorey, A. K. (1999). *Better baby contests: The scientific quest for perfect childhood in the early twentieth century.* Jefferson, NC: McFarlane and Co.

Gold, R. B., & Sonfield, A. (1999). Family planning funding through four federal-state programs FY1997. *Family Planning Perspectives, 31*(4), 176–181.

Gorst, J. (1895). "Settlements" in England and America. In J. M. Knapp (Ed.), *The universities and the social problem* (pp. 1–29). London: Rivington, Percival.

Hogan, A. (1975). A tribute to pioneers. *Journal of Nurse–Midwifery, 20,* 6–11.

Hooker, R. A. (1933). *Maternal mortality in New York City: A study of puerperal deaths 1930–1932.* NY Academy of Medicine Committee on Public Health Relations. New York: Commonwealth Fund.

Hull House. (2002). Retrieved August 10, 2005, from http://www.Spartacus.schoolnet.co.uk/USAhullhouse.htm

Hull-House Residents. (1895). *Hull-House maps and papers: A presentation of nationalities and wages in a congested district of Chicago.* Boston: Crowell & Company.

Josiah Macy, Jr. Foundation. (1968). The midwife in the United States. (Report of a Macy Conference). New York: Author.

Litoff, J. B. (1978). *American midwives, 1860 to the present.* Westport CT: Greenwood Press.

Litoff, J. B. (1986). *The American midwife debate.* Westport, CT: Greenwood Press.

Maternal and Child Health Bureau. (2000). *Maternal and Child Health Bureau (MCHB)* [Fact sheet]. Retrieved August 10, 2005, from ftp://ftp.hrsa.gov/mchb/factsheets/mchb.pdf

Maternal and Child Health Bureau. (2003). *Women's Health USA 2003.* Retrieved February 7, 2006, from http://mchb.hrsa.gov/pages/page_67.htm

Maternity Center Association. (1943). *Maternity Center Association, 1918–1943.* New York: Author.

Meckel, R. A. (1990). *Save the babies: American public health reform and the prevention of infant mortality 1850–1929.* Baltimore, MD: Johns Hopkins University Press.

Meigs, G. L. (1917). *Maternal mortality from all conditions connected with childbirth in the United States and certain other countries*. (Publication No. 19). Washington, DC: U.S. Department of Labor, Children's Bureau, Government Printing Office.

Mosher, W. D., Martinez, G. M., Chandra, A., Abma, J. C., & Willson, S. J. (2004). Use of contraception and use of family planning services in the United States: 1982–2002. *Advance Data from Division of Vital Statistics*. (CDC No. 350). Atlanta, GA: Centers for Disease Control and Prevention.

Mullan, F. (1989). *Plagues and politics. The story of the United States Public Health Service*. New York: Basic Books.

Mustard, H. S. (1945). *Government in public health*. New York: Commonwealth Fund.

Office of Budget. (2005). *FY 2005 President's Budget for HHS*. Retrieved August 10, 2005, from http://www.hhs.gov/budget/docbudget.htm

Office of Population Affairs. (n.d.). *Office of Family Planning*. Retrieved February 7, 2006, from http://opa.osophs.dhhs.gov/titlex/ofp.html

Office of Population Affairs. (2005). *Office of Family Planning, OFP references*. Retrieved February 7, 2006, from http://opa.osophs.dhhs.gov/titlex/ofp_references.html

Prevention of infant mortality 1909. (1909, November 11–12). Paper presented at the Conference on Prevention of Infant Mortality, New Haven, CT.

Price, G. M. (1919). *Hygiene and public health*. New York: Lea & Febiger.

Putnam, W. L. (1925). Letter of transmittal. *Why the appropriations for the extension of the Sheppard-Towner Act should not be granted*. Boston, MA.

Raisler, J., & Kennedy, H. (2005). Midwifery care of poor and vulnerable women, 1925–2003. *Journal of Midwifery and Women's Health, 50*(2), 113–121.

Rooks, J. P. (1997). *Midwifery and childbirth in America*. Philadelphia: Temple University Press.

Rooks, J. P., Weatherby, N. L., Ernst, E. K., Stapleton, S., Rosen, D., & Rosenfield, A. (1989). Outcomes of care in birth centers. The National Birth Center Study. *New England Journal of Medicine, 321*(26), 1804–1811.

Roosevelt, T. (1909, January 25). *First White House conference on the care of dependent children*. Retrieved August 10, 2005, from http://libertynet.org/edcivic/whoukids.html

Rosen, G. (1975). *Preventive medicine in the United States, 1900–1975. Trends and interpretations*. New York: Science History Publications.

Rosen, R. L. (2003). *Reproductive health—reproductive rights: Reformers and the politics of maternal welfare 1917–1940*. Columbus: Ohio State University Press.

Rude, A. E. (1922). *The Sheppard-Towner Act in relation to public health*. Washington, DC: Government Printing Office.

Rude, A. E. (1923). The midwife problem in the United States. *Journal of the American Medical Association, 8*, 989–990.

Shoemaker, M. T. (1947). *History of nurse–midwifery in the U.S.* Washington, DC: Catholic University of America Press.

Smilie, W. (1949). *Public health administration in the United States*. New York: MacMillan.

Soule, E. S., & MacKenzie, C. (1940). *Community hygiene*. New York: MacMillan.

Thomas, M. W. (1942). Social priority no. 1: Mothers and babies. *Public Health Nursing, 34*(8), 442–445.

Thomas, M. W. (1965). *The practice of midwifery in the United States*. (U.S. Department of HEW, Children's Bureau Publication No. 436). Washington, DC: Government Printing Office.

Tom, S. A. (1982). The evolution of nurse–midwifery. *Journal of Nurse Midwifery, 27*(4), 4–13.

Trattner, W. I. (1970). *Crusade for the children: A history of the National Child Labor Committee and child labor reform in America*. Chicago: Quadrangle Books.

U.S. Department of Agriculture, Food and Nutrition Service. (2006). *WIC program annual summary*. Retrieved June 13, 2006, from http://www.fns.usda.gov/pd/wisummary.htm.

U.S. Department of Health, Education, and Welfare. (1979). *Healthy people*. Washington, DC: U.S. Printing Office.

U.S. Public Health Service. (1997, April). *50 years at the Division of Nursing United States Public Health Service*. Retrieved August 12, 2005, from http://bhpr.hrsa.gov/nursing/50years.htm

Van Blarcom, C. C. (1914). Midwives in America. *American Journal of Public Health, 4*, 197–207.

Van Inger, P. (1921). The history of child welfare in the United States. In Ravenel, M. P. (Ed.), *A half century of public health: Jubilee historical volume*. New York, NY: American Public Health Association.

Wattenberg, B. (n.d.). *Infant and maternal mortality: How Julia Lathrop and the Children's Bureau tried to save the babies*. (First Measured Century Program Segments 1900–1930). Retrieved August 10, 2005, from http://www.pbs.org/fmc/segments/progseg3.htm

Williams, J. W. (1911). The midwife problem and medical education in the United States. *Transactions of the 2nd annual meeting of the Association for the Study and Prevention of Infant Mortality* (pp. 165–194, November 16–18, 1911, Chicago, IL). Baltimore, MD: Franklin Printing Company.

Williams, J. W. (1912). Medical education and the midwife problem in the United States. *Journal of the American Medical Association, 58*, 1–7.

CHAPTER 4

Midwifery Accreditation and Education

Diane Boyer, CNM, PhD, FACNM
Lynette Ament, RN, CNM, PhD, FACNM

Learning Objectives

1. Discuss the purpose of accreditation in higher education.
2. Describe a brief history of the ACNM Division of Accreditation.
3. Discuss the purpose and the benefits of accreditation by the ACNM Division of Accreditation.
4. Discuss the difference between programmatic and institutional accreditation.
5. Describe the DOA accreditation process.
6. Compare the ACNM Division of Accreditation and the Midwifery Education Accreditation Council.
7. Discuss current issues facing the ACNM Division of Accreditation.
8. Discuss the components of the core competencies.
9. Describe the types of midwifery educational programs in the United States, including the evolution of the CM.
10. Identify innovative learning modalities in midwifery: modular learning, distance education, and community-based education.
11. Discuss past and future challenges for midwifery education.

In the United States, no single national agency has regulatory control over institutions of higher education. Individual states exercise varying degrees of authority over postsecondary education. Because colleges and schools have considerable autonomy in their operations and educational offerings, quality can vary widely. Accreditation has evolved as a means of assuring that educational institutions and programs meet certain quality standards. Private accrediting agencies develop criteria and conduct periodic evaluations to assess whether those criteria are met. Although voluntary, most schools, and many programs within those schools, seek the peer evaluation offered by accrediting agencies. Such agencies can be regional or national in scope, and are often formed by professional organizations. The United States Department of Education (U.S. DOE) does not accredit educational institutions, but does have criteria and a process for recognizing accrediting agencies as institutional and/or programmatic accreditors. Recognized agencies can be viewed at www.ed.gov.

According to the U.S. DOE (2005), some functions of accreditation are:

- Verifying that an institution or program meets established standards
- Assisting prospective students in identifying acceptable institutions
- Assisting institutions in determining the acceptability of transfer credits
- Helping to identify institutions and programs for the investment of public and private funds
- Protecting an institution against harmful internal and external pressure
- Creating goals for self-improvement of weaker programs and stimulating a general raising of standards among educational institutions
- Involving the faculty and staff comprehensively in institutional evaluation and planning
- Establishing criteria for professional certification and licensure and for upgrading courses offering such preparation
- Providing one of several considerations used as a basis for determining eligibility for Federal assistance

History of Accreditation in Midwifery Education

History of the ACNM Division of Accreditation (DOA)

In many other countries of the world, midwifery education is regulated by a national governmental agency. In the United States, quality assurance in midwifery education has followed the private, professional model described above. The American College of Nurse–Midwifery was formed in 1955. One of its objectives was to evaluate and approve nurse–midwifery services and education (American College of Nurse-Midwives [ACNM], 2004). After the American College of Nurse–Midwifery joined with the American Association of Nurse–Midwives in 1969 to form the American College of Nurse–Midwives (ACNM), a Committee on Curriculum and Approval was formed. This committee received requests to develop an evaluation procedure for midwifery education programs, and consequently conducted a comprehensive survey about midwifery education and practice. The results of this survey were used to develop the first *Criteria for Accreditation of Basic Certificate, Basic Graduate and Pre-Certification Nurse–Midwifery Education Programs.* Subsequently, a *Policies and Procedures Manual* was written to specify the policies and processes to determine whether education programs were meeting these criteria. Revisions of *Criteria* documents and the *Policies and Procedures Manual* are made every 5 years, with input from the midwifery profession.

The Division of Approval was formed as a separate division of the ACNM in 1974. In 1984, the name was changed to the Division of Accreditation (Carrington & Burst, 2005). Recognition by the U.S. DOE as a programmatic accrediting agency was granted in 1982 and has been renewed every 5 years since then. Such recognition requires that an accrediting agency be legally separate from the professional organization. The DOA pays for office space and staff at the ACNM National Office and is administratively and financially separate from the ACNM. The name, Division of Accreditation, may cause some confusion in the midwifery community and among the public about the relationship of the DOA to the ACNM. The term "Division" is also used in naming other groups, such as the Division of Education, which actually are a part of the ACNM, the professional organization.

In 1989, the DOA was charged by the ACNM Board of Directors to explore non-nursing routes to midwifery education. In 1994, the DOA completed a lengthy process to determine what competencies obtained from nursing education were essential prerequisites to midwifery education. These competencies and essential prerequisite courses were compiled in the document *Skills, Knowledge, Competencies and Health Sciences Prerequisite to Midwifery Practice.* Subsequently, accreditation criteria were modified to accommodate accreditation of non-nurse midwifery education programs, and this expansion of scope was recognized by the U.S. DOE in 2001. Currently, two such programs are accredited by the DOA (ACNM, 2004).

The DOA has been recognized by the U.S. DOE as a specialized accrediting agency since 1982, accrediting postbaccalaureate and higher nurse–midwifery and midwifery certificate and graduate programs, as well as precertification programs for professional midwives from other countries who are RNs in the United States. The DOA is not yet recognized as an institutional accreditor. Accreditation of an institution by an accrediting agency recognized by the U.S. DOE makes students in that institution eligible to apply for federal student loans available through the Higher Education Act. Requests by several midwifery education programs for the DOA to become an institutional accrediting agency were the impetus for the process that the DOA began in 2001 to explore petitioning for expansion of scope to become an institutional as well as a programmatic accrediting agency. This endeavor was supported by the ACNM members present at the annual meeting in 2003. The document *Criteria for Institutional Accreditation of Freestanding Institutions of Higher Education with Nurse–Midwifery/Midwifery Education and Related Health Education Programs* was published in January 2004. The first institutional accreditation was granted in January 2005, and the DOA will apply to the U.S. DOE for recognition as an institutional accrediting agency in 2006. In order to apply for recognition, an accrediting agency must have gone through the process of accrediting an institution. If such recognition is granted, students in freestanding institutions offering midwifery education that are accredited by the DOA could become eligible for federal student loans. The ability of the DOA to accredit freestanding institutions that offer midwifery education could promote the development of innovative educational routes into midwifery practice. Readers are referred to the comprehensive review of the history of the DOA by Carrington and Burst (2005).

As of January 2005, the DOA lists 39 accredited midwifery education programs and 1 accredited institution. Two additional programs have received pre-accreditation status and have accepted their first classes of students.

History of the Midwifery Education Accreditation Council (MEAC)

In a meeting at the ACNM Annual Meeting in 1982, called by ACNM president Sister Angela Murdaugh, the Midwives' Alliance of North America (MANA) was formed

(Davis-Floyd, 1998). MANA has developed into an organization with a broad-based membership that includes direct-entry midwives, CNMs and CMs, and members of the public. One of the purposes of MANA was to "set educational guidelines for the training of Midwives" (Midwives' Alliance of North America [MANA], 1985). In 1987, MANA created the North American Registry of Midwives (NARM, which has developed a certification process for the credential of Certified Professional Midwife (North American Registry of Midwives [NARM], 2004). In 1991, the Midwifery Education Accreditation Council (MEAC) was established to "accredit direct-entry midwifery education programs and institutions" (Midwifery Education Accreditation Council [MEAC], 2005). MEAC has been recognized by the U.S. DOE as a programmatic and institutional accrediting agency. As of February 2005, MEAC had accredited 11 programs (Baul, 2005).

Structure and Function of the ACNM Division of Accreditation

The purpose of the DOA is to plan, implement, and evaluate the accreditation process for programs or institutions that offer midwifery education. The DOA is the official accrediting body of the American College of Nurse–Midwives (ACNM). To maintain autonomy, the DOA is administratively and financially independent from the ACNM. Except for a part-time paid staff member, all DOA activities are carried out by dedicated volunteers.

The Structure of the DOA

The DOA consists of four units:

- The Governing Board is responsible for the administration of the DOA's activities, the formulation of policy, and the development of the criteria used by the Board of Review in determining accreditation status.
- The Site Visitor Panel arranges, conducts, and evaluates accreditation visits to midwifery education programs or institutions.
- The Board of Review (BOR) is responsible for review of an applicant's Pre-accreditation Report or Self-Evaluation Report and the Site Visit Report (SVR), and for determination of accreditation status.
- The Advisory Committee, composed of members representing nursing, medicine, education, and the public, as well as the immediate past chair of the DOA, advises in the development of policy and evaluation of the DOA.

The Goals of the DOA

The goals of the DOA are the following:

- Assist midwifery education programs in assessing the achievement of their stated purposes and outcomes in keeping with DOA pre-accreditation or accreditation criteria.
- Foster the continuous development and improvement in the quality of midwifery education programs throughout the United States, its territories, and the District of Columbia.

- Assure the institution, the education program, the administration and faculty, the students, and the public that the highest possible standards of education and professional competence are maintained by serving as an interested outside observer.
- Bring together CNMs and CMs in service and in education in an activity directed toward improving educational preparation for midwifery practice.
- Promote an understanding and ongoing evaluation of the accreditation process among institution administrators, faculty, students, and general membership of the ACNM.
- Provide an external peer review process for programs and institutions that offer midwifery education.

The Process of Programmatic Accreditation

If an accredited institution of higher education wishes to start a midwifery education program or an already-existing program wishes to apply for continuing accreditation, the CEO of the institution contacts the chair of the DOA to initiate the process.

A number of documents are used to guide the accreditation process. The most important are:

- The *Policies and Procedures Manual* specifies procedures to be followed by the institution and the DOA, lists the possible outcomes of the Board of Review deliberations, and describes the appeal process that is available.
- The *Criteria for Programmatic Pre-accreditation of Programs in Nurse–Midwifery and Midwifery with Guidelines for Elaboration and Documentation* lists the criteria that a new program must address in a Pre-accreditation Report (PAR) and that must be met in order to receive pre-accreditation status from the Board of Review. After graduation of its first class of students, a pre-accredited program is eligible to apply for full accreditation.
- The *Criteria for Programmatic Accreditation of Education Programs in Nurse–Midwifery and Midwifery with Guidelines for Elaboration and Documentation* lists the criteria that an established program must address in a Self-Evaluation Report (SER) and that must be met to receive accreditation status from the Board of Review. Both *Criteria* documents are organized into six sections: Introduction, including an overview of the program and the process of preparing the SER/PAR; Organization and Administration; Faculty and Faculty Organization; Students; Curriculum; and Resources, Facilities, and Services.
- The program must describe how its philosophy is congruent with the *Philosophy of the American College of Nurse–Midwives.*
- The *ACNM Core Competencies for Basic Midwifery Practice* describes all of the hallmarks and competencies of midwifery practice that must be addressed in the curriculum of the program seeking accreditation.

After the program prepares its PAR or SER, dates for a site visit are arranged with the coordinator of the Site Visitors Panel. The coordinator recruits two site visitors, one of whom is designated as the senior site visitor. During the site visit, usually lasting $2^{1}/_{2}$ days, the site visitors conduct interviews with administrators, faculty, and students; review documents; and visit classes, clinical facilities, and other resources. The purpose of the site visit is to clarify, verify, or amplify information that the program has presented in its PAR or SER and to summarize that information in a report that the site visitors prepare for the Board of Review. The site visitors do not make decisions about whether accreditation is to be granted.

The Board of Review, which meets twice per year, carefully reviews all of the information submitted by the program and the site visitors, and makes a decision about pre-accreditation or accreditation. The maximum length of accreditation granted is for a period of 10 years. The BOR may grant accreditation without recommendations or with recommendations that are not mandatory, grant accreditation pending submission of satisfactory progress reports that are mandatory, or deny accreditation.

The DOA also monitors programs between accreditation intervals and requires the submission of annual reports. Substantive changes in programs must be reported to the DOA and are evaluated by the Board of Review to determine if any action is necessary. A list of accredited programs can be found on the ACNM Web site (http://www.midwife.org/edu/schools.cfm).

Although the preparation of a SER and the process of accreditation are time-consuming and costly endeavors for education programs, they also are valuable activities. They provide an opportunity for intensive, detailed, periodic assessment by a program of its curriculum and all other aspects of its program. Accreditation fosters the continuous development and improvement of midwifery education, and assures the public that accredited programs meet consistent standards. Graduates of DOA-accredited programs are eligible to take the American Midwifery Certification Board (AMCB) certification examination.

The Process of Institutional Accreditation

The criteria and processes for institutional accreditation are new for the DOA. However, the processes parallel those of programmatic accreditation. Specific criteria must be addressed by the institution in an SER. A site visit is then conducted, and a decision about accreditation is made by the Board of Review. For institutional reviews, the site visitor team and the Board of Review must include members who are experienced in institutional accreditation.

Structure and Function of the Midwifery Education Accreditation Council

Readers are referred to the MEAC Web site for further information about the structure and function of this accrediting agency (http://www.meacschools.org).

Current and Emerging Issues in Midwifery Accreditation

Financial Issues

The DOA must be financially separate from ACNM to maintain recognition by the U.S. DOE. The large majority of income for the DOA comes from fees paid by accredited programs, with a small amount from the sale of DOA documents. The DOA recognizes that in order for education programs to survive, costs must be kept to a minimum. With a small budget, the DOA has limited resources to fund new activities, such as the development of institutional accreditation. However, in 2003, a mechanism was approved for the DOA to be able to receive donations through the ACNM Foundation, Inc. This is another potential source of revenue for the DOA to fund new and innovative endeavors.

Maintaining the Integrity of a Separate Accreditation Process

Formal midwifery education in the United States has been closely allied with nursing education, and most education programs that the DOA accredits are located within schools of nursing. In addition, many midwifery education programs and midwifery students have received funding from federal programs for advanced nursing education. Thus, although most midwives believe that nursing and midwifery are separate disciplines and that nursing is not the only legitimate route into midwifery, continuing to maintain good relationships with schools of nursing is in the best interests of the DOA and the programs it accredits. The DOA believes that its accreditation criteria and processes, which are independent of the accrediting agencies that accredit nursing education programs, have contributed substantially to the excellent quality of midwifery education that exists today. Many administrators in schools of nursing, concerned about the costs of accreditation, would like to see accreditation of all programs located in their schools subsumed under the umbrella of one of the nursing accrediting agencies, such as the Commission on Collegiate Nursing Education. Believing that it is in the best interests of midwifery education, the DOA is committed to maintaining its separate accreditation process, while at the same time collaborating with schools of nursing and other schools that have midwifery education programs in order to streamline and reduce the costs of accreditation. For example, the DOA has developed guidelines for conducting joint site visits with other accrediting agencies to decrease the time and cost of such visits.

International Issues

With increasing mobility of health care professionals from country to country, and with the development of distance learning methodologies, accrediting agencies are increasingly faced with quality assessment issues affecting students and educational institutions internationally. Education across international borders is increasing, and some U.S. accrediting agencies are already accrediting programs located in other countries. Although the DOA has no immediate plans to expand its activities internationally, it is open to exploring such possibilities. It has already received a request from a midwifery student to use a preceptor who is a licensed midwife in another country, and the DOA expects that similar issues will surface with increasing frequency.

Governmental Issues

The Higher Education Act (HEA) Reauthorization, introduced in May 2004 and as of February 2005 pending before Congress, contains several provisions that are of concern to accrediting agencies. If passed in its current form, the HEA would require, among a number of other increased demands on accrediting agencies and institutions, that such agencies make summaries of their findings public when they make a decision about accreditation status. Institutions currently are assured a degree of confidentiality during the accreditation process, and leaders in higher education fear that the new requirements would motivate schools to conceal their problems from accrediting agencies. The HEA would also mandate that accreditors ensure that institutions supply certain required data to the federal government, thus making private accrediting agencies "into a data-collection arm of the government" (Bollag, 2004, p. A22). The Council for Higher Education Accreditation (CHEA), a large membership organization that advocates for voluntary accreditation and quality assurance, states that "the bill goes far beyond the proper balance of the federal role and the self-regulation of higher education through voluntary, private accreditation" (Council for Higher Education Accreditation [CHEA], 2004). Whatever the form of the HEA that ultimately is approved by Congress, provisions that affect accreditation will affect the DOA as well as all other accrediting agencies in the United States.

Summary

- Higher education accreditation in the United States is largely a voluntary activity conducted by private, professionally associated accrediting agencies. Accreditation serves a number of functions aimed toward quality assurance in higher education.
- The ACNM Division of Accreditation was formed in 1974, and was recognized by the U.S. Department of Education as a programmatic accreditor in 1982.
- The Midwifery Education Accreditation Council, formed in 1991, is another accrediting agency for midwifery education programs in North America.
- The DOA has developed detailed criteria that programs that it accredits must meet, in a process that involves periodic programmatic self-evaluation, site visits, evaluation by the DOA Board of Review, and annual reports by accredited programs.
- The DOA is in the process becoming an institutional as well as a programmatic accreditor, and plans to petition the U.S. Department of Education for recognition of this expansion of scope.
- The DOA is facing a number of issues, including limited financial resources; maintaining the integrity of a separate accreditation process from nursing while at the same time maintaining good relationships with schools of nursing; increasing education across international borders, which may offer opportunities for international collaboration; and potential increased government demands on accrediting agencies.

Midwifery Education

History

Sharp (1983) identified three development stages in the growth of the midwifery profession and midwifery education in the United States. The first stage is trailblazing, whereby pioneers identify a need in society and move forward to find a solution. The second stage is fence building. Fence building begins when the pioneers have found a solution and want to solidify its place in society. The last stage, tower building, is the identification of the profession's process in helping society. Sharp believes that for midwifery, the 1930s through the 1950s were trailblazing times, the 1960s and 1970s were fence-building times, and the late 1970s began the tower-building stage.

Trailblazing began in the 1930s with the creation of midwifery education programs. The first school to educate graduate nurses in midwifery was the Manhattan Midwifery School, which began in New York City in 1925 and closed in 1931 (Cassells, 2000). Concurrently in 1925, Mary Breckinridge established the Frontier Nursing Service (FNS) (Fondiller, 2000). Seven years later in 1932, the Lobenstine Midwifery School, Maternity Center Association, New York City, began (Burst, 2003; Sharp, 1983). While the first director of the Lobenstine Midwifery School was Hattie Hemschemeyer, the Frontier Nursing Service lent Rose McNaught to the Lobenstine Midwifery School as the first midwifery faculty member (Burst, 2003; Sharp, 1983). Hattie Hemschemeyer was a student in her own program and graduated in its first class of 1933 (Burst, 2003). Subsequently, in 1939, the Frontier Graduate School of Midwifery opened, with Rose McNaught as its first director (Burst, 2003).

All nurse–midwifery education programs can trace their origins back to either the Lobenstine Midwifery School or the Frontier Graduate School of Midwifery (Burst, 2003). The State University of New York Downstate Medical Center (SUNY Downstate) is a direct descendent of the Maternity Center Association midwifery program (Burst, 2003). During the trailblazing and fence-building stages between 1941 and 1963, 12 nurse–midwifery programs were started. Of these 12 programs, only 4 are in existence today (Columbia University, Yale University, University of Puerto Rico, and University of Utah). The first university affiliated program, the Flint-Goodrich School of Nurse–Midwifery and Dillard University in New Orleans, was a certificate program and was open for only one year (Burst, 2005). Beginning in 1947, Catholic University School of Nursing/Catholic Maternity Institute was the next university affiliation (Burst, 2005). There were three programs established in the 1950s: Columbia University (1955), Johns Hopkins University (1956), and Yale University (1956). Each of these three programs was based in university medical centers (Burst, 2003).

The advent of the tower-building stage in the 1970s was the result of societal recognition of nurse–midwifery. There were growing numbers of nurse–midwifery practices and nurse–midwifery education could not meet the demand for nurse–midwives in those practices (Sharp, 1983). The number of nurse–midwifery educational program doubled during the 1970s (Hsia, 1982). Then the 1980s brought growing pains to nurse–midwifery education. In 1986, Murphy wrote: "Nurse–midwifery education is in a state of crisis" (p. 1). The nursing shortage of the 1980s brought a decline in the numbers of qualified applicants to nurse–midwifery programs (Raisler, 1987). Concurrently there was also a malpractice crisis. In addition, university budgets were tight and clinical resources were limited, as was the supply of nurse–midwifery educators (Hsia, 1987). As a result, the 1980s brought promotion of creative approaches to nurse–midwifery education.

Educational Innovations

The development of the modular curriculum at the University of Mississippi in 1972 is credited as one of the most innovative approaches to midwifery education (Carr, 2003; Hsia, 1982). The foundation for the modular curriculum is mastery learning, which assumes that all or almost all students can master what they are taught (Hart & Marsico, 1975). In the mastery learning model, students are active learners and must demonstrate measurable objectives in both theoretical and clinical areas (Hart & Marsico, 1975; Hsia, 1982). The University of Mississippi held workshops on the modular curriculum in 1973 and 1974 (Long, Anderson, Hamel, & Shiers, 1975), and the concept was adopted by many nurse–midwifery educational programs.

Although not a new concept, the advent of technology brought a growth in distance learning modalities in nurse–midwifery. Before technology, several nurse–midwifery programs needed to send their students to clinical sites out of state because of limited availability near their educational home, and other programs attempted to create access for those students who did not live an easy distance from a nurse–midwifery educational program (Burst, 2005). In 1980, the Educational Program Associates (EPA) created the first modular distance-learning curriculum using asynchronous education (Carr, 2003). This program closed in the late 1990s. In 1989, through a joint effort with the Maternity Center Association, Frontier Nursing Service, Case Western Reserve, and the National Association of Childbearing Centers, the community-based nurse–midwifery education program (CNEP) began (Treistman, Carr, & McHugh, 1993). The Frontier School of Midwifery and Family Nursing, CNEP's home, was designed so students could use computers for class assignments, case studies, self-assessments, and student support (Brucker & Reedy, 2000). The impetus for the CNEP program was a growing difficulty in finding clinical learning sites for the traditional Frontier midwifery education program. Now, the program attracts self-directed students who attend classes in their own homes, work at their own pace, and finish at different times (Fondiller, 2000). The development of the CNEP program is detailed by Osborne, Stone, and Ernst (2005). Today there are several midwifery programs with distance education components.

Another response to declining numbers of nurse–midwifery students in the 1980s was the ACNM Board of Directors' charge to the Division of Accreditation to develop criteria for evaluating non-nurse professional midwifery educational routes (Rooks, Carr, & Sandvold, 1991). This resulted in the ACNM position paper on professional midwifery (ACNM, 1991). Although this position was not seen by the ACNM as a move to do away with nursing licensure as a prerequisite to midwifery (Rooks et al., 1991), some saw this as a strong movement to remove nursing from midwifery (Muzio, 1991). It wasn't until 1996 that the Division of Accreditation pre-accredited the first direct entry program of midwifery education for candidates who already possessed undergraduate degrees in non-nursing disciplines (Fullerton, Shah, Schechter, & Muller, 2000). Five direct-entry students were admitted into the State University of New York Health Science Center at Brooklyn in a partnership program with North Central Bronx Hospital (Fullerton, Shah, Holmes, Roe, & Campau, 1998).

In 1992, the ACNM BOD created the National Commission on Nurse–Midwifery Education to increase the numbers of graduates of nurse–midwifery programs. Members of the commission included representatives from nursing, obstetrics, pediatrics, public health, funding organizations, and liability insurance groups (ACNM, 1993). Some findings of the commission that had educational implications included the following: nurse–midwifery education is well-positioned for growth; current levels of funding for nurse–midwifery education are inadequate to meet present and future needs; and restrictions on nurse–midwifery practice limit the development of clinical teaching sites for students (pp. 11–12). The commission's recommendations are current today: increase support for nurse–midwifery education; promote universal acceptance of full-scope nurse–midwifery practice; monitor the need, demand for, and supply of nurse–midwives over time; and gradually adjust nurse–midwife/physician ratios within maternity care (pp. 14–17).

The master of science in midwifery degree was a natural progression and complement to the direct-entry midwifery movement. The degree was designed as a new educational model with a focus on the critical evaluation of clinical research and its application to practice (Carr, 2003). Philadelphia University opened its master's degree completion program in 1998, offering a master of science in midwifery (Farley & Carr, 2003). Philadelphia University offers its program in conjunction with the Institute of Midwifery and Women's Health (Carr, 2003). The State University of New York Health Science Center at Brooklyn also offers a master of science in midwifery degree. Both of these programs are distance-based education programs.

Johnson and Fullerton (1998) conducted a study of midwifery education program directors to explore trends in educational approaches. Forty-four of the 45 existing program directors responded. At the time of their study, the majority of programs were traditional (in-class sessions on campus) and were using a synchronous method of teaching. Nine percent used asynchronous learning, 32% incorporated distance education, 23% used a combination of traditional and distance education, and 61% used a modular curriculum.

Although it may or may not be considered an innovation, one of the educational characteristics that sets midwifery education apart from other advanced practice nursing educational programs is its competency-based outcomes. In sharp contrast to our nurse practitioner colleagues, who must complete a prescribed number of clinical hours, student midwives must have sufficient numbers of clinical experiences to attain the program objectives, theoretical and clinical, parallel with the core competencies. Student midwives must demonstrate competency in preconception care, antepartum care (both initial and return visits), labor management, birth management, postpartum care (0–5 days and 4–8 weeks), newborn assessment, breastfeeding support, primary care common health problems, family planning, gynecological care, and perimenopausal/postmenopausal care.

ACNM Core Competencies

While some nurses-midwives advocated for a core curriculum (ACNM, 1973), the ACNM BOD charged the ACNM Education Committee with the responsibility to develop a set of core competencies expected of graduates of nurse–midwifery programs (Avery, 2000,

2005). Led by Sister Nathalie Elder, CNM, Chair of the Education Committee, and Helen Burgess, CNM, Chair of the Subcommittee on Core Competencies, the *Core Competencies in Nurse–Midwifery: Expected Outcomes of Nurse–Midwifery Education* was approved by the BOD in 1978 (Avery, 2000, 2005; ACNM, 1978).

The core competencies document has been revised four times: in 1985, 1992, 1997, and 2002 (ACNM, 1985, 1992, 1997, 2002a; Avery, 2005). Each revision has been in response to the changing practice of midwifery and/or the changing health care system. Even through revisions, the core competencies have maintained a constant framework: concepts essential to midwifery practice, midwifery management of care, basic components of midwifery care, and professional responsibilities (Avery, 2005). The 2002 Core Competencies revision identified the scope of newborn care as the first 28 days of life, reorganized basic competencies into a section of "Fundamentals," clarified the scope and nature of primary health care, updated terms and definitions, and added some key statements (Roberts, 2002). The articles by Avery (2000, 2005) in the *Journal of Midwifery & Women's Health* are excellent reviews of the history and evolution of the core competencies. For more information about how the core competencies affect clinical practice, see Chapter 8.

Midwifery Education Faculty

In the formative years of midwifery education, the nurse–midwifery education program directors were leaders not only in education, but also in the profession. Many held visible leadership positions within ACNM and were strong representatives of midwifery to other health care professions. In 1976, midwifery education program directors began convening annual meetings, primarily as a support group for each other (Burst, 2005). This group was and continues to be their own group and not an official division, committee, or standing group within ACNM. As issues within the profession that also affected midwifery education began arising, the program directors began structuring formal meeting agendas that included such persons as the ACNM executive director, the ACNM president, the DHHS Division of Nursing representative (who is a CNM), and the ACNM senior policy analyst. The program directors typically meet twice a year, at the ACNM Annual Meeting and at a fall meeting. During the fall meeting they meet in conjunction with the Service Directors Network and meet both together and separately. Together, the two groups discuss issues including, but not limited to, student education and new graduates, such as availability of clinical sites and readiness of new graduates for employment.

In 2000 the program directors reorganized, including the development of bylaws and structured voting for officers, into the Directors of Midwifery Education (DOME). The purpose of DOME is to "advance midwifery education through the national network of midwifery education program directors to provide a forum for information exchange, peer support, mentorship and advisement on issues, policies and trends pertinent to midwifery education" (Directors of Midwifery Education, 2004).

The ACNM Division of Accreditation works to ensure that faculty participating in the education of midwives are qualified to provide students instruction, supervision, and evaluation that are compatible with safe practice and student learning needs (ACNM, 2004). Midwifery faculty in DOA pre-accredited or accredited programs must:

- Be certified by ACNM, ACC, or AMCB.
- Have a minimum of a master's degree.
- Demonstrate proficiency in the 2002 Core Competencies appropriate to their teaching responsibility.
- Have preparation in teaching (didactic and clinical, as appropriate).
- Have 1 year of clinical midwifery experience prior to teaching.

A more recent challenge for midwifery faculty in academic institutions has been the requirement of a master's degree in nursing. This requirement not only impacts full-time midwifery faculty members, but also midwifery clinical preceptors, who are considered members of the midwifery faculty. The requirement for a master's degree in nursing comes from the National Council of State Boards of Nursing (NCSBN) recommendations, which state that faculty in advanced practice nursing programs have a minimum of a master's degree in nursing (2004), and the accrediting bodies of nursing schools: the National League for Nursing Accrediting Commission (NLNAC) and the Commission on Collegiate Nursing Education (CCNE). The latest revision of the NLNAC guidelines for accreditation state that faculty should possess a minimum of a master's degree in nursing (NLNAC, 2004); the CCNE accreditation criteria state that faculty must be academically and experientally qualified (CCNE, 2003). The ACNM QuickInfo on faculty degree requirements in schools of nursing provides more background and advice for ACNM members attempting to address this situation (ACNM, 2005).

Student Demographics

In 2002, the ACNM conducted a Web-based student education survey. A total of 274 of 830 enrolled midwifery students responded, for a response rate of 33%. At that time, 74.45% of respondents were enrolled in a master's degree midwifery program and 24.45% were enrolled in a certificate program ($n = 271$ responses). When asked if financial constraints delayed entry into midwifery school, 42.65% were not delayed by finances ($n = 272$), but 86% needed financial assistance for their midwifery education. Results showed that 39.71% received financial assistance from loan repayment and 26.47% received assistance from scholarships and loan repayment; 10.81% received National Health Service Corps (NHSC) scholarships and less than 1% received Indian Health scholarships ($n = 111$). Of those responding 55.35% worked 21 or more hours per week, while 44.65% worked 20 hours or less during school ($n = 215$).

The 2003 ACNM annual membership survey (Schuiling, Sipe, & Fullerton, 2005) indicated that the mean age of student midwives was 34.88 with a range of 23 to 58 years. The survey showed that 43.7% were Caucasian/Euro-American, 0.7% were American Indian/Inuit, 1.6% were Asian/Pacific Islander, 5.2% were Black/African American, 1.7% were Hispanic/Latina, and 47.2% were other/missing. The majority of midwifery students had bachelor's degrees as their highest academic degree (48.2%), while 0.5% had diplomas, 1.6% had associate degrees, 1.7% had master's degrees, and 0.9% had doctorates. It is of note that the number of students responding in 2000 was 728 and in 2001 was 811, but in 2002 and 2003 the rate decreased to 697 and 579 respectively.

In 2004, Carr, Schuiling, and Williams conducted a survey of midwifery education pro-grams to gather data on nurse–midwifery education (ACNM, 2005). Thirty-two of the then 45 programs responded (71%). Eighteen programs responded that the cost of midwifery education at their institution ranged from $10,000 to $30,000, and nine programs cost more than $30,000. Debt load of graduates ranged from $10,000 to over $50,000. Forty-seven percent of the programs responded that their enrollment had decreased, 25% re-mained constant, and 25% increased enrollment. Overall, there has been a decline in the number of midwifery students graduated annually, from a high of 587 in 1997 to approx-imately 330 in 2004.

Future Challenges

One of the more controversial issues in the history of midwifery education in the United States is whether the master's degree should be the initial degree for entry into practice. At the 1967 nurse–midwifery education workshop (there have been six education workshops: 1958, 1967, 1973, 1977, 1980, 1992 [Burst, 2005; Sharp, 1983]), a major result was the statement that "professional nurse–midwifery education should be at the master's level, while experimentation for technically prepared nurse–midwives should continue" (Sharp, 1983, p. 19). When enrollments declined in the 1980s, Rooks, Carr, and Sandvold (1991) advocated that nurse–midwifery education should "remain and become more accessible to nurses without baccalaureate degrees" (p. 126). The rationale provided for their argument was that there is no evidence to support that nurse–midwives with master's degrees are safer or more effective than nurse–midwives with certificates. On the other hand, Carrington and Decker (1997) argued that with the advent of managed care and health care competition, the ACNM must respond by calling for the master's degree as the entry-level credential for nurse–midwives. Today the ACNM continues to maintain that entry into practice should be at the baccalaureate level (ACNM, 1998).

The most current report of the ACNM membership survey (2005) indicates that of the 6345 members who responded, the highest academic degree earned by members was: 4.4% diploma, 4.6% associate's degree, 27.7% bachelor's degree, 53.8% master's degree, and 4.5% with an earned doctorate. Members earned master's degrees in categories such as business, counseling, education, science, and sociology. Only 0.6% of respondents indi-cated their master's degree was in midwifery, and 4.1% received master's degree in public health.

Another challenge for midwifery education is the Institute of Medicine's call for a new vision for health professions education:

> All health professionals should be educated to deliver patient-centered
> care as members of an interdisciplinary team, emphasizing evidence-
> based practice, quality improvement approaches, and informatics.
> (Institute of Medicine, 2003, p. 3)

This call is a direct result of the 2001 Institute of Medicine report *Crossing the Quality Chasm: A New Health System for the 21st Century*. Medical errors lead to thousands of pa-tient injuries and deaths each year, and health professions educators must respond to the call to examine how we prepare practitioners for the future. *Charting a Course for the 21st Century: The Future of Midwifery* (Pew Health Professions Commissions, 1999), in its recommendations for education, also recommended that midwifery education programs "should provide opportunities for interprofessional education and training experiences, . . . which requires intra- and interprofessional collaboration between colleges, universities, and education programs to develop affiliations and complementary curriculum pathways" (p. 33). Neither ACNM nor DOME has developed a formal response to this challenge.

Last, in response to growing concerns that the future supply of CNMs/CMs will not meet the expanding need for women's health in the United States, particularly for vulnerable populations, the ACNM convened a midwifery educational summit in September 2005. This was the first midwifery education workshop since 1992. The objectives for the 2005 summit included: 1) to describe the need for midwifery education in the United States; 2) to delineate the problem(s) facing the education of midwives, including but not limited to declining enrollment, decreased funding, accreditation, evolving requirements for licensure, and retaining clinical sites; 3) to analyze the broad context affecting midwifery education in the United States; 4) to define the core values that will provide a foundation for the recommendations to be developed by the summit; and 5) to develop the recommendations that address the problems delineated by the summit (N. Dickerson, personal communications, July 21, 2005, and August 18, 2005). Topics for discussion included the Doctor of Nursing Practice (DNP), baccalaureate versus master's degree as entry into practice, funding for midwifery education, and trends for other APNs.

Summary

As of August 2005, the ACNM lists a total of 43 accredited or pre-accredited midwifery education programs (N. Dickerson, personal correspondence). Four of these programs offer postbaccalaureate certificates and 39 offer a master's degree (MA, MN, MSN, MPH, or MS). Of those offering a master's degree, two solely offer the MPH degree, and one of these programs is closing. Frontier School of Midwifery and Family Nursing is accredited as a freestanding institution of higher education, in addition to being accredited as a midwifery program. Three of these programs will be closing in 2005–2006. Two programs offer midwifery education programs in conjunction with nurse–midwifery education programs: Baystate Medical Center and SUNY Downstate Medical Center.

As we emerge into the 21st century, midwifery education has a solid curricular base due to the work of the ACNM DOA. In addition, CNM/CM education has a rich and varied history of curricular innovations and positive outcomes. As the mutual forces of health care systems, technology, and supply and demand of CNMs/CMs continue to evolve, so will midwifery education and its innovations.

References

American College of Nurse–Midwives. (1973). *Responding to the demands for nurse–midwives in the United States: A workshop report.* Washington, DC: Author.

American College of Nurse–Midwives. (1978). *Core competencies in nurse–midwifery.* Washington, DC: Author.

American College of Nurse–Midwives. (1985). *Core competencies in nurse–midwifery.* Washington, DC: Author.

American College of Nurse–Midwives. (1991, May/June). Position paper on professional midwifery. *Quickening,* 8.

American College of Nurse–Midwives. (1992). *Core competencies for basic nurse–midwifery practice.* Washington, DC: Author.

American College of Nurse–Midwives. (1993). *Educating nurse–midwives: A strategy for achieving affordable, high-quality maternity care. Executive summary.* Washington, DC: Author.

American College of Nurse–Midwives. (1997). *Core competencies for basic midwifery practice.* Washington DC: Author.

American College of Nurse–Midwives. (1998). *Mandatory degree requirements for midwives.* Washington, DC: Author.

American College of Nurse–Midwives. (2002a). *Core competencies for basic midwifery practice.* Washington, DC: Author.

American College of Nurse–Midwives. (2002b). *Student education survey.* Washington, DC: Author.

American College of Nurse–Midwives. (2004). *Division of Accreditation policies and procedures manual.* Washington, DC: Author.

American College of Nurse–Midwives. (2005). *Faculty degree requirements in schools of nursing. QuickInfo.* Silver Springs, MD: Author.

Avery, M. (2000). The evolution of the Core Competencies for Basic Midwifery Practice. *Journal of Midwifery & Women's Health, 45*(6), 532–536.

Avery, M. (2005). The history and evolution of the Core Competencies for Basic Midwifery Practice. *Journal of Midwifery & Women's Health, 50*(2), 102–107.

Baul, M. A. (2005). *A message: Who are we and why does it matter?* Retrieved February 18, 2005, from http://www.meacschools.org/FAQ/Summary/summary.html

Bollag, B. (2004). Opening the door on accreditation. *Chronicle of Higher Education, 50*(45), A22.

Brucker, M. C., & Reedy, N. J. (2000). Nurse–midwifery: Yesterday, today, and tomorrow. *MCN: The American Journal of Maternal/Child Nursing, 25*(6), 322–326.

Burst, H. V. (2003). Genealogic origins of nurse–midwifery education programs in the United States. *Journal of Midwifery & Women's Health, 48*(6), 464–472.

Burst, H. V. (2005). The history of nurse–midwifery/midwifery education. *Journal of Midwifery & Women's Health, 50*(2), 129–137.

Carr, K. C. (2003). Innovations in midwifery education. *Journal of Midwifery & Women's Health, 48*(6), 393–397.

Carr, K. C., Schuiling, K., & Williams, D. (2005). *Challenges and opportunities for nurse–midwifery education.* Paper presented at the 2005 Education Summit, September 9, 2005, Arlington, VA.

Carrington, B. W., & Burst, H. V. (2005). The American College of Nurse–Midwives' dream becomes reality: The Division of Accreditation. *Journal of Midwifery & Women's Health, 50*(2), 146–153.

Carrington, B. W., & Decker, B. (1997). A master's degree for entry-level ACNM-certified midwives: An option or necessity? *Journal of Nurse–Midwifery, 42*(4), 360–366.

Cassells, J. (2000). *The Manhattan Midwifery School*. Master's thesis, Yale University School of Nursing, New Haven, CT.

Commission on Collegiate Nursing Education. (2003). *Standards for accreditation of baccalaureate and graduate nursing programs*. Washington, DC: Author.

Council for Higher Education Accreditation. (2004, May 26). CHEA letter to Congress on HR 4283.

Council for Higher Education Accreditation. (2005, February 11). *House Republicans repeat their 2004 bill. CHEA Update*. Retrieved February 19, 2005, from http://www.chea.org/Government/HEAupdate/CHEA_HEA19.htm

Davis-Floyd, R. E. (1998). The ups, downs, and interlinkages of nurse- and direct-entry midwifery: Status, practice, and education. In J. Rosenberg, J. Southern, & J. Tritten (Eds.), *Pathways to becoming a midwife: Getting an education*. Eugene, OR: Midwifery Today.

Directors of Midwifery Education. (2004). *Bylaws*.

Farley, C., & Carr, K. C. (2003). New directions in midwifery education: The master's of science in midwifery degree. *Journal of Midwifery & Women's Health, 48*(2), 133–137.

Fondiller, S. (2000). In the footsteps of Mary Breckinridge: A glorious 75th anniversary celebration. *Nursing and Health Care Perspectives, 21*(3), 112–114.

Fullerton, J. T., Shah, M. A., Holmes, G., Roe, V., & Campau, N. (1998). Direct entry midwifery education: Evaluation of program innovations. *Journal of Nurse–Midwifery, 43*(2), 102–105.

Fullerton, J. T., Shah, M. A., Schechter, S., & Muller, J. H. (2000). Integrating qualified nurses and non-nurses in midwifery education: The two-year experience of an ACNM COA accredited program. *Journal of Midwifery & Women's Health, 45*(1), 45–52.

Hart, E., & Marsico, T. (1975). Mastery learning: An approach to individualized learning. *Journal of Nurse–Midwifery, 20*(3), 17–19.

Hsia, L. (1982). Fifty years of nurse–midwifery education: Reflections and perspectives. *Journal of Nurse–Midwifery, 27*(4), 1–3.

Hsia, L. (1987). Social and demographic challenges: Nurse–midwifery education must respond. *Journal of Nurse–Midwifery, 32*(5), 275–276.

Institute of Medicine. (2001). *Crossing the quality chasm: A new health system for the 21st century*. Washington, DC: National Academy Press.

Institute of Medicine. (2003). *Health professions education: A bridge to quality*. Washington, DC: National Academy Press.

Johnson, P. G. & Fullerton, J. T. (1998). Midwifery education models: A contemporary review. *Journal of Nurse–Midwifery, 43*(5), 351–357.

Long, P. J., Anderson, E. E., Hamel, A., & Shiers, R. D. (1975). Meeting specialized problems with creative solutions: An experience with faculty exchange. *Journal of Nurse–Midwifery, 20*(3), 22–24.

Midwifery Education Accreditation Council. (2005). *Supporting quality and innovation in midwifery education*. Retrieved February 18, 2005, from http://www.meacschools.org

Midwives' Alliance of North America. (1985, July). *History of MANA*. Retrieved February 18, 2005, from http://www.mana.org/history.html

Murphy, P. (1986). Nurse–midwifery education: Challenges ahead. *Journal of Nurse–Midwifery, 31*(1), 1–2.

Muzio, L. G. (1991). Midwifery education and nursing: Curricular revolution or civil war? *Nursing and Health Care, 12*(7), 376–379.

National League for Nursing Accrediting Commission. (2004). *NLNAC accreditation manual.* New York: Author.

North American Registry of Midwives. (2004, March 4). *NARM mission statement.* Retrieved February 18, 2005, from http://www.narm.org/htb.htm

Osborne, K., Stone, S., & Ernst, E. (2005). The development of the community-based nurse–midwifery education programs: An innovation in distance learning. *Journal of Midwifery & Women's Health, 50*(2), 138–145.

Pew Health Professions Commissions and the University of California, San Francisco Center for the Health Professions. (1999). *Charting a course for the 21st century: The future of midwifery.* San Francisco, CA: Center for the Health Professions.

Raisler, J. (1987). Nurse–midwifery education: Issues for survival and growth. *Journal of Nurse–Midwifery, 32*(1), 1–3.

Roberts, J. (2002). The evolution of midwifery as reflected in the 2002 revisions of the ACNM's core competencies. *Journal of Midwifery & Women's Health, 47*(5), 301–302.

Rooks, J. P., Carr, K. C., & Sandvold, I. (1991). The importance of non-master's degree options in nurse–midwifery education. *Journal of Nurse–Midwifery, 36*(2), 124–130.

Schuiling, K. D., Sipe, T. A., & Fullerton, J. (2005). Findings from the analysis of the American College of Nurse–Midwives' membership surveys: 2000–2003. *Journal of Midwifery & Women's Health, 50*(1), 8–15.

Sharp, E. (1983). Nurse–midwifery education: Its successes, failures, and future. *Journal of Nurse–Midwifery, 28*(2), 17–23.

Treistman, J. M., Carr, K. C., & McHugh, M. K. (1993). Community-based nurse–midwifery education programs: Distance learning in nurse–midwifery education. *Journal of Nurse–Midwifery, 38*(6), 358–365.

U.S. Department of Education. (2005). *Accreditation in the United States.* Retrieved January 30, 2005, from http://www.ed.gov/print/adminis/finaid/accred/accreditation.html

Table 4–1: For Your Professional Files   95

Table 4–1 For Your Professional Files: Essential Documents for the ACNM Division of Accreditation

- *ACNM Division of Accreditation Policies and Procedures Manual*, January 2004
- *ACNM Division of Accreditation Criteria for Programmatic Preaccreditation*, October 2003
- *ACNM Division of Accreditation Criteria for Programmatic Accreditation*, October 2003
- *ACNM Division of Accreditation Criteria for Institutional Accreditation*, January 2004
- *ACNM, The Core Competencies for Basic Midwifery Practice*, May 2002
- ACNM Division of Accreditation, *The Skills, Knowledge, Competencies and Health Sciences Prerequisite to Midwifery Practice*, October 2000
- ACNM QuickInfo, *Recruiting Future Midwives*, 2002
- *Standards for the Practice of Nurse–Midwifery*, March 2003
- *Philosophy of the American College of Nurse–Midwives*, September 2004

CHAPTER 5

Certification and Licensure in Midwifery

Carol Howe, CNM, DNSc, FACNM
Nancy K. Lowe, CNM, PhD, FACNM, FAAN

Learning Objectives

1. Discriminate between certification and licensure.
2. Compare and contrast the mission of the professional organization with the mission of the certification organization.
3. List the significant milestones in the development of midwifery certification.
4. Identify major responsibilities of licensing agencies.
5. Identify the individual's responsibility for maintenance of professional competence.

In the United States, the overall objective of protecting the public welfare for those in the health professions is accomplished through three primary interdependent mechanisms: 1) a prescribed, accredited course of study; 2) national certification; and 3) governmental, usually state or other jurisdiction, licensure (**Figure 5–1**). As illustrated, program accreditation in nurse–midwifery is the responsibility of the American College of Nurse–Midwives (ACNM) Division of Accreditation (DOA). Certification is the responsibility of the American Midwifery Certification Board (AMCB), which requires completion of an ACNM DOA-accredited educational program in nurse–midwifery or midwifery to be eligible for certification. Finally, licensure is regulated by the state or other jurisdiction, which may or may not depend on ACNM DOA program accreditation of midwifery programs or AMCB certification.

It is critical that midwives understand the difference between these three forms of regulation. The first two generally are the responsibility of the profession itself. In principle, certification is usually nongovernmental and voluntary (Schoon & Smith, 2000), although the voluntary certification may be required to obtain a state license to practice. National certification is a profession's means of recognizing individuals who achieve specified standards in the profession at the entry or advanced level. Licensure is the mechanism by which the state attempts to protect the public from unsafe practice by individuals.

Figure 5–1 The interrelationships of education, certification, and licensure for public protection.

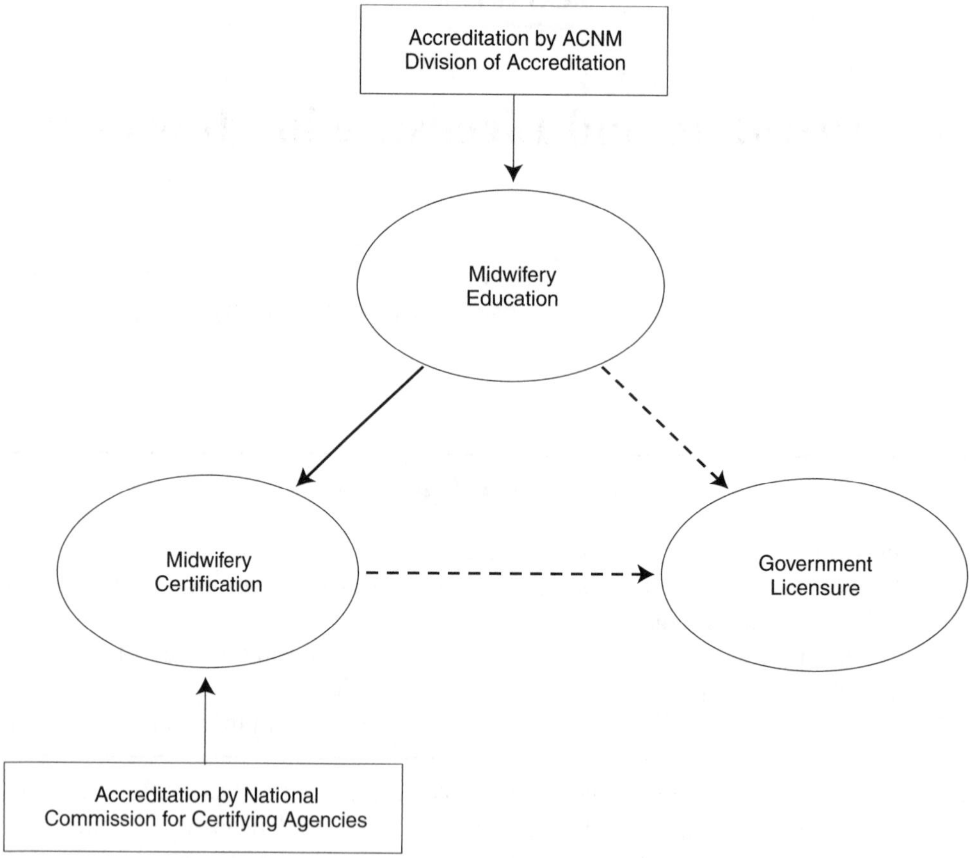

It should be noted that in addition to direct regulation through accreditation organizations, certification organizations, and state licensing boards, professions are regulated indirectly through other institutions, including professional organizations, funding agencies, and the like. These organizations set criteria for the education and practice of health professionals that strongly influence the criteria for certification and licensure. An example of indirect regulation is the fact that current funding for midwifery education flows through the United States Department of Health and Human Services, Division of Nursing, which now funds only master's-level programs in nurse–midwifery. Although the AMCB and the ACNM recognize the legitimacy of the postbaccalaureate certificate in midwifery, the number of certificate programs has declined markedly due to lack of access to federal funding. Similarly, the National Council of State Boards of Nursing continues to advocate for the master's requirement for licensure. As more states adopt the master's requirement, graduates of certificate programs will find their ability to practice limited to fewer and fewer states. The impact on educational and certification requirements in midwifery of the American Association of Colleges of Nursing's (AACN) 2004 adoption of a policy to require the Doctorate of Nursing Practice for entry level into advanced practice nursing by 2015 is not yet clear.

This chapter reviews the process and history of certification as first established by the ACNM and now handled by the AMCB, formerly the ACNM Certification Council (ACC). In addition, issues related to state licensure of Certified Nurse–Midwives (CNMs) and Certified Midwives (CMs), including the agencies that license midwives, the requirements for licensure, scope of practice, and prescriptive privilege, will be discussed.

Certification in Nurse–Midwifery/Midwifery

Purpose of Certification

The process of certification is inextricably tied with the members of the profession. However, certification is not a function of the professional organization. The missions of a professional organization and a certification organization are very different, and their stakeholders are dissimilar as well. The purpose of a professional organization is to serve its membership, through policy, advocacy, and professional services. Its stakeholders are the members of that profession. Therefore, the purpose of the AMCB is to serve midwives.

The mission of a certification organization is to protect the public recipients of the profession's services. All policies and decisions of the AMCB are made with the welfare of women and infants served by midwives as its first priority. Public protection is accomplished by a process that provides:

1. Evidence of entry-level competency in the profession
2. Evidence of continuing competency in the profession
3. A mechanism through which individuals practicing unsafely or unscrupulously can be disciplined

It is important to distinguish between entry-level certification and certification for excellence. The AMCB offers entry-level certification in midwifery, which is appropriate for professionals who have just completed their educational requirements and need to demonstrate mastery of the fundamental expectations of safe practice. Certification for excellence is typified by the specialty and subspecialty certifications offered in medicine after the physician has completed education over and above what is required for licensure and has practiced for several years in the specialty. In addition to written and oral examinations, documentation of patient care outcomes is required. However, physicians also demonstrate entry-level competence in medical practice through the three steps of the United States Medical Licensing Examination (USMLE) taken during the second, fourth, and internship years of medical education. The American Board of Obstetrics and Gynecology (ABOG) awards specialty certification in obstetrics and gynecology on successful completion of 1) a standardized written examination, usually taken at the end of the 4-year residency in obstetrics and gynecology; and 2) an oral examination based on the presentation of cases by the candidate a year or more after the written examination. The physician who successfully completes both elements is designated board-certified in obstetrics and gynecology.

Although the primary purpose of certification remains to protect the public welfare, there are professional benefits as well. Foremost among those benefits is the fact that the reputation of the profession is enhanced when substandard practitioners are screened out. Not all individuals who successfully complete an accredited educational program will attain national certification. This is true across the professions and is validation of the independence of certification from education in the triad of public protection mechanisms previously illustrated in Figure 5–1. An excellent and rigorous certification process lends credence to the credential offered by the organization. In the case of midwifery, the Certified Nurse–Midwife (CNM) and the Certified Midwife (CM) titles represent a nationally recognized level of excellence. The AMCB holds federal title protection over these titles, and no other organization can authorize or restrict the use of these credentials.

Certification is often required for other professional necessities, including state licensure, prescriptive privilege, hospital staff privileges, or inclusion in health plan provider panels. Furthermore, federal and state reimbursement for Medicare and Medicaid also depend upon certification.

Process of Certification

The concept of certification is most closely identified with national examination. The national certifying examination (NCE), however, is only a part of the certification process. Each certifying organization must first determine the criteria that applicants must meet in order to be a candidate to sit for the NCE. For midwifery, these criteria include successful completion of an ACNM DOA-approved program in midwifery or nurse–midwifery and the program director's documentation that the student has successfully completed all program requirements. Therefore, the DOA and the individual midwifery programs are integral components of the certification process. Candidates for the CNM must also document current licensure as a Registered Nurse.

The NCE is, of course, the most recognizable aspect of certification. The AMCB examination is based primarily upon a periodically conducted task or job analysis of basic midwifery practice. The task analysis is a survey of newly practicing (< 5 years) midwives to determine the nature of the knowledge and skills required of recent graduates. In addition to the task analysis, the examination is also informed by the ACNM Core Competencies for Basic Midwifery Practice (2002), the ACNM Standards for the Practice of Midwifery (2003), and current literature in the field. It is a 175-question multiple-choice examination, now offered in computer-based testing (CBT) format through a commercial testing vendor. A complex scoring process ensures equitable results among differing forms of the examination. A more detailed description of examination development is provided later in this chapter.

Candidates who complete the examination successfully are entitled to use either the title Certified Nurse–Midwife (CNM) or Certified Midwife (CM), depending upon their nursing background. Individuals seeking certification as nurse–midwives or midwives must take the NCE within 12 months and achieve certification within 30 months of completion of their midwifery programs. If a candidate fails the examination on the first attempt, 30 days must elapse before the candidate may retake the exam. If the second attempt is unsuccessful, retakes may occur no more frequently than every 90 days during the 30 months of eligibility for certification. If certification is not accomplished within 30 months of midwifery program completion, the individual is no longer eligible for AMCB certification; eligibility can only be gained by again completing a nurse–midwifery or midwifery program accredited by the ACNM DOA.

The certification process also includes periodic recertification. In the AMCB, recertification is coordinated through the Certificate Maintenance Program (CMP). Recertification occurs in 8-year cycles and may be accomplished through two different routes. The certificant may choose to retake the NCE in the seventh year of the cycle, or to complete three CMP-prepared self-learning modules (with post-test) and 10 hours of ACNM or continuing medical education (CME) approved continuing education during the 8 years.

Evolution of Certification

The certification process in nurse–midwifery/midwifery is among the most rigorous and respected in the health professions. Recognizing early in the development of professional midwifery that certification was a critical need, leaders in nurse–midwifery education established a testing committee of the American College of Nurse–Midwives in the 1960s (Foster, 1986). The committee's purpose was to develop, validate, administer, and evaluate a national certification examination for nurse–midwives. Early chairpersons of the committee included nurse–midwives Joy Cohen, Ann Hempey, Joyce Cameron Foster, and Joan Imhoff. After completion of an initial task analysis, the first NCE was offered in 1971 and the CNM credential by examination conferred. The first examinations were in modified essay format and required 8 hours to complete. In addition, for the first 2 years of the certification process, a clinical examination was conducted as well. Analysis of the results of these two different evaluation mechanisms revealed that the clinical component offered no new data. Candidates who did well on the written examination did well on the clinical examination. Candidates who did not perform well on the written examination also performed poorly on the clinical examination. Further, the assessment of clinical competency by the candidate's educational program director, who had observed the student throughout her midwifery education, was more valid than a 2-hour clinical observation. The clinical component was therefore discontinued in 1974 since it was an expensive endeavor without additional benefit.

As the certification process was further developed and refined, responsibility was transferred in 1975 to a new division of the ACNM, the Division of Examiners. Chairs of this Division included nurse–midwives Helen Varney Burst, Sally Yeomans, Joyce Thompson, and Sarah Cohen. In addition, Judith Fullerton, CNM, provided critical expertise in certification and psychometrics and conducted the first task analysis that formed the basis for the NCE.

In 1990, recognizing the inherent difference in mission and the potential conflict of interest in maintaining the certification function within the professional organization, the ACNM Board of Directors transferred the certification responsibility to a new and separately incorporated organization, the ACNM Certification Council (ACC). Under the leadership of its first president, Sarah Cohen, this new organization developed its own Articles of Incorporation and Bylaws, formed its own Board of Directors, and established a separate office to discriminate clearly between the functions of the professional organization and those of the certification organization. Responsibility for midwifery certificates, both previously and newly issued, came under the purview of the new organization.

In 1994, Carol Howe, CNM, became president of ACC. By this time, the increasing number of midwifery graduates each year had made the modified essay format of the examination untenable. Although an excellent form of testing, the modified essay format required at least two readers to agree on the grading of the exam and a third if there was significant disagreement. It required 80 examinations to be completed before the exam could be validated psychometrically. Therefore, in addition to being a very expensive form of testing, it was also time consuming and required that 80 candidates complete the test developed for a given year before scores could be released. The decision was made to move to a multiple-choice format for the NCE.

Although clearly a necessary move, this transition required the ACC Exam Committee members to become skilled in the development of multiple-choice questions and the development of a test bank sufficiently large to support three different forms of the examination each year. The first multiple-choice examination was offered in December 1996. Although this format was less expensive and allowed for earlier release of results, security concerns dictated that the examination was offered only three times per year. It was difficult to identify dates for the examination that met the needs of a variety of midwifery programs with different times of graduation.

Three additional major changes to the certification process were also introduced during the late 1990s. First was the recognition that a recertification process was needed. Although the initial certification in midwifery was rigorous, the credential was bestowed for a lifetime. As the ACC followed evolving professional standards of certification, it was clear that recertification was becoming a national expectation of the certification process. In 1996, the ACC began issuing time-limited certificates that required recertification every 8 years.

In 1986, the Continuing Competency Assessment (CCA) program was introduced by the ACNM as a partial answer to the continuing competency issue. The CCA process requires the documentation of either 1) successfully passing the current national certification examination provided by AMCB, or 2) completion of five continuing education units (CEUs) (50 contact hours) over a 5-year cycle. Initially, the CEUs had to be ACNM approved, but Accreditation Council for Continuing Medical Education (ACCME) CEUs are also now acceptable. Early in the CCA program, equal numbers of CEUs were required in each of the areas of midwifery scope of practice (antepartum, intrapartum, postpartum, newborn, and well-woman care). This requirement became untenable as CNMs had difficulty identifying continuing education programs that were accessible, affordable, and met the requirements. Currently, the CEUs may be obtained in any area related to midwifery and a variety of other activities, such as the completion of a formal educational course relevant to midwifery, and can be used for documentation of currency in lieu of CEUs (see http://www.midwife.org/edu/cca-alternatives.cfm). The CCA process documents attendance at CEU programs or completion of other relevant activities and has no relationship to the maintenance of the CNM/CM credential.

In the context of adopting time-limited CNM/CM certification in 1996, the ACC developed the Certificate Maintenance Program (CMP). All certificants since that time are required to enroll in the CMP. Those whose certificates were initially granted in perpetuity are not required to participate. The CMP initially was met with a great deal of controversy. Those who were required to enroll to maintain their certificate felt it unfair not to require all CNMs to participate, and those who had been granted their certificate with no expiration date felt that it was unfair to change their requirements. As midwives certified early in the process retire, the proportion of CNMs/CMs with time-limited certification increases and the principle of recertification becomes more universal in the health care fields, these issues and disagreements are becoming less important.

During the late 1990s, the issue of a professional disciplinary process was also considered. For many years, the ACNM had maintained a disciplinary process to address concerns regarding midwives who were practicing unsafely, unethically, or beyond their scope of practice. Unlike many professions, this process was actively implemented by the ACNM. When grievances were filed, they were reviewed. If deemed potentially serious by the president of ACNM, they were investigated and reviewed. Several nurse–midwives had actions on their certificate, including suspension and decertification. When responsibility for certificates was transferred to ACC, the disciplinary process was discontinued by the ACNM. Initially, ACC did not establish a disciplinary process due to concerns about liability issues resulting from taking negative actions upon certificates. However, it became clear that liability could be incurred for failing to discipline as well, and in 1998 a new disciplinary policy and procedure was adopted. These documents are available from the AMCB website at http://www.amcbmidwife.org.

Also in the 1990s, significant discussion was occurring about the relationship of nurse–midwifery and direct-entry midwifery. The ACNM participated with the Midwives Alliance of North America (MANA) in working groups to determine areas of congruence and divergence on significant issues related to education and practice. Although both organizations agreed on philosophical issues related to issues such as the normalcy of birth and the empowerment of women, there were significant and irreconcilable difference in views on professional education and standards of practice. As a result, the ACNM embarked upon a process of encouraging the development of professional education programs, affiliated with institutions of higher learning, for the education of midwives without a nursing background. The DOA developed accreditation criteria for these programs. And after extensive study and debate, the ACC agreed to certify graduates of these programs as Certified Midwives (CMs).

This decision created considerable controversy within the nursing profession. Many nursing leaders vehemently disagree with such a tangible demonstration that although the disciplines of nursing and midwifery are closely related, they are not identical and can be considered separately. This tension continues as requirements for Advanced Practice Nursing programs and licensure continue to have an impact on the education and licensure of nurse–midwives. Although the AMCB grants certification to CMs, in many states these midwives have no mechanism to become licensed, and their ability to practice is restrained.

Nancy Lowe, CNM, became president of ACC in 2000. Issues addressed during her tenure have included the accreditation of the ACC by the National Commission for

Certifying Agencies (NCCA), the move to computer-based testing (CBT), refinement and implementation of the disciplinary process, and reorganization and renaming of the organization. External validation of the credibility of the ACC's certification process was achieved in 2001 with the ACC's accreditation by NCCA. A process begun by Carol Howe, NCCA accreditation was granted on the basis of the ACC's documentation of meeting NCCA's (2004) the *Standards for the Accreditation of Certifying Agencies* through the submission of a detailed self-study report. NCCA accreditation provides objective evidence that ACC, now AMCB, meets established standards for the conduct of a competency assurance certification program.

CBT was a goal to which the ACC aspired for many years. The primary advantage is the ability to offer the examination in multiple sites throughout the nation according to the convenience of the candidate. Furthermore, results of the exam are available immediately and the security of the examination is assured. However, the small number of candidates tested annually compared to larger professions made transition to this form of testing financially impossible until improved technology and commercial vendor development brought the cost within the reach of midwifery graduates. The first computer-based testing was offered in February 2005.

The need for reorganization and renaming of the organization reflected the growth and increasing responsibilities of the organization. In particular, it became clear that many CNMs and CMs did not understand that the ACNM and the ACNM Certification Council were not the same organization. Although reasonable at the time of its founding, the incorporation of the initials *ACNM* into the ACC's name created confusion even among the most knowledgeable midwives. As a result, when a midwife changed her personal information, such as name or address, with one organization she assumed that both entities were informed; or when midwives had questions or concerns about either organization, those communications frequently went to the inappropriate organization. Therefore, in 2005, the name of the ACC became the American Midwifery Certification Board (AMCB) to clearly distinguish it from the ACNM.

In summary, the development of professional certification in nurse–midwifery and midwifery was born within the ACNM and has evolved over more than 30 years. The strong foundation for a rigorous certification process provided by nurse–midwifery leaders through the ACNM firmly established the credibility of the CNM credential. Sarah Cohen expertly guided the transition to a separate credentialing organization, which allowed the continued evolution of a certification mechanism that serves its stakeholders well. Since the formation of the ACC in 1990, midwifery's independent certification body has accomplished eight major initiatives: 1) the retirement of the essay examination and the initiation of the multiple choice examination; 2) the adoption of time-limited certification; 3) the development of the CMP; 4) the certification of midwives who are not nurses; 5) the adoption of a professional discipline policy and procedure; 6) the accreditation of the organization by the NCCA; 7) the implementation of CBT; and 8) the renaming of ACC to AMCB. The process of certification continues to evolve along with the midwifery profession. The profession is fortunate in that its members have continuously supported rigorous and meaningful professional standards that include meticulous program accreditation and stringent certification requirements.

American Midwifery Certification Board (AMCB)

The AMCB is a nonprofit corporation whose mission is "to protect and serve the public by providing the certification standards for individuals educated in the discipline of midwifery (AMCB, 2005)." The AMCB fulfills its mission through three primary activities: initial certification in nurse–midwifery and midwifery through an NCE, recertification through the certificate maintenance program, and professional discipline.

The AMCB is governed by an 11-member Board of Directors composed of the AMCB's three officers (president, treasurer, secretary), the four chairpersons of each of its standing committees (except for the Finance Committee, whose chairperson is the treasurer), three professionals from other health care disciplines with experience in certification, and one consumer. Although all officers and committee chairpersons must be CNMs or CMs, the inclusion of other professionals and a consumer on the board helps to guard against professional self-interest that may interfere with the AMCB's public protection responsibility. The balancing of AMCB's board with individuals within and outside of the profession is a powerful public statement about the corporation's commitment to public protection in its certification, recertification, and discipline functions. Each board member is elected for a 3-year term and may be re-elected once for a maximum of 6 consecutive years on the board. The current members of AMCB's board can be found on the organization's Web site at http://www.amcbmidwife.org. All officers, chairpersons, directors, and committee members serve the organization as unpaid volunteers. AMCB's executive director and a representative from the ACNM Board of Directors serve as ex officio members of the board.

Standing committees of the AMCB are the Credentials, Administration & Reporting (CAR) Committee; the Certificate Maintenance Program (CMP) Committee; the Examination Committee; the Research Committee; and the Finance Committee. Each committee has a number of volunteer committee members who are appointed by the board on recommendation of the respective committee's chairperson. The CAR Committee is responsible for the development and implementation of policies related to the credentialing of applicants for certification, the administration of the NCE, and the reporting of examination results to the individual. The CMP Committee is responsible for all aspects of the certificate maintenance program, including the development of the self-study modules and the policies related to recertification. The Examination Committee conducts all activities related to the development of the NCE, including the construction of all questions that are part of the examination item bank and the psychometric analysis of examination results. The Research Committee conducts the periodic task analysis that provides the primary data for the construction of the NCE test plan and other research about the performance of certification candidates across time. Finally, the Finance Committee advises the board about the corporation's budget and pricing for AMCB services.

AMCB's professional staff is led by its executive director at its headquarters in Linthicum, Md. The examination program is administered in collaboration with Applied Measurement Professionals, Inc. (AMP), who provide the testing sites for the NCE in midwifery. AMP test sites are available across the nation, providing candidates access to testing 5 days per week.

NCE in Nurse–Midwifery and Midwifery

The NCE tests candidates for entry-level competence to practice nurse–midwifery/ midwifery using a standardized multiple-choice examination format. The AMCB Examination Committee, composed of CNMs and CMs practicing in a variety of settings around the country, is responsible for all aspects of the construction and evaluation of the examination. Working with a professional testing consultant, the committee develops the content blueprint, detailed content outline, and individual questions used to construct each examination. Currently, the examination is composed of 175 multiple-choice questions, a portion of which are being pretested for psychometric evaluation prior to their use as scored items.

The most important characteristic of an NCE is its content validity or correspondence to competence in the profession (Henderson, 1996). The primary data that inform the development of the NCE are the findings of the most recent job or task analysis survey of practicing CNMs and CMs in the United States. AMCB's Research Committee periodically conducts the task analysis (Oshio, Johnson, & Fullerton, 2000). The data generated are used to determine the knowledge, skills, and abilities essential to safe midwifery practice and to develop the test blueprint. The test blueprint is a topical outline of content across the domains of midwifery practice (see **Table 5–1**). It also specifies the percentage of specific content that should be tested in relationship to the effect of the content on safe professional practice (Fullerton, Parker, & Severino, 1997).

The generation of individual test items to represent the many elements of each aspect of test content is an ongoing activity of the AMCB Examination Committee. Individual committee members draft potential items in their specified areas of expertise and provide validation with current peer-reviewed, professional literature. The items are reviewed individually by the committee as a whole and revised as needed until the item is deemed acceptable. A standard is set for performance on each item using a modification of the criterion-referenced method originally described by Nedelsky (Fullerton, Greener, & Gross, 1989; Gross, 1985) that results in a minimum pass index (MPI) for each item. A criterion-referenced methodology means that item and exam results are evaluated against a pre-established criterion rather than against the cohort of individuals who took the exam. A new item is pretested and psychometrically evaluated before it is included in the pool of items scored on the examination. Pass rates for first-time takers of the NCE typically range around 85%. This rate is comparable to that of other reputable certification organizations in health care fields.

Certification Maintenance Program in Nurse–Midwifery/Midwifery

All CNMs/CMs certified by ACC/AMCB since 1996 must participate in the CMP to maintain their certification. Philosophically, the CMP is designed to assure the public that certificants maintain safe, minimal competencies as described by the ACNM Core Competencies for Basic Midwifery Practice (American College of Nurse-Midwives [ACNM], 2003). Further, AMCB believes that every CNM/CM is responsible for maintaining competency as specified in the ACNM Standards for the Practice of Nurse–Midwifery (ACNM, 2002). The objectives of the CMP are to keep CNMs/CMs' certifications valid and current, foster critical review of recent advances in midwifery practice, and provide documentation of CNMs/CMs' certification status as required to credentialing/licensing authorities.

Certificates can be maintained through the CMP by one of two methods. The first is the Certificate Maintenance Module Method. This method requires that the CNM/CM successfully completes 3 certificate maintenance modules and 20 contact hours (2.0 CEUs) of ACNM or ACCME Category 1–approved continuing education units during the 8-year certification cycle. One CMP module must be completed in each of the three practice areas of antepartum, intrapartum/newborn, and postpartum/gynecology/primary care. Each CMP module includes objectives for the topics of the module, a reference list related to the objectives, the option to purchase an article reprint package of the reference list, and an open-book multiple-choice exam with answer sheet. When completed, the answer sheet is returned to AMCB for scoring, with successful module completion requiring a score of 75% or higher.

The second method of certificate maintenance is the Reexamination Method, which requires the CNM/CM to take the current NCE no sooner than the seventh year of the 3-year cycle and to complete 20 hours of continuing education as previously described. Regardless of which method of certificate maintenance is chosen, the CNM/CM must submit an annual report of her certificate maintenance activities.

Licensure in Nurse–Midwifery and Midwifery*

Unlike most countries, licensure to practice in the health professions in the United States is a responsibility delegated to the individual states, as previously presented in Figure 5–1. Licensure does not occur at the federal level, and thus state licensing boards, their standards, scopes of practice, and requirements vary. This is a difficult concept for foreign educated health professionals, and also for many students, to accept. It is a confusion that the process of certification attempts to make easier, although with limited success. Although the National Council of State Boards of Nursing (NCSBN) has attempted to rectify this problem by developing the APRN Uniform Licensure/Authority to Practice Requirements (National Council of State Boards of Nursing [NCSBN], 2004), these uniform standards have not yet been adopted by most state legislatures; hence, licensure requirements continue to vary from state to state. In addition, these uniform requirements specify the master's degree as preparation for advanced practice nursing, a standard that nurse–midwifery/ midwifery has not adopted.

Licensure in midwifery is even more varied than in most professions for a variety of reasons. Foremost among those reasons is the fact that the profession of midwifery exists both with and without a nursing requirement—nurse–midwifery and direct-entry midwifery, respectively. Further, within direct-entry midwifery there are those who are educated in programs accredited by the AMCB DOA and certified by the AMCB, those who are educated

---

*Nurse–midwives practice in all 50 states as well as U.S. territories and the District of Columbia. For purposes of the chapter, the word "state" encompasses all of these jurisdictions, and numbers may therefore not add up to 50.

through routes approved by the Midwives Alliance of North America (MANA) and certified by the North American Registry of Midwives (NARM), and those who have no formal education and no certification. Recognition of those various pathways is widely divergent at the state level.

Professional certification is often required for licensure, but as noted earlier, it is a very different form of professional regulation. Professional organizations and certifying bodies assist licensing boards to understand the educational and certification standards of the specific profession, as well as its scope of practice. However, the requirements of the state are governed by the legislative body that enacts the statutory authorization and by the boards themselves that develop specific rules to implement the law. The state is not obligated to accept the profession's approved educational routes, its certification process, or its defined scope of practice.

Licensing Agencies

Nurse–midwifery is recognized in every state as well as the U.S. territories and the District of Columbia. In 42 states, nurse–midwifery licensure is in the purview of the state board of nursing. However, other licensing bodies for nurse–midwifery include the medical licensing board (2 states), the board of health (4 states), a board of advanced practice nursing (1 state), and a board of certified nurse–midwifery (1 state). In 5 states, CNMs are regulated jointly by the boards of nursing and medicine. In only 1 state (New York) are nurse–midwifery and direct-entry midwifery combined into one licensing board for professional midwifery (ACNM, 2001). New York regulations were developed based upon the standards promulgated by the ACNM.

In many states, the CNM is viewed as a category of nurse practitioner (NP) or advanced practice nurse (APN). In 18 states, the CNM is recognized as a distinct specialty separate from NPs or APNs (Reed & Roberts, 2000).

The ability of direct-entry midwives to be licensed ranges from full recognition to explicit denial of the right to practice in the state. In 9 states, the practice of direct-entry midwifery is legally prohibited. In 7 states, although not illegal by statute, regulations effectively prohibit the practice of direct-entry midwives. In 16 states, direct-entry midwifery is both recognized and regulated. The requirements for direct-entry licensure vary; some states require MANA certification as a Certified Professional Midwife (CPM) and others have less or more stringent requirements. In 13 states, direct-entry midwifery is legal, but not regulated; that is, the state does not recognize direct-entry midwifery, but does not consider its practice an infringement upon medical or nurse–midwifery licensure. Only in New York are CNMs and CMs licensed by the same board, with the same scope of practice and standards of care. The CM is not formally recognized elsewhere at this time. For purposes of the remaining discussion, therefore, nurse–midwifery will be the focus.

The licensing board that is ultimately responsible for oversight of midwifery practice is determined by statute. The fact that state legislators are responsible for the decision underscores the political nature of the choice. As noted, in most states midwifery licensure rests within nursing. Only two states have a separate midwifery or nurse–midwifery board. As the practice of nurse practitioners (NPs) has advanced, it has often been beneficial to align with the larger group in order to exert more political power for greater independence in practice, prescriptive privileges, third-party reimbursement, and the like. The disadvantage has been that CNMs in those states are often subject to requirements that have not been endorsed by the ACNM, particularly degree requirements. In addition, in states in which midwifery is licensed under nursing (or medicine), midwives are rarely represented on the board itself. A final consideration in the placement of regulatory authority is the fact that in most states, licensing boards are required to be self-supporting through licensing fees. Some states with several dozen or even a few hundred CNMs, as compared to thousands of nurses, could find the costs of licensure prohibitive by a midwifery board under those circumstances.

Requirements for Licensure

Requirements for licensure in health professions typically involve documentation of an approved educational pathway, successful completion of a licensing or certification examination, and if not a new graduate, demonstration of currency in practice through continuing education or recent practice experience. In some cases, mandatory degree requirements exist. Those who have practiced elsewhere prior to application for licensure can expect to be questioned regarding any history of negative actions upon a previous license, felony convictions, or health deterrents to safe practice. It is likely that the licensing board will query the National Practitioner Data Bank (NPDB). Established by the Health Quality Improvement Act of 1986, the NPDB serves as a national reservoir of information regarding physicians, nurse practitioners, midwives, nurses, and other health professionals. Information reportable to the NPDB includes negative actions on licenses or certifications (e.g., suspensions or revocations), loss or curtailment of institutional practice privileges, and judgments in malpractice suits.

In some states the CNM must have a master's degree, and several of those states require the master's degree be in nursing. Some states continue to recognize graduates of certificate programs in nurse–midwifery, but increasingly, especially in states in which licensure is under boards of nursing, the requirement is for a graduate degree. In 2004, when 24 states required master's degree preparation, the American Association of Colleges of Nursing (AACN) called for the requirement of a Doctorate of Nursing Practice (DNP) for all advanced practice nurses, including nurse practitioners, clinical nurse specialists, and nurse–midwives by 2015. Whether state boards of nursing will ultimately adopt this requirement is not yet clear.

National certification is a typical, but not universal, requirement for licensure. Nine states have no requirement at all for national certification of nurse–midwives. Some continue to review educational programs rather than recognize national certification, citing concerns regarding the quality of the certification process in some nurse practitioner specialties. Twenty-four states require ACC/AMCB certification. Nine states require certification and mention ACC/AMCB specifically, but not exclusively. Seven states require certification but stipulate no particular organization, while nine require certification but do not mention any organization explicitly. New graduates may practice temporarily in 40 states while awaiting the results of their certification examination. However, even when licensed by the state, practice of new graduates is frequently limited by the inability to obtain hospital privileges and to be credentialed by health plans without certification results.

Scope of Practice

In addition to establishing requirements for minimum competency, licensure boards also typically establish the scope of practice for the health professional *in that state.* Scopes of practice may be more or less restrictive than those established by the profession itself. In fact, one of the primary mechanisms by which scopes of practice evolve is effort by practitioners at the state level to broaden the scope of practice in their practice act. When a critical number of states adopt a new aspect of scope of practice, educational programs are forced to incorporate new content and skills to keep pace with state law. A prime example of this process is the incorporation of prescriptive privileges. In 1976, Oregon became the first state to allow independent prescriptive privilege, requiring 30 hours of pharmacology, including pharmacokinetics and instruction on how to write a prescription. More states followed suit with variations on the amount of content required and midwifery educational programs were required to incorporate more formal pharmacological content so that their graduates could meet state requirements for prescriptive privileges. In 2001, 48 states, the District of Columbia, Guam, and American Samoa allowed CNMs prescribing authority, although in some jurisdictions limitations continue to exist. These limitations may restrict the prescription of controlled substances or require supervision/delegation from the physician.

In addition to prescriptive authority, the most common aspect of scope of practice that is addressed is the level of independence with which midwives can function. Although 11 states have no specific requirements for physician/CNM relationships, 28 states require some level of specified physician collaboration, consultation, and referral. Twelve states require physician supervision or direction. Four states stipulate the number of CNMs that a physician can supervise. The number ranges from 3 in Alabama, Nevada, and South Carolina to 4 in South Dakota. Five states limit the number of CNMs *with prescriptive authority* that a physician can supervise. Louisiana requires a 2:1 ratio; Ohio requires 3:1; California, Oklahoma, and Virginia specify 4:1; Colorado stipulates 5:1. No state requires the physician's presence at the time of delivery.

Although all states recognize the general nurse–midwifery scope of practice (antepartum, intrapartum, postpartum, newborn, and well-woman care), specific restrictions may be placed on various aspects of care. For example, California regulations (State of California, 2001) stipulate "all birthing complications shall be referred to the physician immediately." They further state "the practice of nurse–midwifery does not include the assisting of childbirth by any artificial, forcible or mechanical means, nor the performance of any version." CNMs in California may perform and repair episiotomies and suture lacerations (first and second degree only) in hospitals or birthing centers in which the supervising physician has privileges. New York (State of New York, 2004) requires a written agreement for physician consultation and referral that must "provide guidelines for the identification of pregnancies not considered normal and address the procedures to be followed." New York rules further stipulate that if there is a dispute with regard to the judgment of normal pregnancy, "the physician shall prevail." In contrast, the scope of practice in Oregon rules is adopted directly from the American College of Nurse–Midwives: "The independent management of women's health care, focusing particularly on pregnancy, childbirth, the postpartum period, care of the newborn, and the family planning and gynecological needs of women" (Oregon State Board of Nursing, 2005).

Data presented here regarding licensure were obtained through the ACNM legislative resource documents and are current to 2001 (ACNM, 2001). State regulation, however, is an ever-changing landscape, and all midwives have a professional responsibility to know and practice within the requirements of the jurisdiction in which they work. They have a further responsibility to work actively within their jurisdiction to develop statutes and rules that allow midwives to practice to the fullest extent of their education and professional scope.

Chapter Exercises

1. Visit the AMCB Web site to review current requirements for the NCE and CMP.
2. Obtain the relevant practice act for midwifery in the state or other jurisdiction in which you intend to practice or in which your midwifery program exists.
3. List five key messages about your professional responsibilities regarding certification and licensure.

References

American College of Nurse–Midwives. (2001). *Nurse–midwifery today: A handbook of state laws and regulations.* Washington, DC: Author.

American College of Nurse–Midwives. (2002). *Core competencies for basic midwifery practice.* Retrieved January 24, 2005, from http://www.midwife.org/prof/display.cfm?id=137

American College of Nurse–Midwives. (2003). *Standards for the practice of midwifery.* Retrieved January 24, 2005, from http://www.midwife.org/prof/display.cfm?id=138

American Midwifery Certification Board. (2005). *Home page.* Retrieved June 22, 2006, from http://www.amcbmidwife.org.

Foster, J. C. (1986). Ensuring competence of nurse–midwives at entrance into the profession: The national certification examination. In J. Rook & J. E. Haas (Eds.), *Nurse–midwifery in America* (pp. 14–16). Washington, DC: American College of Nurse–Midwives.

Fullerton, J. T., Greener, D. L., & Gross, L. J. (1989). Criterion-referenced competency assessment and the national certification examination in nurse–midwifery. *Journal of Nurse–Midwifery, 34,* 71–74.

Fullerton, J. T., Parker, K. W., & Severino, R. (1997). Development and outcomes of the multiple-choice format national certification examination in nurse–midwifery and midwifery. *Journal of Nurse–Midwifery, 42,* 349–354.

Gross, L. J. (1985). Setting certification cutoff scores on credentialing examinations: A refinement in the Nedelsky procedure. *Evaluation and the Health Professions, 8,* 469–493.

Henderson, J. P. (1996). Job analysis. In A. H. Browning, A. C. Bugbee, & M. A. Mullins (Eds.), *Certification: A NOCA handbook* (pp. 41–66). Washington, DC: National Organization for Competency Assurance.

National Commission for Certifying Agencies. (2004). *Standards for the accreditation of certifying agencies.* Retrieved March 17, 2005, from http://www.noca.org/ncca/docs/STANDARDS904.pdf

National Council of State Boards of Nursing. (2002). *Advanced practice registered nurse compact.* Retrieved January 26, 2005, from http://www.ncsbn.org/nlc/aprncompact.asp

National Council of State Boards of Nursing. (2004). *APRN uniform licensure/authority to practice requirements.* Chicago: Author.

Oregon State Board of Nursing. (2005). *Nurse Practice Act. Division 50. Nurse practitioners.* Retrieved March 17, 2005, from http://egov.oregon.gov/OSBN/pdfs/npa/Div50.pdf

Oshio, S., Johnson, P., & Fullerton, J. T. (2000). *Task analysis of American nurse–midwifery and midwifery practice: A project report and survey analysis of the practice of nurse–midwifery and midwifery within the United States. 1999–2000.* Landover, MD: ACNM Certification Council.

Reed, A., & Roberts, J. E. (2000). State regulation of midwives: Issues and options. *Journal of Midwifery and Women's Health, 45,* 130–149.

Schoon, G. G., & Smith, I. L. (2000). *The licensure and certification mission.* New York: Professional Examination Service.

State of California. (2001). *The certified nurse–midwife.* Retrieved March 17, 2005, from http://www.rn.ca.gov/practice/pdf/npr-b-31.pdf

State of New York. (2004). *Midwifery.* Retrieved January 15, 2005, from http://www.op.nysed.gov/midwif.htm

Table 5–1 AMCB Test Content Outline for the National Certification Examination in Nurse–Midwifery and Midwifery

I. Primary Care (WH)
   A. Physiology/pathophysiology
   B. Pharmacology (includes alternative/complementary therapies)
   C. Assessment of the well woman
      1. History
      2. Physical examination
         a. HEENT
         b. Heart and lungs
         c. Breast
         d. Abdomen/CVAT
         e. Pelvic exam (bimanual/speculum)
         f. Skin/extremities
         g. Neurologic
         h. Vital signs
      3. Cultural factors
   D. Health promotion and assessment
      1. SID counseling
      2. Breast self-exam
      3. Immunizations
      4. Substance abuse (smoking, ETOH, street drugs)
      5. Domestic violence
   E. Laboratory tests and procedures (order/obtain/interpret)
      1. Routine assessments
      2. Those indicated by status of woman
      3. Diagnostic/screening tests for the older woman (e.g., mammography, bone density studies, hormonal, lipid and cholesterol levels)
   F. Assessment and management of deviations from normal
      1. Identification of deviations
         a. Cardiovascular/anemia
         b. Dermatologic
         c. Endocrine (obesity, thyroid)
         d. Eye, ear, nose, and throat
         e. Gastrointestinal
         f. Musculoskeletal
         g. Neurologic
         h. Respiratory
         i. Urinary
      2. Development of a management plan
      3. Consultation, co-management or referral, as indicated

II. Antepartum Care (AP)
   A. Physiology/pathophysiology
      1. Pregnancy
      2. Genetic, embryology, fetal development

continues

Table 5–1 AMCB Test Content Outline for the National Certification Examination in Nurse–Midwifery and Midwifery *continued*

  B. Diagnosis of pregnancy
   1. Presumptive, probable, and positive indicators of pregnancy
   2. Laboratory tests
   3. Ultrasound
   4. Counseling regarding pregnancy options
  C. Collection of data base for pregnancy
   1. Historical data (family, personal, medical-surgical, obstetrical, gynecological, sexual, social, present pregnancy)
   2. Exposures and habits (medications, drugs, smoking, alcohol, caffeine, toxins, work hazard)
   3. Genetic risks, counseling and/or referral
   4. Physical examination
    a. Vital signs
    b. Pelvic examination
    c. Clinical pelvimetry
  D. Calculation of current gestational age and estimated date of birth
  E. Baseline laboratory tests (order/obtain/interpret)
   1. Serum tests
   2. Pap smear and cultures
  F. Management of pregnancy
   1. Internal assessments to evaluate status of pregnancy
    a. Vital signs/urine
    b. Weight gain patterns
    c. Leopold's maneuvers
    d. Auscultation of the fetal heart (fetoscope or Doppler)
    e. Assessment of fetal movement (includes fetal movement counts)
    f. Assessment of fundal height
   2. Laboratory tests (order/obtain/interpret)
   3. Diagnostic tests and procedures
    a. Nonstress testing
    b. Contraction stress testing (includes nipple stimulation)
    c. Ultrasound
    d. Amniotic fluid index/biophysical profile
   4. Counseling regarding normal pregnancy
    a. Common discomforts, including use of alternative and complementary therapies
    b. Health promotion and disease prevention (includes exercise, hygiene, prenatal Rh immune globulin)
    c. Nutritional assessment and counseling
    d. Psychologic/emotional response to pregnancy (includes family relationships)
    e. Referral to community resources (WIC, nutrition and social services, domestic violence and substance abuse counselors)
  G. Patient and family education to prepare for childbirth and parenthood
   1. Informed childbirth methods/pain management options/birth plan/assisted delivery techniques
   2. Counseling/preparation of woman for external breech version

3. Counseling regarding vaginal birth after cesarean
4. Infant nutrition (includes breast- and bottle-feeding)/parenting skills
H. Assessment and management of deviations from normal pregnancy
   1. Identification of deviations
   2. Development of a management plan
   3. Consultation, co-management, or referral, as indicated

III. Intrapartum Care (IP)

A. Physiology/pathophysiology of labor
B. Assessment for admission to labor
   1. Update personal history and health status
   2. Vital signs
   3. Physical examination to determine labor status (contraction pattern, cervical exam)
   4. Fetal status
      a. Auscultation/initial monitoring of fetal heart rate
      b. Presentation
      c. Position
   5. Diagnosis of rupture of membranes
C. Fetal monitoring
   1. Manual
      a. Palpation
      b. Auscultation
   2. Electronic
      a. Uterine activity
      b. Fetal heart rate
      c. Indications/techniques for internal monitoring
D. Labor support
   1. Nonpharmacologic support techniques and measures
   2. Analgesia
   3. Anesthetic techniques
      a. Epidural (co-management)
      b. Paracervical
E. Labor management
   1. Assessment and management of progress in labor—first stage
   2. Assessment of woman's physical response to labor (e.g., I & O, vital signs, laboratory tests)
   3. Assessment of fetal status following AROM
   4. Assessment and management of second stage labor
F. Monitoring/co-management of woman receiving pharmacologic therapy during labor
   1. Cervical ripening/induction agents
   2. Group B streptococcus prophylaxis
   3. Tocolytics
   4. Magnesium sulfate
G. Management of the perineum
   1. Perineal preparation and support
   2. Local anesthetic techniques (including pudendal)
   3. Episiotomy
H. Conduct of delivery
   1. Hand maneuvers/mechanisms of labor

continues

Table 5–1 AMCB Test Content Outline for the National Certification Examination in Nurse–Midwifery and Midwifery *continued*

      a. Occiput anterior

      b. Occiput posterior

      c. Nonvertex presentations

    2. Maternal position at delivery

    3. Management of the umbilical cord (including nuchal cord)

    4. Shoulder dystocia

  I. Third stage labor

    1. Determination of placental separation

    2. Delivery of the placenta

    3. Inspection of the placenta (includes cord vessels)

  J. Fourth stage labor/immediate postpartum period

    1. Examination of cervix, vagina, and perineum

    2. Repair of episiotomy or laceration

    3. Diagnosis of hemorrhage/estimated blood loss

    4. Control of hemorrhage

      a. Fundal massage/initiation of breastfeeding/laceration repair

      b. Pharmacologic management (oxytocics)

      c. Bimanual compression

      d. Manual exploration of uterus/manual removal of the placenta

  K. Assessment and management of deviations from normal labor and delivery

    1. Identification of deviations

    2. Development of the management plan

    3. Consultation, co-management, referral, or transport, as indicated

IV. Postpartum (PP)

  A. Physiolgy/pathophysiology

    1. Postpartum

    2. Lactation

  B. Postpartum physical assessment

    1. Uterine involution

    2. Perineum

    3. Lochia

    4. Urinary bladder

    5. Extremities

    6. Vital signs

  C. Management of the normal postpartum period

    1. Breast care (management and prevention of engorgement, sore nipples)

    2. Physical adaptation/recovery (includes diastasis recti, uterine involution, exercise, nutrition)

    3. Family planning/resumption of sexuality

    4. Psychosocial adaptation/parental–infant relationship

    5. Postpartum Rh immune globulin/immunizations

  D. Six-week postpartum examination

  E. Laboratory tests (order/obtain/interpret)

  F. Assessment and management of deviations from normal in the postpartum period

    1. Identification of deviations

     2. Development of a management plan

     3. Consultation, co-management, or referral, as indicated

V. Neonatal Care (NB)

  A. Physiology/pathophysiology of the newborn

  B. Assessment and management of transition to extrauterine life

     1. Assignment of the Apgar score

     2. Support of normal transition

       a. Suction

       b. Stimulation

       c. Temperature maintenance

     3. Intervention

       a. CPR of the newborn

       b. Medications used in resuscitation

       c. Transfer/transport

  C. Newborn assessment

     1. Physical examination

     2. Newborn reflexes

     3. Gestational age assessment

  D. Infant nutrition

     1. Support and instruction for breastfeeding

     2. Support and instruction for bottle-feeding

  E. Newborn care and interventions

     1. Eye prophylaxis

     2. Administration of medications (e.g., vitamin K, immunizations)

     3. Circumcision counseling

     4. Education of family for infant care

  F. Laboratory tests (order/obtain/interpret)

     1. Routine assessments and interventions (e.g., PKU)

     2. Those indicated by status of newborn (e.g., bilirubin)

  G. Assessment and management of deviations from normal in the newborn period

     1. Identification of deviations

     2. Development of a management plan

     3. Consultation, co-management, or referral, as indicated

VI. Family Planning/Gynecology (GYN)

  A Physiology/pathophysiology

     1. Menstruation, interconceptional period

     2. Peri- and postmenopausal period

  B. Family planning

     1. Collection of a data base for the provision of contraceptive options

       a. Screening for contraindications

       b. Teaching and counseling concerning available methods

     2. Provision of contraceptive methods and devices

       a. Natural family planning

       b. Barrier methods (e.g., condoms, diaphragm, cervical cap)

       c. Oral contraceptives

       d. Injectable contraceptives

continues

Table 5–1 AMCB Test Content Outline for the National Certification Examination in Nurse–Midwifery and Midwifery *continued*

        e. Intrauterine devices

        f. Subdermal implants

        g. Sterilization counseling

        h. Emergency contraception

     3. Management of contraceptive method problems and complications

     4. Fertility promotion

        a. Preconceptional counseling

        b. Initial assessment and diagnostic procedures/referral for infertility

  C. Well-womanl/perimenopausal care

     1. Laboratory tests and procedures (order/obtain/interpret)

        a. Screening (e.g., Pap smear)

        b. Diagnostic (e.g., wet mount, colposcopy)

        c. Ultrasound

     2. Assessment and management of specific concerns

        a. Vaginitis

        b. Signs/symptoms of menopause

        c. Hormone replacement therapy (includes alternative therapies)

        d. Sexuality

        e. Sexual abuse/sexual assault

  D. Assessment and management of deviations from normal

     1. Identification of deviations

     2. Development of a management plan

     3. Consultation, co-management, or referral, as indicated

VII. Professional Issues (MI)

  A. Midwifery practice

     1. Scope of practice

     2. Development of clinical practice guidelines

     3. Development of patient education materials

     4. Patient records/charting

     5. Interdisciplinary relationships

     6. Ethics

  B. Health care system and its relationship to midwifery practice

     1. Equal access to health care/cultural sensitivity

     2. Administrative structure of agencies (hospitals, birth centers, HMOs)

     3. National health care policy (e.g., WHO Baby Friendly Hospital Initiative)

     4. Barriers to midwifery practice (restraint of trade, limited access, reimbursement issues)

  C. Legal issues

     1. Statutes/regulations that affect midwifery practice

     2. Medical malpractice/legal liability issues

     3. Birth registration

  D. Maintaining standards of care

     1. Evidence-based practice/review of practice-related literature

     2. Peer review/quality improvement

     3. Continued competency activities

Approved by the CNM Certification Council Board of Directors, November 17, 2000

CHAPTER 6

Legal Bases for Midwifery Practice, Negligent Practice, and Liability Reduction

Cecilia Jevitt, CNM, PhD

Learning Objectives

1. Describe various levels of standards and regulation in midwifery practice.
2. List the elements required for negligent practice.
3. Describe the tort claim process following an accusation of malpractice.
4. List methods for reducing liability risk.
5. List types of liability insurance or special protection plans available to midwives.

Legal Basis for Midwifery Practice

Health care professions are the most regulated occupations in the United States. Multiple layers of regulation are meant to protect the public from careless practitioners. Midwives must follow standards and regulations that range from the national level to the individual area of practice, such as a hospital labor and delivery unit.

National Standard of Practice

Midwifery practice is defined by various levels of legal regulations and standards. At the macro level, national standards provide an expectation of care delivery. The increasing mobility of health care providers and their multi-state practices have led to the increasing importance of national standards (Furrow, Greaney, Johnson, Jost, & Schwartz, 2001). The American College of Nurse–Midwives publishes the *Core Competencies for Basic Midwifery Practice*, which outlines entry-level knowledge and skills that all midwives should possess (American College of Nurse–Midwives [ACNM], 2002a). The Core Competencies are used by midwifery educational programs to assure that all new nurse–midwives can safely deliver care within the scope of usual midwifery practice. The

ACNM Standards for the Practice of Midwifery (ACNM, 2003a) is another example of national, professional standards which define midwifery practice. The ACNM also issues clinical bulletins, such as "Limited Obstetrical Ultrasound in the Third Trimester" (ACNM, 1996), that provide practice standards. Because midwives work interdependently with other health care professionals, particularly physicians, other standards of care may apply. For example, the American College of Obstetricians and Gynecologists (ACOG) issues regular practice bulletins, committee opinions, and educational bulletins that become standard of practice for American obstetrical and gynecological care. Bulletins on induction of labor, shoulder dystocia, and gestational diabetes are examples of ACOG guidelines that apply to midwifery practice. Utilizing guidelines such as ACNM and ACOG statements can unify practice within a group and assure evidence-based practice.

State Licensure

At the next level, midwifery practice is regulated in the state of practice through licensure to practice. If a midwife practices in two states, she must be licensed by both states. Standard I of the ACNM Standards for the Practice of Midwifery requires that the midwife "is in compliance with the legal requirements of the jurisdiction where the midwifery practice occurs" (ACNM, 2003a). State licensure is meant to protect the consumer by ensuring that the clinician has appropriate education for the profession and has a history of providing safe care. States have different methods for licensing midwifery practice. In some states, nurse–midwives are licensed as advanced practice nurses (or advanced registered nurse practitioners). Other states, such as New York, have boards of midwifery that supervise midwifery practice separate from nursing. Some states regulate nurse–midwives under boards of nursing through the nurse practice act while having separate midwifery statutes that regulate midwives who are not nurses. Whatever the state mechanism for licensure, the midwife must be licensed to practice within the state where she provides care and she must adhere to any limitations set by state law. A state may, for example, require that a midwife file a written protocol signed by the consulting physicians each year and have malpractice liability insurance. A midwife not filing protocols or not having current malpractice insurance would be practicing illegally in that state.

Community Standards

Community standards once formed the base of reasonable practice. Customary practice and available resources still vary from one midwifery community to another. Community standards dictate that a midwife's duty must be objectively evaluated according to the availability of medical and practical knowledge that would be used in the treatment of like or similar patients under like or similar circumstances by minimally competent midwives, given the facilities, resources, and options available (Furrow et al., 2001). As an example of community standards changing midwifery duty, consider the midwife working in a level-one hospital where cord blood gas analysis is not available compared to a midwife working in a level-three hospital where cord blood gas analysis is available 24 hours a day.

The midwife working in the level-one hospital has no duty to document cord blood gases when the technology is not available.

Employment Agreements/Contracts

Related to the standard of care and scope of practice is the issue of responsibility for care in midwifery practice. Employment agreements or contracts help to define individual midwifery practice. The midwife has a responsibility to provide standard of care within her scope of practice. Clients' needs often exceed the scope of practice for independent midwifery. The midwife must then document how she provided ongoing care for her client through consultation, collaboration, or referral. Documentation of interdependent care is essential for smooth communication between providers and defense of practice if it is legally challenged. This documentation is found in written practices guidelines (ACNM, 2003a) and the written medical record.

Responsibility for care may also be defined by the employment status of the midwife. A midwife who is self-employed and refers all high risk clients to a consulting obstetrician may be less responsible for a bad outcome than a midwife who is employed by the obstetrician and continues to participate in the care of the high risk client. Midwives and physicians who are separately employed by a hospital corporation have a different legal relationship than midwives who are employed by a physician-owned practice corporation (Rubsamen, 1999).

Practice Guidelines or Protocols

Standard V of the ACNM Standards for the Practice of Midwifery (ACNM, 2003a) requires that, "Midwifery care is based upon knowledge, skills, and judgments which are reflected in written practice guidelines." The practice guidelines describe the parameters of independent and collaborative midwifery practice and when transfer of care will be needed. Ideally, practice guidelines address each specialty area within midwifery, such as the primary care of healthy women and newborn care. The practice guideline for each section should include:

- Client selection criteria
- Parameters and methods for assessing health status
- Parameters for risk assessment
- Parameters for consultation, collaboration, and referral
- Appropriate interventions including treatment, medication, and devices

Practice guidelines should be written broadly so that they cover a range of treatments and practices. They demonstrate a responsible mechanism for providing care when a woman's needs exceed the scope of midwifery practice.

Practice guidelines were traditionally called protocols. A protocol is a code of conduct or correct procedure. A protocol is more rigid than a guideline. Some state practice acts use the word *protocol* instead of *practice guideline*.

Practice guidelines or protocols define practice at the individual practice level. Ideal practice guidelines are evidence-based. Guidelines based on national standards or a body of research demonstrate that the midwife practices within the standard of care. It is critical that midwifery practice follow the written practice protocols. A midwife who initiates and manages tocolytics to stop a preterm labor when this is not permitted by the group practice guidelines has worked outside the scope of practice defined by her practice guidelines. If, however, her practice guidelines permit physician consultation and collaboration for preterm labor, and the midwife documents consultation or collaborative management of the preterm labor, she has practiced within the scope of practice guidelines. Practice guidelines can support midwifery practice in malpractice claims or can be used by the plaintiff to support negligence if the midwife hasn't followed the practice guidelines (Furrow et al., 2001).

Institutional Policies

Institutional-level policies may also define the scope of midwifery practice. Midwives working in hospitals are governed by hospital staff bylaws. Standard IV of the ACNM Standards for the Practice of Midwifery requires that the midwife practice "in accord with service/practice guidelines that meet the requirements of the particular institution or practice setting" (ACNM, 2003a). When applying for hospital practice privileges, midwives will have to provide evidence of education and experience. Like state licensure, this level of review is meant to assure that quality clinicians are available to clients; assuring quality clinicians also limits the liability of the hospital regarding malpractice by incompetent staff. Hospital medical staff applications provide skill lists for each type of clinician that broadly define practice. Midwives, for example, can expect to have approval to manage uncomplicated labor and vaginal birth and provide immediate newborn care. With appropriately documented education and supervision, a midwife might have use of a vacuum extractor or repair of a fourth-degree laceration added as hospital-approved skills. Performance of cesarean sections would be limited to the obstetricians' skills list.

The midwife working within a hospital should also review the policies of the units on which midwifery care is provided. A labor and delivery unit might have policies that limit midwifery practice. A hospital policy might state that the order to initiate oxytocin must be made by a physician. If the midwife writes an order to start oxytocin under her own name, she is technically practicing outside of hospital policy. Hospital policies are easier to change than professional standards or state practice acts. A midwife who finds that a hospital policy unreasonably constrains her practice should work with the unit management and medical staff to revise the policy.

Liability Insurance Policy Restrictions

Medical liability insurance policies may also limit midwifery practice. The midwife must know what practice the policy covers. A policy purchased through an employing corporation most likely will not cover hours worked with another practice. Some policies have clauses to limit the insurer's liability, such as clauses preventing the midwife from using vacuum extractors or attending home births. A liability policy might also prohibit use of recording devices such as video cameras in the birth suite.

Figure 6–1 summarizes the legal bases for midwifery practice. If a midwife works outside of the legal bases for practice and has a poor care outcome, she may be placing herself in a position of being accused of professional negligence.

Medical Malpractice in Midwifery

Professional Negligence

Medical malpractice is a legal error committed by medical personnel (Furrow et al., 2001). In legal terms, this error is a tort—a civil wrong that injures a person. The law allows an injured person to seek damages from the wrongdoer to remedy the tort. If a tort is intentional, it becomes the crime of assault or battery. Negligence, a form of malpractice, is an unintentional tort. Professional negligence is conduct that falls below a professional standard of care. The law expects that all professionals have a defined standard of minimum knowledge and ability. For midwifery, these standards are codified in midwifery core curricula, state licensure statutes, and standards from professional organizations. (Refer to the section "Legal Basis for Midwifery Practice".)

Figure 6–1 The Legal Bases of Midwifery Practice

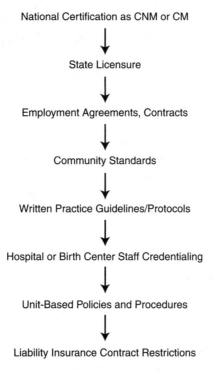

National Certification as CNM or CM

↓

State Licensure

↓

Employment Agreements, Contracts

↓

Community Standards

↓

Written Practice Guidelines/Protocols

↓

Hospital or Birth Center Staff Credentialing

↓

Unit-Based Policies and Procedures

↓

Liability Insurance Contract Restrictions

To prove a negligent tort occurred, four elements must be identified:

1. *A duty must exist between the injured party and the professional accused of wrongdoing.* In midwifery, this duty begins by the client initiating care. Duty demands that the midwife provide standard of care screening and treatment for the client.

2. *A breach of duty must have occurred.* The midwife must have practiced outside the standard of care for a breach to occur. Although breach of contract involves a duty, it is regulated separately within contract laws.

3. *The breach of duty must be the proximate cause of the claimed injury.* A claimant cannot charge that the midwife failing to do an episiotomy caused a rectovaginal fistula; however, a woman might claim that the midwife's improper repair of a fourth-degree perineal laceration caused a rectovaginal fistula.

4. *There must be damages or injuries to the claimant that are recognized by the law and compensable.* A claimant could sue for the additional costs to repair a rectovaginal fistula and wages lost during the repair and recovery, but could not sue for pain and suffering due to a prolonged birth that was managed within the standard of care, even though the labor experience did not meet the expectations of the patient.

Negligent actions include errors of commission or omission. In errors of commission, the defendant does something that another ordinary, reasonable, and prudent person of the same profession would not do. A midwife who ruptures membranes to stimulate labor while the presenting part is out of the maternal pelvis has committed an error of commission. When this amniotomy is followed by a prolapsed umbilical cord, the amniotomy is the proximal cause of the resulting injuries, which include fetal hypoxia, emergency cesarean delivery, and a prolonged stay in the neonatal intensive care unit for the newborn.

A midwife who forgets to do third trimester screening for diabetes during a pregnancy has committed an error of omission. An ordinary, reasonable, and prudent midwife would follow national standards and recommend that the client have a 1-hour diabetic screening during the early third trimester. Errors of omission are common in busy, large organizations. Systems developed to protect patient safety often have a focus of reducing errors of omission.

If the defendant's actions were seen as malicious or intentionally harmful, the claimant can seek punitive damages in addition to other awards. Punitive fines are meant to be strong deterrents to unprofessional behavior.

What constitutes the professional standard of care for midwifery is defined by many institutions. Taken together, these standards form the concept of what a reasonable and prudent midwife would do.

The Liability Claim Process

Disputed Outcome

When a client perceives that she has been injured, she may consider suing the midwife for malpractice. Americans who carry individual health insurance that has co-pays and deductibles have an incentive to sue to recover the costs of their health care. Clients may also sue for lost wages when unable to work or for emotional damages. A client must demonstrate damages to initiate a claim. A client initiating a malpractice claim is called a plaintiff.

Not all perceived damage is disputable. For example a woman contacted an attorney claiming a midwife had incorrectly prescribed Monistat Cream for a case of vaginitis. The vaginitis did not resolve and the client went to another provider who diagnosed bacterial vaginosis and prescribed metronidazole. The metronidazole treatment resolved the symptoms. The client claimed that the midwife's initial treatment caused her unnecessary pain and suffering and that she lost a half day of work in seeking the second opinion. Although the client may have had prolonged symptoms and lost wages, there was no way to prove that the midwife misdiagnosed the vaginitis. There was no permanent injury and the attorney declined the case.

The Complaint

When a client has a permanent injury caused by the midwife, the plaintiff's attorney writes and files a complaint, also known as a declaration, at the local court. The complaint includes allegations, the legal basis for the claim, and a request for damages.

Table 6–1 contains some allegations common to midwifery malpractice claims. Once the complaint is filed, the court issues a summons to the defendant or defendants. The midwife may be named as the sole defendant. Because of the interdependent nature of midwifery practice, most midwives are not sole defendants, but are one of several parties named in the claim. Other practice members, consulting physicians, and any hospital staff involved in the disputed care may be summoned as co-defendants. A hospital, professional corporation, or birth center employing the nurse–midwife or serving as a site of practice may also be sued for damages in a claim. A summons may be delivered to the midwife by a local deputy or a process server, or may be mailed depending on the jurisdiction.

Once a summons has been received, the midwife must notify her liability insurance carrier. The carrier will begin investigation of the claim and assign a defense attorney. Generally, the midwife does not have a choice of an attorney. The insurer hires attorneys who are experienced and are most able to defend their insured, thereby preserving corporate funds. Communications between the midwife and the defense attorney are privileged, that is, they cannot be admitted as evidence in a trial. Communications between the midwife and the insurer are not privileged. The midwife should limit information given to the insurer.

Many midwives are distraught when confronted with a malpractice claim. One of the prides of midwifery is the relationship with the client. This relationship seems violated when a client files a liability claim. The midwife must remember that the claim is more concerned with the client's financial needs than the care rendered or the relationship formed during the care. Faced with accusations of malpractice, midwives instinctively turn to other midwives for support. The midwife must refrain from discussing the case with professional colleagues. This is not privileged information. Colleagues with knowledge of a case could be subpoenaed into court to give testimony about the midwife's statements.

Midwives must refrain from changing or adding to a record when a summons is received. Forensic techniques easily detect altered records. Altered records make a case

Table 6–1 Common Malpractice Allegations in Midwifery

Allegations	Risk Reduction Measures
Failure to recognize risk factors for shoulder dystocia and prevent the dystocia by arranging for a cesarean birth	• Document excessive prenatal weight gain and nutritional advice given • Document estimated fetal weight • Document consult with physician if macrosomia is suspected • Assess progress of labor; consult for any deviations; document consultation
Failure to correctly perform the maneuvers to disimpact a shoulder dystocia and extract the fetus in a timely manner	• Review maneuvers with labor nurse before birth • Document maneuvers used and time elapsed
Management involvement beyond midwifery scope of practice, including involvement in pre-eclampsia, pregnancy-induced hypertension, premature birth, birth of a multiple gestation, or insulin-dependent diabetes	• Delineate scope of practice in protocols • Follow protocols • Consult as needed and document consultations • Have referral mechanism in place if skill needed exceeds ability or availability of obstetrician (e.g., mothers with cardiac disease)
Practice outside of limits set by practice protocols, hospital protocols, or hospital policy	• Know legal base of practice • If protocols and policies don't reflect regular practice, correct them • Have consistent wording in protocols and policies
Failure to arrange for cesarean birth earlier in labor process including labors complicated by fetal distress, cephalo-pelvic disproportion, shoulder dystocia, and hemorrhage	• Assess and document progress of labor • Consult for lack of labor progress; document consultation and management plan
Failure to correctly manage and contain postpartum hemorrhage	• Recognize risk factors; be prepared • Know standard of care treatments • Document management completely
Failure to correctly manage birth complicated by amniotic fluid containing meconium	• Document resuscitation measures • Document ancillary help summoned for resuscitation (i.e., nursery staff)
Misinterpretation of fetal heart rate tracing	• Attend and document regular fetal monitoring updates • Consult obstetrician and document plan • Document assessment, treatment, and plan for fetal heart rate abnormalities
Failure to diagnose cancer	• Know and perform cancer screening components of a complete physical exam, such as a breast exam • Know and use cancer screening guidelines from national organizations • Provide follow-up for testing or consultations ordered; document attempts to reach noncompliant patients

Allegations	*Risk Reduction Methods*
Failure to call obstetrician for assistance in a timely manner	• Assure that protocols define when a physician should be notified • Document all consultations • Provide a mechanism to obtain consultation or surgery when primary physician is unavailable
Excessive and/or prolonged pitocin stimulation of labor leading to fetal compromise	• Assess progress of labor • Consult obstetrician for lack of labor progress; document consultation • Follow hospital policy for pitocin use • Maintain neonatal resuscitation certification

indefensible. Lost or irretrievable records also made defense difficult. A midwife has a responsibility to assure that her sites of practice, including office, clinic, birth center, and hospital, follow state laws for the preservation of medical records and can do accurate record retrieval. Original records always remain at the practice site or hospital. Copies are sent to the attorneys after appropriate consent is obtained from the client.

The court allows the defense attorney 30 days to respond to the summons. If the midwife, through her insurer and defense attorney, fails to respond within the 30 days, a default occurs. A default is considered an admission of guilt.

The Discovery Period

When the defense attorney responds to the summons, a time called the discovery period is initiated. During the discovery period, attorneys send questions to each other regarding the case and their clients. These lists of questions are called interrogatories. Interrogatories must be answered and are done under oath. Requests are made for an admission of facts, a series of factual statements concerning the incident and the practitioner(s) involved. Documents, such as medical records, are identified as genuine through the request for genuineness of documents during the discovery period. Documents related to the case from prior or subsequent treatment, such as treatment for breast cancer, are also certified as genuine. The certification of documents speeds their admission as evidence during a trial. The discovery period is limited, generally up to 90 days. The discovery period is also the time when expert witnesses are arranged for the plaintiff and the defense. The discovery period is meant to be a period of fair fact-finding for both sides of a case, preventing concealment of facts important to the proceedings.

Once the discovery period ends, a case may be settled by the insurer. A case may be settled when a mistake by the midwife is evident. Sometimes, a midwife is named in a suit as a member of her group practice. If she were uninvolved in the client's care, she may be dropped from the case after the discovery period. In some cases, the insurer may decide to settle a claim when the midwife did no incorrect action. In such a case, the defense attorney and insurance administrators may decide that in the long run, the settlement would cost less than a trial. The midwife may have little say in a settlement even if she wants to prove her innocence and good practice in court. It is the responsibility of the insurer to preserve funding that might be needed to defend other insured practitioners.

If the insurer, the defense attorney, and expert witnesses think the claim is defendable and that the defense is financially reasonable, they will request a trial following the discovery period. During preparation for trial, depositions are taken to discover undocumented facts about the case and its outcome. Depositions are question and answer periods taken under sworn oath. The defense and plaintiffs' attorneys attend depositions along with the person being deposed. Attorneys may cross-examine each other's witnesses during a deposition. The deposition is recorded by a court recorder who produces a written transcript of the proceeding. Depositions:

- Obtain statements by opposing parties to the claim
- Lock in testimony by witnesses
- Identify other potential witnesses
- Identify facts and conflicts within the claim

Following the collection of depositions from all involved parties and expert witnesses, the defense or plaintiff's attorney has another opportunity to make a settlement with release of further claim. The plaintiff's attorney may move for settlement if it is doubtful that the case would be supported in court. If the dollar amount of the settlement sought by the plaintiff will be lower than trial costs, the defense might agree to a settlement at this point. Any financial settlement paid on behalf of an individual following a malpractice claim must be reported to the National Practitioner Data Bank by the insurer, regardless of the guilt or innocence of the midwife. (See the section on the National Practitioner Data Bank.) **Table 6–2** outlines reasons the plaintiff, the defendant, or the insurance company might favor a settlement over trial.

Some states have developed methods of alternative dispute resolution, including arbitration and mediation, to settle claims before initiating the trial process. In arbitration, an arbitration board may have a single judge instead of a jury. Some boards additionally have five to six members who serve in place of a jury. The attorneys present evidence to the arbitration board and the board makes settlement recommendations. Mediation is a process in which a trained mediator works with the plaintiffs and defendants to seek dispute reso-

Table 6–2 Reasons Favoring Claim Settlement

Insurance Company/Defendant	*Plaintiff*
• A favorable jury verdict is doubtful.	• A favorable jury verdict is doubtful.
• Avoids a verdict that might exceed the limits of the liability insurance.	• Compensation to the client is assured. The delay in compensation is limited, that is, the client has funds when they are most needed for treatment and rehabilitation.
• Limits the loss of time and resources during trial preparation and the trial.	• Limits the loss of time and resources during trial preparation and the trial.
• Expert witness case review does not support the midwife's practice.	• Expert witness case review does not support the plaintiff's claim.
	• Attorney's fees are assured.
	(Attorney's fees come from the damages award.)

lution. If a settlement is reached through arbitration or mediation, the cost of trial is avoided. The settlement fee is reported to the National Practitioner Data Bank. If the arbitration board finds in favor of the defendant, no damages are awarded and no report is made to the National Practitioner Data Bank.

Nationally, approximately 95% of liability claims are settled before trial (U.S. General Accounting Office [GAO], 2003). The Government Accounting Office estimated in 2003 that 70–86% of claims going to trial were settled in favor of the defendant. A claim might be settled the evening before the trial opens. If, however, the defense attorney thinks the midwife would prevail in court and the cost of trial is bearable, the defense attorney will insist on a trial. The time from summons to trial varies state to state, but often takes as long as 5–10 years (GAO, 2003).

Trial

A trial is assigned a judge and a date in the court docket. A jury is selected through review of potential jurors by the defense and plaintiff's attorneys. The trial begins with opening statements by both the plaintiff's attorney and the defense attorney, which is followed by presentation of evidence by both sides. Parties to the claim, the plaintiff, and any care providers named are interviewed as witnesses. Both the plaintiff and the defense will interview expert witnesses including midwives, physicians, and nurses to support their claims. Expert witnesses for the defense and the plaintiff will give evidence regarding standards of practice and community standards of care. The judge or jury makes a decision based on the evidence presented, whether or not the midwife's actions met the standard of care.

Following the testimonies, both the plaintiff's attorney and the defense attorney give closing arguments. The judge then gives instructions to the jury about their options for a verdict. The jury meets, makes a decision for either the plaintiff or the defendant, and gives the judge the verdict. The jury can recommend a claim amount, but the judge makes the final decision on the claim amount. If the plaintiff prevails, known as a plaintiff's verdict, the midwife's insurer must pay the claim. This verdict and payment must be reported to the National Practitioner Data Bank. If the defendant prevails and there is a defense verdict, no report is made to the National Practitioner Data Bank. In some states, if there a defense verdict, the plaintiff must pay the attorney's fees and court costs for the defendant. This serves as a disincentive for spurious claims.

Following a plaintiff's verdict, the defense attorney has the right to ask the trial court to set aside the verdict and grant a new trial. The defense attorney can also request that the trial court change the verdict and enter a judgment in the defendant's favor. The defense also has the right to request a reduction in the amount of the damage award. An attorney might choose this option if prevailing in an appeal seems unlikely but the current damages awarded are excessive. The defense may request that the plaintiff's attorney reopen settlement negotiations. This might occur if the defense thought it would prevail in trial, lost, and the midwife has insufficient insurance and assets to pay the damages awarded by trial. The defense attorney may also file an appeal.

Following a defendant's verdict, the plaintiff's attorney has similar rights. The plaintiff's attorney may ask the trial court to set aside the verdict and grant a new trial or ask the trial court to change the verdict and enter a judgment in the plaintiff's favor. The plaintiff's attorney may request that the amount of damages awarded be increased and may also request that the defense reopen negotiations to provide a settlement. The plaintiff's attorney also may file an appeal with the court. Few malpractice cases move to appeal either by the plaintiff or the defense. **Figure 6–2** summarizes the liability claim process.

Aggressive Incident Management

Immediate attempts to settle a potential claim are called aggressive incident management. Following a fetal death during labor, for example, where it appears that the midwife and nursing staff failed to recognize recurrent late decelerations, the hospital's insurer and the liability insurance carrier for the midwife may offer the parents a monetary settlement that precludes further legal action.

The movement for aggressive incident management was popularized during 2004, but has its roots in the voluntary arbitration laws passed by some states in the 1970s (GAO, 1992). Aggressive incident management saves time for all involved parties, saves trial costs, and avoids excessively high jury awards.

The Department of Health and Human Services (HHS) initiated an early resolution program in 2004 to speed the resolution of claims and decrease the cost of litigation (U.S. Department of Health and Human Services [HHS], 2004). The Early Offers Program is available to clients who are treated by practitioners employed by federal community health centers and the Indian Health Service. Participation by the injured client is voluntary. A plaintiff who has filed a claim against HHS receives a letter from them with information about the Early Offers Program and an offer to negotiate a settlement for a specified dollar amount. The injured client has 90 days to accept the negotiation offer. HHS may make a settlement offer stating the dollar amount of the compensation it is willing to provide. The plaintiff and HHS make their offers confidentially through an independent third party who compares the offers and determines if a settlement has been achieved.

Experience with aggressive incident management demonstrated that most clients want more than monetary remuneration; they want an apology and want to know that measures have been taken to prevent similar incidents from occurring in the future (Liebman & Hyman, 2004). New research and writing about early incident resolution focuses on honest communication with clients, admission of error, apology, and incident investigation that is problem-solving rather than blame-seeking (Vincent, 2003).

Woods and Rozovsky (2003) give examples of open communication with patients following an unanticipated obstetrical outcome. Some of the steps they advocate include:

1. Communicate with the client and family members immediately and frequently after an unanticipated outcome. Too often, practitioners are shocked and hurt and fear that the patient may express anger, so they avoid patient contact. They worry about making the situation worse. The client, not seeing the practitioner, thinks the worse and assigns blame where none is due. Communication is a learned skill. Active listening is an essential component of open communication. Communication

Figure 6–2 The Liability Claim Process

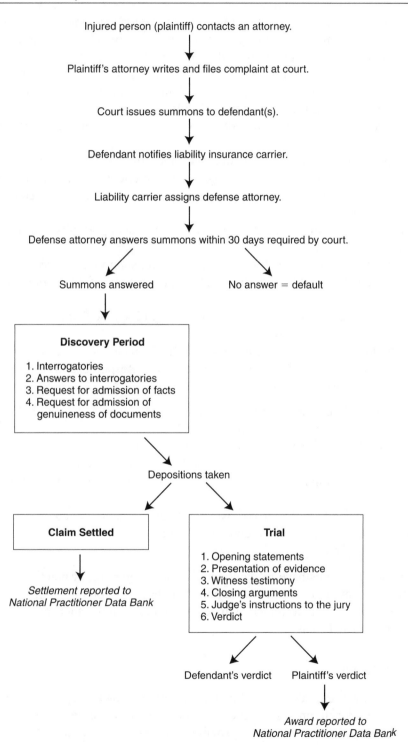

Injured person (plaintiff) contacts an attorney.

Plaintiff's attorney writes and files complaint at court.

Court issues summons to defendant(s).

Defendant notifies liability insurance carrier.

Liability carrier assigns defense attorney.

Defense attorney answers summons within 30 days required by court.

Summons answered   No answer = default

Discovery Period

1. Interrogatories
2. Answers to interrogatories
3. Request for admission of facts
4. Request for admission of genuineness of documents

Depositions taken

Claim Settled

Settlement reported to National Practitioner Data Bank

Trial

1. Opening statements
2. Presentation of evidence
3. Witness testimony
4. Closing arguments
5. Judge's instructions to the jury
6. Verdict

Defendant's verdict   Plaintiff's verdict

Award reported to National Practitioner Data Bank

should take place in an environment where all parties are physically comfortable and there will be no interruptions.

2. New practitioners may want to bring a more experienced practitioner with them as they learn to talk about unexpected outcomes. Experienced practitioners should offer to help a newer practitioner through initial client contact.

3. The practitioner should review the facts of the case and the outcomes with the patient and any family members the patient wants included in the discussion. Offering the facts and admitting errors may clarify the situation for the client and reduce client anger that results from confusion about the incident or unanticipated outcome.

4. The practitioner should say, "I am sorry," and offer condolences if necessary.

5. The practitioner should look for anger from the client and validate the anger. The practitioner might say, for example, "A problem like this can make feelings intense. I understand your anger."

6. The client and family should be given an additional opportunity to state their questions and feelings.

7. The practitioner arranges for follow-up care and support as needed.

8. The practitioner needs to do thorough documentation of interactions with clients and families.

Readers are encouraged to study Woods and Rozovsky (2003) so that they are prepared for the eventual unanticipated outcome.

The Colorado liability insurance company, COPIC, instituted an early resolution program in 2002 called the 3Rs Program: Recognize, Respond, and Resolve (COPIC Companies, 2002). The 3Rs Program uses these steps:

- Recognize the injury or complication and respond immediately (within 72 hours).
- Contact COPIC Risk Management.
- Communicate with the patient in an empathetic manner.
- Ensure that the patient receives prompt evaluation and consultation.
- Arrange for additional care or services the patient might need as a result of the injury or complications.
- Resolve the episode in the most satisfactory manner, including compensating the patient for lost work days and unreimbursed medical expenses. (COPIC has some limits on reimbursement.)

Early resolution programs have recognition of error, assumption of practitioner responsibility, honest apology, and prompt attention to client needs in common. Further experience with aggressive incident management will be needed to reveal whether early resolution decreases tort claims and trials.

The Expert Witness

The expert witness is a practitioner who uses education, knowledge, skill, and experience to assist the case triers to understand the facts and issues of the case (Furrow et al., 2001). Both the defense and plaintiff's attorneys will hire expert witnesses to support their cases.

The ideal expert witness is experienced, is in active practice, and can testify about the education of midwives and standards of practice.

Expert witnesses are identified during the discovery period. The expert witness reviews background documents for the case and makes a statement regarding the case called an affidavit. The affidavit from an expert witness defending a midwife might say, for example, that the defendant appropriately followed national standards of care and provided the same care that any reasonable and prudent midwife would. The expert witness must provide documentation to support any claims.

Expert witnesses will read records from the case and depositions from other parties involved in the case, and will be deposed under oath. If the case goes to trial, the expert witness may give testimony in court. Expert witness fees are paid by the liability insurance carrier.

The National Practitioner Data Bank

The National Practitioner Data Bank (NPDB) was proposed as a federal solution to the problem of incompetent practitioners avoiding licensure suspension by moving from state to state. Mandated by the Health Care Quality Improvement Act of 1986 (Title IV, PL 99-660), the NPDB became operational in September 1990 (HHS, National Practitioner Data Bank Guidebook). The NPDB collects information on nurse–midwives and non-nurse midwives. All financial payments made in the name of a midwife by an insurer must be reported to the NPDB whether a settlement is made outside of the court system or the case has a plaintiff's verdict with damages awarded. Additionally, any practitioner who is excluded from Medicaid or Medicare reimbursement is reported to the NPDB by the Centers for Medicare and Medicaid. The Drug Enforcement Agency must report any practitioner whose registration is revoked to the NPDB. The Department of Defense, the Veterans Administration, the Department of Justice Bureau of Prisons, the Public Health Service, and the Department of Health and Human Services are all required to report adverse actions to the NPDB.

Detailed information about the operations of the NPDB and its data can be found at http://www.npdb-hipdb.com.

Although state boards are not required to report actions against midwifery licenses to the NPDB, they may do so. Hospitals, health maintenance organizations, and other organizations must report actions taken against physicians that adversely affect their practice for more than 30 days. These organizations may, but are not required to, report actions against midwives. **Table 6–3** lists examples of actions reported to the NPDB. Reports to the NPDB from one malpractice claim may affect a practice through its midwives and physicians (HHS, National Practitioner Data Bank Guidebook). No midwife should be surprised by information contained in the NPDB. The NPDB is required to notify a midwife any time a report is made in her name. There is an appeals process if the midwife thinks the report is erroneous.

The NPDB contains public access files that list the types of malpractice occurrences and the number of these occurrences each year. The files of individual practitioners are not open to the general public. A state board might, for examples, use NPDB files to research the types of obstetrical malpractice occurring within the state and the range of damages

---

Table 6–3 Actions Reportable to the National Practitioner Data Bank

- Practice beyond the scope of practice
- Incompetence, negligence, malpractice
- Settlements/damages paid on behalf of a practitioner
- Fraud (e.g., fraudulent billing)
- Unsafe practice related to substance use
- Violation of drug statutes

---

awarded. The NPDB does original research from its files and publishes data about medical malpractice and disciplinary action.

State boards check the NPDB files of individual midwives when processing licensure applications. Hospitals and insurers can also access the files of a midwife during the credentialing process. The NPDB prevents midwives from concealing past malpractice or actions against their licensure and credentialing. NPDB data are confidential. Fraudulent use of NPDB data and confidentiality breaches are subject to criminal prosecution, fines, and imprisonment.

Liability Insurance

Insurance is purchased protection against unforeseen events. Home insurance, for example, protects against occurrences that do not happen regularly such as fire, theft, and hurricanes. When purchasing insurance, the insured is one of many who pay premiums into a pool. Insurance premiums are set by actuaries, who calculate, based on history, how often maloccurrences will require coverage. Not all individuals within the pool will have a maloccurrence generating a claim each year. The accumulated funds ensure coverage for the few individual who will use the insurance each year. The insurance company uses the fund dollars to earn money. Funds are conservatively invested in bonds and the stock market. State insurance departments regulate the investments of insurers and the surpluses they are mandated to keep on hand for claims payment. Required surpluses generally equal one year of premium collections (GAO, 2003).

Premiums colleted and return on investments (investment income) form the earnings of the insurance company. With investment income, insurers can pay out more in claims than they collect in premiums. Earnings are also paid to shareholders as dividends. Insurance companies are corporations whose duty is to earn a profit for the shareholders, while providing insurance for policy holders. Due to the long lag between incidents and verdicts, insurance companies must hold huge payment reserves.

As professionals, midwives can be held personally liable for breaches of duty. Midwives can purchase liability protection insurance. This is often called medical malpractice insurance. A midwife may obtain liability coverage by:

- Purchasing her own policy
- Being covered as a member of a corporation or group practice
- Being part of a self-insured organization such as a hospital or a university
- Being covered by state sovereign immunity or the Federal Tort Claims Act

Insurance premiums must be available and affordable. Insurers can offer discounts to the insured or add surcharges to the policy (GAO, 2003). Midwives attending vaginal births after cesarean sections, for example, might be charged an additional premium if the insurer has evidence that this will increase its financial liability. Physicians have had surcharges added to their insurance policies if they supervise midwives (ACNM, 1994b). State insurance departments regulate insurance premiums. The number of insurers offering liability coverage to midwives has decreased in the last two decades as the number of claims against midwives rose and the amount of awards made by juries increased, making liability insurance a less profitable business. Data on midwifery claims and judgments have not been gathered; however, the malpractice experiences of midwives mirrored those of obstetricians, and these phenomena are documented for obstetricians (GAO, 2003).

Liability insurance has limits both on individual claims and the amount that will be paid out in a single year. These are known as policy limits. A policy may cover an individual claim at $250,000 and no more than $750,000 worth of claims in a single year. This is often abbreviated as $250,000/$750,000 coverage. If a midwife has a verdict that awards more than $250,000 in one case, she is personally liable to pay the damages above $250,000. Another common level of coverage is $1 million/$3 million. The higher the coverage, the higher the premium paid. When claims are paid by the insurance company on behalf of the midwife, the cost of liability insurance to that individual midwife increases. Because an insured is part of a protection pool, the cost of pay-outs will also be spread around the pool in the form of increased premiums.

The larger the number of insured a liability corporation has, the greater the collection of premiums and the greater the payment reserves. In eras when investment income is high, companies may be able to pay damages out of income. Companies then may lower premiums below the cost of claim payouts to attract more policy purchasers and form larger pools. This occurred in the 1990s. Stock earnings fell precipitously in 2000 and 2001, just as more claims were filed than ever before and the dollar amount of jury awards reached record highs (GAO, 2003). Insurers were caught without sufficient damage payment reserves. This drove many liability insurers out of business. Those remaining made steep increases in premiums, sometimes tripling the cost of premiums in a single year. Although average liability premium costs for midwives have not been researched, the Government Accounting Office reported in 2003 that annual liability premiums for obstetricians ranged from $36,000 in Northern California to $201,000 in Miami, Florida. Although the exact dollar amounts are not available, midwifery liability premiums vary similarly between states with tort reform laws (California) and areas of high litigation and settlement costs (Miami). Changes in the insurance market since 1990 made liability insurance less available to midwives and less affordable. For most midwives, liability insurance is an unavoidable part of the cost of doing business.

Some states require that a midwife provide evidence of liability insurance before licensure. This is meant to assure that the consumer has a means of obtaining damages for proven malpractice. Some hospitals have bylaws that stipulate a level of coverage. A medical staff might rule, for example, that any provider practicing within the hospital carry at least $1 million/$3 million coverage. Setting a minimum level of coverage prevents some providers from having more insurance than others, thereby becoming targets for malpractice claims ("deep pockets").

When the market for liability insurance has availability and affordability problems, some organizations and states change rules to allow providers to practice "bare," that is, without liability insurance. Without liability insurance, a midwife would be personally responsible for any court-awarded damages against her. Being bare may make a provider less attractive to sue because the damages a single provider could pay out are limited. Before going without coverage, a midwife must decide what she would lose if a claim was settled against her, such as savings, house, car, vacation home, and retirement funds. Some states have laws that limit what a professional can lose when damages are awarded. In Florida, for example, a midwife might use all her personal savings and assets to pay awarded damage payments; however, by law, she cannot lose her primary residence or vehicle. Practicing without coverage raises the ethical issue of a midwife being responsible for her professional practice and the protection of her clients.

The Insurance Contract

An insurance policy is a contract regulated by the insurance laws of individual states. The individual protected by the policy, the insured, purchases coverage from an insurance company, the insurer. Policies are purchased through agents. Through the insurance contract, the insurer assumes a defined amount of risk (liability) on behalf of the insured. With liability insurance, the insurer makes payments for the insured for damages awarded for negligence whether or not, in fact, the insured was negligent. That is, payments are made based on jury awards and not actual practitioner guilt or innocence.

Policy premiums vary with the individual midwife applicant. Those new to practice who have no prior claims may expect lower premiums than experienced midwives who have been involved in suits. Many factors are involved in the calculation of an insurance premium (**Table 6–4**). A midwife's premiums with one insurer generally do not decrease over time, even if the midwife has no claims made against the policy. However, the midwife might shop for a less expensive policy. The midwife must compare policies carefully to determine that less expensive policies provide the coverage needed.

A liability policy may pay other costs related to liability claims, including investigation costs, attorney's fees, and expert witness fees. The midwife needs to know what the contract covers and what is not covered. For example, a policy might cover a negligence claim through trial and settlement; however, it might not cover a report of negligent practice to a state board. The report to the state board will require investigation and defense by an attorney on behalf of the midwife. If not covered in the liability policy, the midwife may pay thousands of dollars in attorney's fees to defend her license to the state, and in addition, may pay thousands of dollars in fines to the state board. Examples of areas that some liability policies do not cover include:

- Work done at a second employer (moonlighting)
- Births where recording equipment is used (Weiss, Miranda, & Hess, 2004)
- Home births

Table 6–4 Factors Included in Premium Rate Calculations

- Size of the corporate premium pool
- Number of insured/policy contracts
- Corporate profits from premiums collected
- Investment income profits
- Underwriting costs, marketing costs, administrative costs
- Corporate taxes
- Corporate losses (i.e., claims payouts)
- State insurance regulations
- Competition in the insurance market
- The claim history of the individual applicant
- The practice of the individual applicant (midwives providing only well-woman gynecology may have lower premiums than those attending births)
- The regional claims history (claims are more frequent and damages awarded are higher in some regions than others)

- Use of vacuum extractors by midwives
- Work time and wages lost during a malpractice trial

In addition, some insurers, finding that medical errors increase as the number of births attended by one practitioner each year increases, have capped the number of births the policy will cover each year. In 2004, some insurers capped covered births per provider at 125 per year.

The insurance contract covers a limited time period, which is generally a year. This is the policy period or time in force. Incidents occurring before or after the contract period are not covered. There are two types of liability contracts: occurrence and claims made.

Occurrence Policies

Occurrence policies are rarely available to midwives now; however, they provide the best long-term practice coverage. Occurrence policies cover any incident that happens during the policy period. Events are covered regardless of when the damages are discovered, when the claim is filed, or whether the policy contract is still in force.

As an example, a midwife had an occurrence liability policy that was in force from 1/1/00 through 12/31/02. In May 2001, the midwife repaired a fourth-degree perineal laceration following a birth. The midwife took a new job in October 2002 with a state health department and became covered by state sovereign immunity. No longer needing the occurrence liability policy, she stopped payments and let that contract lapse. In July 2003, the midwife was served notice of a claim against her by the client who sustained the fourth-degree laceration. The woman claimed that the midwife had negligently delivered a macrosomic infant instead of arranging for a cesarean section, and improperly repaired the fourth-degree laceration. She further claimed that the midwife's negligence was the proximal cause of her anal sphincter damage and subsequent incontinence. Unknown to the midwife, the woman had had two failed sphincter repairs since the birth. The midwife's former client was suing for the costs of attempted repairs, lost wages, and emotional damages. Even though the midwife was no longer paying on the occurrence liability contract, the incident happened during the policy period. The policy covered the cost of investigation, trial, and settlement. This case demonstrates how the lag time in claim filing and the unpredictability of claims makes the administration of occurrence policies impractical and prohibitively expensive.

Claims Made Policies

A claims made policy covers only incidents that occur while the policy is in force and the claim must be initiated while the policy is in force. Claims made policies are inexpensive in the first years of practice, and therefore are attractive to the midwife new to practice. Premiums increase annually as the midwife accumulates practice liability. As premiums increase, the policy matures and, in time, reaches a stable "mature" premium. Claims made policies may take 5 to 10 years to mature. Midwives purchasing new claims made policies need to know the average time for a policy to mature and how much premiums are expected to increase each year. This increase must be budgeted into the cost of practice. Insurers changed from selling occurrence policies to claims made policies in the 1970s and 1980s in order to be better able to predict claims expenses (GAO, 2003). Claims made policies are the only policy types currently available to midwives. They are less expensive than occurrence policies, but pose distinct disadvantages for midwives.

Midwives, particularly those early in their practice careers, may change employment every several years. Switching employment often means changing liability coverage for a midwife. If the midwife is covered with a claims made policy through an employer, the new employer is not likely to continue the same liability policy. Once the midwife stops payment on the claims made policy, all responsibility from the insurer to the midwife ends. Frequent causes of midwifery liability claims, such as a child who fails to meet developmental milestones after a difficult birth or unrecognized cancers, may take years to become evident. While these cases develop, the midwife may change insurers and lose her coverage for the claims made policy period.

To provide coverage past the policy period, insurers offer extended reporting periods (ERP). These endorsements to the original contract are commonly called "tail" coverage. Extended reporting periods generally must be chosen within 30 days of canceling the liability contract. Some insurers limit extended reporting periods to 5 years. If a state allows up to 18 years for a claim involving a birth injury to be made, the midwife could be faced with 13 years of uncovered liability. This is one of the reasons many states have limited the periods for filing birth-associated claims. Some states require that birth-related suits be initiated within 3 years of the birth.

Extended reporting periods are costly. The ERP premium might equal 3 years of the mature premium or up to 200% of the mature annual premium. The midwife who pays $18,000 per year in liability premiums might have an ERP payment of $54,000. Generally, this must be paid in one lump sum at the end of the policy period.

To maximize the coverage of a claims made policy, the midwife should request that the availability of an ERP be written into the original policy contract. The way the future ERP premium will be calculated should also, ideally, be agreed upon in the original contract. A midwife newly employed by a practice that provides liability coverage through a claims made policy might also negotiate in her employment contract that the practice pay the cost of an ERP should the midwife be laid-off or the practice chooses another insurer. A midwife losing employment with claims made liability insurance who doesn't have contractual protection might negotiate with a new employer for the new employer to pay the cost of the ERP premium. The midwife might receive the ERP payment as a sign-on bonus, gradually repay the cost of the ERP premium to the practice, or have its repayment waived in lieu of performance bonuses over several years. **Example 6–1** illustrates how midwives can be affected by mismanaging liability insurance.

Example 6–1: The Limitations of Claims Made Liability Insurance

Two midwives were employed in a group practice. Half of their practice revenue came from well woman gynecology. After 10 years of practice, one gynecologist retired and the group split. The two midwives were faced with extended reporting period payments of $36,000 on a liability policy that provided $1 million/$3 million coverage. Neither midwife had ever been named in a malpractice claim.

One midwife took a second mortgage on the equity in her home to make the ERP payment that would provide her with another 5 years of coverage. She planned to pay the second mortgage from a sign-on bonus that would be paid to her at the end of her first year with the new group and from savings. The second midwife, knowing of no maloccurrences during her practice years, decided not to purchase extended reporting coverage.

Two years after the group split, both midwives received summons from a claim that alleged they missed a breast cancer growing during provision of prenatal and postpartum 3 years prior. The case went to trial and the jury awarded damages in the amount of $1 million against each midwife. The midwife who paid for the ERP had her attorney's fees, court costs, and awarded damages paid by the insurer. The second midwife faced these expenses alone.

Other Forms of Liability Protection

Self-Insurance

Individuals and organizations can accumulate reserves to pay their own costs of litigation and damage settlements. This is referred to as being self-insured. In 2003, approximately 40% of hospital members of the American Hospital Association were self-insured (GAO, 2003). Midwives directly employed by a self-insured hospital might be covered by the hospital's self-insurance plan.

Some states allow physicians and midwives to post bonds to assure damage payments to injured clients. Personal property, such as a home, secures the bond. This method is less expensive than liability insurance policies, but places the individual practitioner at high risk for losing personal property through malpractice damage awards.

Mutual, Nonprofit Insurances

Following the liability crises of the 1970s, many physicians joined together and formed their own nonprofit insurance companies. Since 1992, physician owned and operated corporations cover 60% of the liability insurance market (GAO, 2003). Nonprofit insurance corporations decrease administrative costs and avoid the profits that for-profit insurers must pay to shareholders.

Joint Underwriting Authorities

To assure availability, many states have chartered joint underwriting authorities. The joint underwriting authorities are sometimes called markets of last resort (GAO, 2003). Joint underwriting authorities are collectives of commercial insurers compelled by the state to offer insurance when it is available from other sources. One company administers the joint underwriters' plan. Midwives will be able to purchase liability insurance through the joint underwriting mechanism; however, the premiums may be high. Joint underwriting authorities may offer other types of insurance, such as catastrophic homeowner's insurance, in addition to liability insurance. The Florida Joint Underwriting Authority offers homeowner's protection as well as liability insurance. When Florida sustains high losses from hurricane activities, midwifery liability premiums through the Joint Underwriting Authority rise.

Arbitration

The Government Accounting Office described 15 states in 1992 that had approved voluntary arbitration as a means of settling medical malpractice claims during or after the malpractice crisis of the 1970s (GAO, 1992). These states included California, New York, Florida, Illinois, and, Virginia. Arbitration reduces claim costs by speeding up the process and avoiding trial. The GAO (1992) found that arbitration settled claims in 19 months on average compared to 33 months for trial. Arbitration allows the plaintiffs earlier access to damages, permitting them to pay bills instead of accumulating debt. The arbitration process typically lasts 2 to 4 days compared to several weeks in trial.

Sovereign Immunity

The concept of sovereign immunity comes from English Common Law and is rooted in the ancient concept of a divine king who can do no wrong. Following the Revolutionary War, American leaders rejected the concept of divine rule and had to create a concept to limit governmental liability ('Lectric Law Library, n.d.). Under federal law the "sovereign is exempt from suit [on the] practical ground that there can be no legal right against the authority that makes the law on which the right depends" (205 U.S. 349, 353). At the federal level, sovereign immunity serves to channel claims speedily to the appropriate venue more than prevent claims. Claims settled against the federal government are paid out of Congressional appropriations. Malpractice claims involving military midwives fall under sovereign immunity and use the federal court system.

States have their own sovereign immunity through the Eleventh Amendment to the Constitution ('Lectric Law Library, n.d.). Sovereign immunity is a defense to liability claims, not a right to be free of tort proceedings, regardless of the quality of practice. Diverse state government employees including the National Guard, volunteer firefighters, and state department of health employees may be covered by sovereign immunity (Sovereign Immunity, 2005).

Federal Tort Claims Act

The Federally Supported Health Centers Assistance Act (FSHCAA) of 1992 and its 1995 reauthorization created a medical malpractice insurance program for federally qualified community health centers that is commonly known as the Federal Tort Claims Act (FTCA). The FTCA provides no cost liability protection to centers that participate (Bureau of Primary Health Care, 2005). In order to participate, a center has to be "deemed" a federal employee for the purposes of medical malpractice. The deeming process includes credentialing of practitioners and querying their files through the National Practitioner Data Bank. Participating centers must use clinical protocols, tracking systems, and medical record review, and have active quality assurance programs. Once deemed, the center becomes immune from prosecution.

Seventy-five percent of community health centers participate in the FTCA program, thereby saving thousands of dollars on medical liability insurance premiums and making that funding directly available for health care (Bureau of Primary Health Care, 2005). Some settlements are made through FTCA. Funds for these are not appropriated through Congress but are made from funds set aside from federal appropriations for health centers.

Special State Funds

Some states have special programs to cover high risk areas of practice. Florida, for example, established the Neurological Impairment Compensation Association (NICA) in 1987 (Florida Statutes 766.301–766.316). NICA is a special insurance pool that covers the health care costs of term infants weighing more than 2500 grams who suffer neurological damage during labor or birth. NICA removes tort claims that satisfy these criteria from the Florida court system. NICA claims are heard and settled by an administrative judge. NICA is financed by collecting $250 from each physician's license renewal. Additionally, each participating physician pays $5,000 a year into the pool. Any physician involved in the birth process may participate in the NICA plan: obstetricians, emergency room physicians, anesthesiologists, and emergency room physicians. Participating nurse–midwives pay annual premiums of $2,500. Hospitals may also pay into the NICA pool for coverage. The pool covers only practitioners and hospitals that pay to participate. Patients must be given written notice that their providers and hospitals are NICA participants. NICA has survived constitutional challenge and almost two decades of claims.

Chapter Exercises

1. **Applying ACNM Risk Reduction Statements to Practice**

   The Professional Liability Section of the ACNM has developed statements to assist the midwife in reducing practice liability. These can be obtained online at www.acnm.org under Strategies for Liability Risk Reduction. The current topics include:

   • Strategies for Liability Risk Reduction
   • Strategies for Liability Risk Reduction in Informed Consent
   • Postdates Risk Reduction
   • Shoulder Dystocia Risk Reduction
   • Preterm Birth Risk Reduction

   Select one of these topics and print out the statement from the ACNM. Compare your usual practice routines to these guidelines. Does your practice follow all the strategies recommended? For example, under shoulder dystocia, routine screening for diabetes is recommended during pregnancy. Is your practice consistently performing and documenting diabetic screening? If not, you have identified an area of risk that your practice can improve.

   Students should work with their clinical site to examine practice routines using a risk reduction statement.

2. **The Annual Liability Policy Check-Up**

   Midwives in practice should know the provisions of their liability coverage as well as they know the provisions of their health or homeowners insurance. Midwifery students should see if their midwifery preceptors will work through this exercise with them using the preceptor's liability insurance coverage.

   Most questions about liability coverage can be answered by reading the face sheet and the liability policy. Although tedious reading, critical facts about coverage are contained in the policy. An employer should be willing to share a copy of the policy with any covered insured. Failure to produce a policy contract is worrisome and cannot be ignored.

   Each year, a midwife should review her liability protection, asking herself the following questions:

   • Is the coverage in the name of the individual midwife?
   • Is the coverage provided under the name of the consulting physician or the practice corporation?
   • Is the coverage provided by a self-insured entity such as a hospital or university on behalf of the individual? Does the self-insured organization have sufficient capital to pay out claims?
   • Is the coverage purchased from an insurance corporation? How long has this insurer been in business?

- When is the policy in force? What are the dates of the contract? (If the contract dates have passed, make sure that the premium has been renewed for the current period.)
- Who is responsible for timely premium payment: the midwife, the employer, the office manager, or the organization's finance office?
- Are premiums current?
- What are the limits of liability for the contract?
- Does the midwife have individual limits of liability, or are limits shared with other practice members?
- Does the liability policy cover attorney's fees, court costs, and the costs to defend and settle any actions by the state board?
- Does the policy cover all midwifery work done during the contract period, or does the contract cover only work done with a specific employer?
- Does the policy contain special exclusions to coverage (for example, use of vacuum extractors by midwives)?
- Does the policy provide for payment of an extended reporting period (ERP) if the midwife changes employment? How will this ERP be financed?

3. **What liability protection can be obtained in your state of practice?**

   In this exercise, the midwife or student midwife should investigate what tort reform laws the state has enacted to protect health care providers from losses in malpractice claims. Some questions regarding this protection include:

   - Are there state board requirements for a midwife to carry liability insurance or be self-insured through a bond?
   - What losses can a midwife suffer following damage awards that exceed coverage by the liability insurance policy? For example, can the midwife's savings be awarded to the plaintiff?
   - Are there state limits on the noneconomic damages (pain and suffering) that a jury can award?
   - Does the state have a special fund to pay for poor obstetrical outcomes?
   - Does the state have a market of last resort for liability insurance, a Joint Underwriting Authority?
   - Does the state limit the number of years following a bad outcome for a claim to be filed?

Table 6–5 For Your Professional Files

These documents from the American College of Nurse–Midwives are used in this chapter or are related to the topics in this chapter. All can be found at www.acnm.org.
- *Core Competencies for Basic Midwifery Practice* (2002)
- *Standards for the Practice of Midwifery* (2003)
- Strategies for risk reduction:
  - *Midwifery Strategies for Liability Risk Reduction* (2003)
  - *Midwifery Strategies for Liability Risk Reduction, Preterm Delivery* (2003)
  - *Midwifery Strategies for Liability Risk Reduction, Postdates Pregnancy/Post Maturity* (2003)
  - *Midwifery Strategies for Liability Risk Reduction, Shoulder Dystocia* (2003)
  - *Midwifery Strategies for Liability Risk Reduction*
- *The Myth of Vicarious Liability* (1994)

References

American College of Nurse–Midwives. (1994a). *Credentialing nurse–midwives*. Retrieved January 17, 2005, from http://www.midwife.org/display.cfm?id=494

American College of Nurse–Midwives. (1994b). *The myth of vicarious liability*. Retrieved January 17, 2005, from http://www.midwife.org/display.cfm?id=495

American College of Nurse–Midwives. (1996). *Limited obstetrical ultrasound in the third trimester* [Clinical bulletin]. Retrieved January 17, 2005, from http://www.midwife.org/display.cfm?id=585

American College of Nurse–Midwives. (2002a). *Core competencies for basic midwifery practice* [Clinical bulletin]. Retrieved January 17, 2005, from http://www.midwife.org/display.cfm?id=484

American College of Nurse–Midwives. (2002c). *Professional liability resource packet*. Retrieved January 17, 2005, from http://www.midwife.org/education.cfm?id=202

American College of Nurse–Midwives. (2003a). *Standards for the practice of midwifery* [Descriptive document]. Retrieved January 17, 2005, from http://www.midwife.org/prof/display.cfm?id=138

American College of Nurse–Midwives. (2003b). *Strategies for liability risk reduction*. Retrieved January 17, 2005, from http://www.midwife.org/prof/strategies.cfm

Bureau of Primary Health Care, Health Resources and Services Administration. (2005). *Federal Tort Claims Act*. Retrieved January 17, 2005, from http://bphc.hrsa.gov/programs/FTCAProgramInfo.htm

COPIC Companies. (2002). A simple way to prevent patient anger, preserve good relationships, and reduce lawsuits. *COPIC Topics, 79*. Retrieved February 22, 2005, from http://www.callcopic.com/publications/ copic_topics/copic_topics_archived_issues_2002

Furrow, B., Greaney, T., Johnson, S., Jost, T., & Schwartz, R. (2001). *Health law: Cases, materials, and problems*. (4th ed.). St. Paul, MN: West Group.

'Lectric Law Library. (n.d.). *Sovereign immunity*. Retrieved January 17, 2005, from http://www.lectlaw.com/def2/s103.htm

Liebman, C.B., & Hyman, C.S. (2004). A mediation skills model to manage disclosure of errors and adverse events to patients. *Health Affairs, 23*(4), 22–32.

Rubsamen, D. (1999). The nurse–midwife: Responsibility and liability. *Physicians Financial News, 17*(15), 33–34.

Sovereign Immunity. (2005). Florida Statute 768.28. Retrieved January 17, 2005, from http://www.leg.state.fl.us/statutes

U.S. Department of Health and Human Services. (2004). *Thompson launches "Early Offers" pilot program to speed compensation to injured patients, help reduce medical costs.* Retrieved February 19, 2005, from http://www.omhrc.gov/omhrc/pressreleases/2004press0921b.htm

U.S. Department of Health and Human Services. Health Resources and Services Administration. Division of Practitioner Data Banks. National Practitioner Data Bank. (n.d.). *2001 annual report.* Retrieved January 10, 2005, from http://www.npdp-hipdb.com/pubs/stats/2001_NPDB_Annual_Report.pdf

U.S. Department of Health and Human Services. Health Resources and Services Administration. Division of Practitioner Data Banks. National Practitioner Data Bank (n.d.). *Fact sheet for attorneys.* Retrieved January 10, 2005, from http://www.npdp-hipdb.com/pubs/fs/Fact_Sheet-Attorneys.pdf

U.S. Department of Health and Human Services. Health Resources and Services Administration. Division of Practitioner Data Banks. National Practitioner Data Bank. (n.d.). *National practitioner data bank guidebook.* Retrieved January 10, 2005, from http://www.npdb-hipdb.com/npdguidebook.html

U.S. General Accounting Office. (1992). *Medical malpractice: Alternatives to litigation.* Retrieved January 10, 2005, from http://archive.gao.gov/d31t10/145592.pdf

U.S. General Accounting Office. (2003). *Medical malpractice insurance: Multiple factors have contributed to increased premiums.* Retrieved January 10, 2005, from www.gao.gov/new.items/d03702.pdf

Vincent, C. (2003). Understanding and responding to adverse events. *New England Journal of Medicine, 348*(11), 1051–1056.

Weiss., P, Miranda, F., & Hess, W. (2004). Lights, camera, (legal) action: Videotaping in the delivery room. *Female Patient, 29*, 19–22.

Woods, J., & Rozovsky, F. (2003). *What Do I Say? Communicating intended or unanticipated outcomes in obstetrics.* San Francisco, CA: Jossey-Bass.

CHAPTER 7

Legislation and Policy Development

Kathryn Shisler Harrod, DNSc, CNM, FACNM
Lisa Hanson, DNSc, CNM
Kathryn Osborne, MSN, CNM

Learning Objectives

1. Discuss the political responsibilities of a midwife.
2. Discuss the role of the individual midwife and the ACNM in affecting legislation.
3. Identify the ACNM legislative agenda and priorities.
4. Outline the process by which a bill becomes law.
5. Describe components of effective communication with legislators.
6. Discuss the role of policy in health care as it relates to midwifery and women's health.

Legislation and Policy Development: Midwifery Practice Depends on It

The practice of midwifery is inherently political. The scope of women's health care contains features that often bring it to the center of controversy. Laws impacting women's healthcare consumers and providers are commonplace and ever changing. Further, legislation governing midwifery practice varies among states. Within states, different types of midwives are regulated and monitored by various boards and bodies. The political responsibilities of midwives are ongoing and critical to practice.

If you were asked why you entered the profession of midwifery, you might answer to catch or deliver babies, or maybe even to be with women. Few midwives would respond that they became midwives for the politics of the profession. However, most of midwifery practice is based on laws, rules, and regulations, which were developed through political activity. This makes the sayings, "all politics are local" and "the personal is political" a reality for midwifery practice. These are much-heard terms in political circles, and the statements are true for each and every midwife.

Historically, nurse–midwives have been involved in many key policy initiatives. The focus of these initiatives is often the right to practice midwifery. Because of the political work done by and for midwives, the ability of midwives to practice has expanded. However, there remain many obstacles and barriers to midwifery practice. Midwives who are actively involved in the process of policy development can change current realities and shape the future of midwifery practice (Ament, 2004; Kingdon, 1995). Policy development includes problem recognition, policy generation, and political activity.

Midwifery in the United States is deeply rooted in nursing. The history of nursing is rich in health policy development and the political action needed to make that policy a reality (Mechanic & Reinhard, 2002). Nurses have been well respected by the general public. Because of this respect, they hold a place of critical importance in ongoing contributions to forming public policy and political action (Wakefield, 2004). Nurses and nursing organizations in the United States are far greater in numbers than midwives and midwifery organizations. Proportionately, certified nurse–midwives/certified midwives (CNMs/CMs) make up a small part of advanced practice nurses/nonphysician providers, but when midwives align with advanced practice nurses a powerful collective is formed. When there is the opportunity to work together with nursing groups, nurses and midwives form a formidable coalition. Leaders of these groups can make a significant impact when they work together on healthcare policy and decision making.

Until the beginning of the 20th century, midwives were viewed as experts in childbirth and the health care of women. Gradually, physician-attended hospital birth became the norm. Now, at the beginning of the 21st century, the powerful position of physicians is beginning to change. Physicians have begun to lose their individual control of medical practice to corporate medicine and payors (Robinson, 1994).

Nurses and midwives may know more about vulnerable populations than any other profession (Wakefield, 2004). As women's health care experts it is the duty of midwives to share their expertise with legislators (Capps, 1998). In spite of this, midwives have remained relatively invisible in the larger health care policy arena. This lack of visibility needs to be changed. One way to change this is to disseminate our knowledge and publish. Nurse–midwives frequently publish on issues relevant to teaching, research, and practice. However, most publish in midwifery or nursing publications. This has the potential of rendering nurse–midwifery research invisible in the health policy arena because policy experts do not read these journals (Mechanic & Reinhard, 2002). To more significantly influence the dialogue on public policy, nurse–midwives would benefit from dissemination in journals frequently read by government leaders, such as the *American Journal of Public Health* and the *New England Journal of Medicine*.

In the recent past, nursing schools had fewer qualified women/men attracted to the profession, due in part to the variety of career options available. However, because of changes in the job market, entrance to nursing programs has once again become very competitive. The academic standard for an entry-level CNM/CM is now a baccalaureate degree, while most CNMs/CMs hold a master's degree or higher. As of the year 2010, completion of a graduate degree will be required for entry into clinical practice as a CNM/CM. An increase in highly educated midwives can lead to increased professional recognition and better access for clients to receive their services (Hartley, 2003). It is important for these highly educated midwives to be placed in positions at the policy tables at both federal and state levels. Becoming involved in policy development is vital because health care policy affects all aspects of midwifery practice. Midwives need to be involved with developing and writing the policies that affect their practice and women's health care (Mechanic & Reinhard, 2002).

Evolving Health Policy

The 1950s and 1960s were a time when medical care was provider driven and the providers were physicians. Physicians held high levels of public trust and were independent fee-for-service providers. Fee-for-service describes a payment system in which providers are paid their requested fee for the service rendered. This era was viewed as a time when individual physicians were the sole decision makers for their patients as well as the entire system of health care. However, as health care systems move more towards managed care, the health care team has become a recognized entity in providing quality patient care. During this transformation, the health care system has seen a growing number of nonphysician providers such as certified nurse–midwives (CNMs), certified midwives (CMs), nurse practitioners (NPs), physicians assistants (PAs), and certified registered nurse anesthetists (CRNAs). These nonphysician providers are presenting a challenge to the older model of physician control. In fact, the number of nonphysician providers doubled during the 1990s (Hartley, 2002). These nonphysician or advanced practice providers are presenting viable alternatives for health care consumers.

As nonphysician providers such as CNMs/CMs become more accepted, the stream of public opinion is changing. It is hoped that with this shift, physicians will accept them as partners in a collaborative system of health care. In the late 19th century and the early 20th century, physicians used both ideological and legal means to eliminate midwifery practice. In fact, physicians banded together and worked to pass state laws to eliminate midwifery services (Leavitt, 1986). As a result, midwifery was almost totally eliminated in the early 1900s, except for those midwives who cared for ethnic minorities and the poor. As state policies regarding medical care and scope of practice for midwives were written to attempt to define nurse–midwifery, laws were included assuring that midwives would care for vulnerable women who remain underserved by physician providers. Today, as in the late 19th and early 20th centuries, certain physician groups are once again working to maintain physician care as the centerpiece of the health care system.

The struggle between physician dominance, the rights of underserved vulnerable populations, and the rights of advanced practice providers to have opportunities to practice exists today. This struggle can be characterized by the actions of the Federation of State Medical Boards (the Federation). The Federation is a national nonprofit association whose membership includes all medical licensing and medical disciplinary boards in the United States and its territories. The Federation acts as a collective voice for medical boards in promoting high standards for medical licensure and practice. Unfortunately, the Federation is also working to stop the growth of autonomy by nonphysician or advanced practice providers (Federation of State Medical Boards of the U.S., Inc., 2003). In April 2003, the Federation's House of Delegates approved a resolution that the Federation establish a special committee to specify issues to be considered by state medical boards and legislative bodies. This special committee will address scope of practice initiatives relating to persons without a license to practice medicine (Federation of State Medical Boards of the U.S., Inc., 2003). Just as they did 100 years ago, some medical groups are still trying to define midwifery practice. However, the midwifery profession predates medicine by centuries and is also the international standard of care for childbearing women. It is critical for midwives to define their own scope of practice, be aware that formal groups exist that are targeting advanced practice providers, and be proactive in assuring client access to midwifery care. It is time for midwives to use midwifery knowledge and successes to define the practice of midwifery.

Current Legislative Status of CNMs/CMs

Physician control remains apparent in many aspects of state and local legislation and rules such as those written into hospital bylaws. Nurse–midwifery is legal in all 50 states; however, state policy regulating midwifery practice varies greatly from state to state (ACNM, 2004). The best example of how state law varies can be seen in requirements for collaborating relationships with physicians. Some states require written guidelines signed by the collaborating physician(s) and midwives whereas some local policies require on-site supervision. Practice also varies according to local policies. For example, one hospital may allow independent admissions by CNMs/CMs whereas a different hospital in the same community may require on-site supervision. Physicians are often responsible for decision making about hospital bylaws that allow midwives to practice. Ironically, this places physicians in the role of "gate keepers"; they hold authority to grant or deny admitting privileges that allow the CNM/CM to function autonomously in the hospital setting. This dependence upon physician "permission" poses a barrier to practice for many CNMs/CMs. Sociologist Heather Hartley (2002) conducted a research study about midwifery practice and physician dominance. She found that state and local policy has an important contextual effect on the presence of CNMs/CMs and their ability to function autonomously.

The American College of Nurse–Midwives: Our Professional Organization

Policy development occurs at many levels, including the federal, state, local, and institutional levels. Midwives can affect policy in multiple ways. For example, you can work within institutions by working on committees, through formal government appointments, and through special interest groups such as the American College of Nurse–Midwives (ACNM). The ACNM is the only professional group to represent and support nurse–midwifery and certified midwifery practice.

Because there is power in numbers, it is imperative for all CNMs/CMs to join the ACNM and present themselves as a unified profession to the political world. Most physician groups such as the American Medical Association (AMA) and the American College of Obstetricians and Gynecologists (ACOG) have high membership rates among the profession. Because of the large mass, these groups have a tremendous amount of money and power. Membership in the ACNM provides an opportunity for political advocacy for issues pertinent to midwives and their practices as well as financial support for the work of the profession.

The ACNM Office of Professional Services fosters policy development and political action at the local, state, and federal levels. Midwives and other professionals support this process. The Office of Professional Services midwives work on issues of practice and policy. In addition, the Office of Professional Services includes a state policy analyst and a federal lobbyist. In addition to these helpful professionals, there is also the ACNM Government Affairs Committee, which grew from the Political and Economic Affairs Section of the ACNM. One of the objectives of the Government Affairs Committee is to provide volunteer leadership at the national level on legislative, regulatory, and economic issues affecting midwifery practice and maternal and child health. The Government Affairs Committee is where ACNM divisions can bring policy issues that members think the ACNM should develop and support. The Government Affairs Committee is composed of a chair and representatives from each of the six ACNM regions. Policy sections within ACNM divisions develop ideas and policy issues. The policy section chairs meet with the Government Affairs chair, the state policy analyst, and the federal lobbyist during the fall ACNM Board of Directors (BOD) and Division and Section Chairs meeting to move forward key issues to the BOD. An example of one of the divisions' policy sections is the Division of Women's Health Policy and Leadership (DOW) Policy and Evaluation Section. The main goal of this section is to improve the health of women at the community level through the development, implementation, and promotion of public policy and public information initiatives (http://www.midwife.org/about/dwhpl.cfm).

Following BOD approval, these policy issues are transcribed into the ACNM State and Federal Policy Agenda, and strategies are developed within the Government Affairs Committee to help move the agenda through political action. The ACNM staff and Government Affairs Committee members serve as resources for member midwives as they work together on the legislative agenda.

The ACNM State and Federal Agenda is reviewed every 2 years. The agenda originates within four divisions (DOW, Division of Research, Division of Standards and Practice, and Division of Education) and the Government Affairs Committee with the help and advisement of the state policy analyst and the federal lobbyist. The agenda then goes to the BOD for final approval. Many of the issues on the legislative agenda are ongoing and occur across multiple years. The main issues on the agenda have been identified to support and promote midwifery practice and health care issues for women and their families across the United States.

At the time of this publication, the first item on the legislative agenda is to work to expand access to the full scope of CNM/CM services. The second item is to support professional liability reforms. In addition, the ACNM wants to increase the pool of primary care providers and preserve antitrust remedies. Finally, the ACNM wants to support consumer protection laws and increase awareness of CNMs/CMs and guarantee direct access to us as women's health care providers. (See **Table 7–1** for the full ACNM legislative policy agenda.)

Table 7–1 ACNM State and Federal Policy Agenda, 2005–2006

Expand Access to Full Scope of CNM/CM Services
- Assure adequate federal funding of Medicaid for the growing costs of the program and ensure midwifery services remain a mandatory benefit under federal law.
- Obtain equitable reimbursement for CNMs/CMs' services under the Medicare program and increase access for women with disabilities.
- Contest requirements for physician supervision, direction, or delegation of CNMs/CMs.
- Pass state legislation that fosters midwifery admitting privileges.
- Support changes to federal regulations within the Emergency Medical Treatment and Labor Act that permit midwives in emergency rooms to discharge women in "false labor" without a physician signature.
- Oppose efforts to circumvent state mandatory benefit laws with the creation of Association Health Plans at the federal level.

Support Professional Liability Reforms
- Support passage of state and federal legislation to reform the professional liability system to include the establishment of limits on noneconomic damages, mandating offsets for collateral sources, limitations on contingency fees, creation of periodic payment of future damages, and establishment of alternative dispute resolutions.

Increase the Pool of Primary Care Providers
- Secure increased funding for nursing and midwifery education.
- Facilitate interstate practice and participation in telehealth by CNMs/CMs.
- Support efforts to train CNMs/CMs within the Indian Health Service.
- Support efforts to expand the impact of midwives within the National Health Service Corp.

Preserve Antitrust Remedies
- Oppose any changes to existing state and federal antitrust laws governing health professions' business practices.
- Encourage strong enforcement of existing laws.

Support Consumer Protections and Awareness
- Guarantee direct access to women's health care specialists.
- Ensure continuity of care for pregnant women.
- Promote a national dialogue on the rising rate of cesarean sections.

Health Care Policy Development or Preparing the Bill

The United States invests more money in health care than any other country in the world. Despite this fact, the United States has the least universal and the most costly health care in the industrialized world (Bodenheimer & Grumbach, 1998). Because health care is a major U.S. expenditure, the industry attracts attention from many sources, including the federal and state governments. One of the most important factors influencing health policy is the current social value system. It is possible to create changes based on the current value system after identifying health issues and developing a plan for change through policy making. Policy making involves creating and carrying through research that provides evidence for health care policies (Boufford & Lee, 2002). Health policy is influenced by many different factors and can be created through legislative and nonlegislative processes. It is an interdisciplinary process. If a profession only looks after its own interests, the profession becomes isolated and is often less effective. Therefore, teams of various health care professionals working together write the best health policy. Policy making is influenced by evidence-based research involving the best practices.

Healthy People 2000/Healthy People 2010

One example of health policy established via the nonlegislative process is Healthy People 2000 and Healthy People 2010. The Healthy People Consortium is composed of more than 350 different organizations, including the ACNM. In addition to 54 state and territorial health departments, the consortium includes national organizations and members at all levels interested in improving the health and well-being of the nation. Members of the consortium come from a cross-representation of the American people. In fact, members of the consortium's organizations represent many special interest groups. These special interest groups are made up of members from groups of older adults, racial and ethnic coalitions, educators, businesses, health care providers, scientists, health care organizations, and many others. Consortium members are also broadly based in terms of the range of activities they undertake to support achievement of the national health objectives. Nearly all member organizations have publicized the Healthy People objectives to their members. Like previous documents, Healthy People 2010 was developed through a broad process, built on the best scientific knowledge and designed to measure programs over a 10-year period.

Trends in Health Policy

Currently there is a shift in paradigm from previous views regarding the formation of health care policies. The treatment of diseases is no longer a high priority. Instead, the contemporary approach uses evidence supporting multiple health determinants such as human behavior, biology, environment, education, socioeconomic characteristics, and medical care and the way in which these influence the health of broader communities and populations (Boufford & Lee, 2002). As a result, the definition of health becomes a reflection of the nation's unified value system. This shift has occurred because the outcomes of the U.S. health care system do not reflect the overall improvement in health status that one might expect to see with an increased utilization of resources. In fact, the health status of Americans ranks poorly worldwide in spite of the amount of money spent. In addition, the United States only met about 15% of the Healthy People 2000 goals, and health disparities between ethnic groups and minorities are worsening rather than improving (Boufford & Lee, 2002). In 2000, the U.S. health system was ranked 37th overall and only 24th on overall health attainment (World Health Organization [WHO], 2000). This finding is troubling. Boufford and Lee (2002) remind us we would not tolerate this position in either education or defense. This low rating should not be tolerated in health care either.

Transformation of Health Care Affects Policy

According to Emanuel (2002), health care priorities are changing at the turn of the 21st century. The social context of health care has changed from a social reform orientation to a conservative and business-oriented approach. The focus has moved from a patient-based outlook to a population-based outlook. In population-based health care, fee-for-service is being replaced by a system of capitation. When health care is capitated, care is refused to some individuals. Because the health of and costs of health care for the population are more important than care for the individual, expensive care for the individual is sometimes refused. An example of this would be when an insurer refuses to provide reimbursement for experimental surgeries or some transplants.

In addition, care decision making is moving from individualized care, planned by the provider, to standardized guidelines and management strategies. In this shift in health care delivery there is also a shift from independent providers to organized delivery systems that integrate all types of providers, the majority being physicians. There is also a shift from peer review through hospital credentialing and morbidity and mortality reviews to more organized, quantitative, quality assessments that are available to everyone who has access to the Internet (Emanuel & Emanuel, 1996; Epstein, 1996; Rodwin, 1994). Population-based health care should lead to improved services for reduced costs. In fact, this type of health care leads to much better preventative services, such as smoking cessation and improved use of screening tests. This paradigm shift is an example of a shift in public policy regarding health care issues.

Policy Development: The Process—How Streams Change

Public policies are authoritarian decisions developed in the legislative, executive, or judicial branches of government. These policies are made at the federal, state, or local levels. Ideas are the foundation of policy development (Leatt & Mapa, 2003). Those who are actively involved in the process of policy development work together to form the policies that shape U.S. health care. The democratic process of policy development involves problem recognition, policy generation, and political activity (Wong, 1999).

Policy-making processes are open systems, described as *streams* by Kingdon (1999). These processes are known as streams because they flow; they are in a continuous state of fluctuation. In fact, as discussed previously, our health care systems are also continually changing (Hartley, 2003). Kingdon's (1995) model describes three streams: the problems, proposals, and politics that flow through and around the government. The first step in the process requires policy makers to recognize and identify certain problems as higher priorities. The priorities are set by the current stream, or in other words, the political atmosphere or environment. After the problems have been identified, proposals are defined and written as (or drafted as) policies (Kingdon, 1995).

Descriptors of Policy Development

There are three main descriptors of policy development in the American political system: incrementalism, pluralism, and federalism (Boufford & Lee, 2002). Incrementalism refers to the manner in which programs develop and evolve throughout the years. Federal health care policy reflects the incremental effects of almost 1000 different health and social programs in the federal government. Most of these programs fall under the direction of the

U.S. Department of Health and Human Services (DHHS). It is the role of DHHS to implement and monitor legislation that is passed by Congress and signed by the president (Boufford & Lee, 2002).

Pluralism is the affirmation of diversity in interest and beliefs in citizens and is the term used when many groups are involved in writing policy. Examples of these groups include the various cabinets, cabinet-level departments, insurers, hospitals, physicians, nurses, health plans, and other special interest groups. All these different groups create a challenging environment for the creation of larger health policy issues (Boufford & Lee, 2002). CNMs/CMs have some presence in the creation of larger health policy, but we need to position ourselves to increase this presence.

Finally, federalism is a term used when federal action creates policy. Historically, the division of responsibilities regarding health care policy between the federal government and states has varied throughout the years. As a result, a complex interdependence between the federal government and each state exists. This makes unilateral federal action almost impossible. It is a daunting task to bring all the players together to work on policy development and unifying health policy.

Writing the Policy

Policy agendas are influenced by the current agenda or atmosphere in the federal government, the state government, or local politics. Each party that wants to influence health care policy comes to the table with its own political agenda. When at the table and participating in policy development, problem recognition occurs first. Once a problem is recognized, the process of actual policy generation begins. Health policy can be generated by the presidential staff and appointees, legislators, and special interest groups like the AMA or the ACNM. This creates challenges because in the Senate there may be 100 different policy agendas and in the House there may be another 500 different policy agendas. In addition to these elected officials, political appointees such as the Secretary of DHHS play a large role in influencing the president's policy issues, ideas, and political agenda. There is a current trend for government officials to look towards renowned academics for solutions to problems that have surfaced and to develop policies (Wong, 1999). These policy issues, ideas, and political priorities become part of each agency's legislative agenda. Other political players such as special interest groups, researchers, congressional staffers, bureaucrats, academicians, and lobbyists work towards their own policy ideas. It is important to remember that government does not act alone. Government officials often delegate decisions to professional organizations. They also look to professional organizations for information to aid in the decision-making process.

The Power in Politics: Money = Power

The stronger the organization, the more likely it will be successful in moving policy through political processes. The organization's strength is often based on the resources available to move the policy. Some of the most important resources are financial in nature (Wong, 1999). In reality, it is the politics of financial resources and a group or individual's personal power, interfaced with agencies that support women and their families, that can develop and move policy (Ament, 2004). The AMA has many more members and a great deal more money than midwifery organizations. It is important to look at the power base of each special interest group, as advanced practice nurses are increasingly brought into competition with physicians (Hartley, 2003). It is vital for midwives to participate in policy creation and the political process, because the ability to work as midwives and to be adequately reimbursed depends on it (Ament, 2004). This is another reason it is imperative for you to be a member of the ACNM and to donate to the Midwives Political Action Committee (PAC). A PAC is a campaign fund of a sponsoring labor, business, or trade organization, or the campaign fund of a group formed primarily or solely for the purpose of giving resources to candidates supportive of your organization. When an organization has a PAC, they contribute finances to the campaigns of issue-friendly politicians. The ACNM PAC contributes donations to campaigns of politicians friendly to midwifery and women's health issues. The list of donations is provided to the ACNM membership on an annual basis.

Policy and Regulating Bodies

To fully understand how health policy is created and carried out you need to understand the DHHS and the executive staff (Boufford & Lee, 2002). The lead federal agency for health policy is the DHHS. As the lead health policy agency, the DHHS serves to make policies, provide financing, and protect the public health. In addition, the DHHS is also responsible for collecting and disseminating information about the health of populations and for directing various health-related federal programs.

The name *iron triangle* is used to describe the interconnections that are formed among senior staff of the various operating divisions, congressional staff, and special interest groups. The White House is involved in many different ways. The Office of Budget and Management (OMB) reviews financial requests and approves budgetary decisions of the various DHHS agencies. Policy priorities are set according to the president's agenda. Another organization, the Office of Policy Development, was established in 1993 to further advise the president and to develop and implement social and economic policies. There are many more offices devoted to policy issues in Washington D.C., but these two are the most likely to be working on policy effecting midwifery practice and issues (Boufford & Lee, 2002).

The resources listed thus far are not enough to move policy by themselves. It also takes organized lobby points and a *window of opportunity*. Talking points are written to assist in explaining the issues. In addition, timing is critical! As the process of policy development progresses, input comes from many places, including the government and special interest groups. Those with special interests are constantly watching for a window of opportunity to move their agendas forward (Leatt & Mapa, 2003). When the window of opportunity opens, government officials are receptive to new ideas. All those with a policy agenda ready to move forward must work fast before the window closes (Kingdon, 2002). Midwives may be interested in changing policy but unless there is a *window of opportunity*, our legislation will not move anywhere.

Lobbyists Help to Move Policy

Lobbyists help to move policy towards legislation. Most organizations need to hire lobbyists for federal, state, and even some local work because it is helpful to have political insiders to help move the policy. Just as you would hire a midwife if you want your birth attended by the most qualified expert, hiring a lobbyist assures guidance through the legislative process by a qualified expert. The characteristics of the right lobbyist are also key (Leatt & Mapa, 2003). The lobbyist needs to have developed relationships with the right legislators who will help promote your desired legislation. Effective lobbyists monitor the public policy environment, including government activities for relevant legislation or for opportunities that present the appropriate timing to introduce policy. To become proactive, the lobbyist needs to do forecasting. The art of forecasting involves continuously looking for trends in health policy. Another example of forecasting is developing possible scenarios or plausible stories about the future (Deber & Williams, 2003).

To aid in moving policy forward it is important to be knowledgeable and to do the necessary homework by performing an internal environment analysis. Examples of internal environmental analyses include investigating financial and environmental resources, marketing, operational, and/or cultural issues. According to Ament (2004), midwives are increasingly learning the importance of research and policy analysis to help move the political agenda. For example, in 2005 in Wisconsin many CNMs would like to pursue third-party reimbursement. However, understanding the political climate, particularly as it pertains to legislative leadership, is important. With a Republican majority in power in both state houses, the Wisconsin CNMs recognize that it is likely that any attempt to pursue an insurance mandate will fail. They also recognize that there are problems with mandating third-party reimbursement. The first problem is that due to the underlying fear that insurance mandates may result in higher premiums, statutorily mandating anything is not currently a popular concept. The second problem is that insurance mandates require reimbursement not only for CNMs/CMs, but also for each health care organization to provide midwifery services. Although this mandate would improve employment opportunities for midwives, there are not midwives available in all areas of Wisconsin to meet the need that would be created by such a mandate.

Congressional Committees and Health Care

Members of Congress are key players in the process of policy development. The Senate and House both have committees that address health care issues. Two types of committees are responsible for health policy. The first type is the committees that provide authorization and the second type is the appropriation committees. Authorization committees approve the content of bills and appropriation committees decide if implementation of the bill is affordable and where the money will be allotted (Boufford & Lee, 2002). The most important health-related committee in the House is the Commerce Committee, which is responsible for Medicare Part B and public health issues. The Ways and Means Committee is also an influential House committee. It is responsible for Medicare Part A and some of Part B and the tax codes. Of the remaining health bills, 8% are managed by the Education and

Economic Opportunities Committee, which has jurisdiction over the Employment, Retirement, and Social Security Act (ERISA).

In the Senate, the two dominant committees overseeing health programs are the Finance Committee and the Labor and Human Resources Committee. The Finance Committee is responsible for Social Security, Medicare, Medicaid, and maternal–child health. The Labor and Human Resources Committee is responsible for public health, biomedical research, health and safety, and ERISA. In the Senate, 20% of all bills go to more than one committee; however, for health-related bills the number is far greater (Boufford & Lee, 2002). Legislation needs a window of opportunity and a vehicle to move it forward. In the 1990s in the federal government, this vehicle was frequently one of the budget bills; on the state level it still is today.

Identify Resources

To move policy to reality it is necessary to build political coalitions, enlist assistance from the public, define the stakeholders, and lobby the right legislators. Some of the stakeholders are supportive allies, and some of them are opponents/enemies. It is really important to identify your friends and your enemies. When these players are identified, you can use this information to help move the policy forward. To move policy, resources are critical. These resources are finances, organizational members, time, knowledge, networking and other supporters, and credibility (Kingdon, 2002; Wong, 1999). People are willing to invest in important ideas. Therefore, it is vital to be able to convince people that your ideas are essential by delivering the right message. One of the best ways to deliver the message is to use talking or bullet points. When you write bullet points you present concise, easy-to-remember remarks. Bullet points are used to elicit support from the public and from legislators.

One approach to eliciting public support is to use polls. Polling is done because public opinion matters. It is done to bring ordinary people into decision making where they would not otherwise have a voice. The results of polls help to explain public opinion and to provide more influence on policy development. When the public voices their demands, they can affect health care policy agenda setting (Kingdon, 2002). Another resource to help enlist supporters is credibility. Nurses are viewed as credible professionals; however, there is not a national understanding of midwives. You need to continuously educate everyone with whom you come in contact. Indeed, it is important for the public to have an understanding of the role of the midwife in women's health and how you differ from physicians.

The Strategy

The next step in moving policy is formulating a strategy. To formulate the strategy you need to use all the resources that have been identified. Part of developing the strategy is establishing a time line. After setting the time line, a leader or leaders need to be designated to implement and monitor the process of the planned strategy. The leader could be legislative committee chairs, a paid lobbyist, or a combination of the two (Deber & Williams, 2004). Part of the strategy is knowing where and when to focus political efforts. It is important to recognize where the power to help move policy actually lies and to use this information in the strategy (Deber & Williams, 2003).

Budgetary Constraints Create Barriers

Policy development is often constrained by budgets. In fact, the government's work is constrained by the federal budget. According to Kingdon (1995), three types of programs are pursued during times of severe budget constraints: programs that attempt to regulate fraud legislation, programs that are seen to be low in cost and not use many resources, and programs that have the potential to save money for the government. Many policies are introduced, but few actually make it to the president's desk for a signature. There are many ways for policies to be stopped along the way (Wong, 1999).

In summary, the steps to influence policy are to organize, be prepared, frame your point of view to appeal to the audience, set up a time line to concentrate your activities, and watch for the window of opportunity (Ament, 2004; Milio, 1984). When these steps have occurred, it is time to move the bill towards becoming a law. Remember, to avoid having legislation stopped, health care organizations and special interest groups need to consider their relationships with various levels of government as they advance in the strategic planning process (Deber & Williams, 2003). When the policy has been approved, rules and regulations will be written to implement the policy.

How a Bill Becomes a Law: Government 101

Policy proposals lead to political action. The proposals that survive to the point of becoming a bill are those that possess the technical ability, are consistent with the dominant moral and value systems, and can be implemented within current budgetary constraints (Kingdon, 1995). If a legislator is supporting a bill, the stronger the legislator's influence, the more likely the bill will make it to and through committees. As mentioned previously, one of the most prestigious of the House committees is the Ways and Means Committee. Members of this committee are often the most senior and influential members of Congress. Policy is more likely to move through the legislative process if there is powerful support behind the legislation by either influential legislators or many legislators supporting the same legislation. To move policy forward it takes time, the right political climate, people who are willing to do the work, and few or no constraints. If a bill is attached to a more powerful bill it is more likely to move. This is known as *using a vehicle* to move legislation (Wong, 1999).

The national mood, government, and organized physical forces influence politics. Again, it is imperative to identify both your allies and your enemies. We need to mobilize ourselves, our allies, and any other supporters in order to pass policy on to legislation. To help add to the midwife power base, you also need to mobilize your clients, colleagues, and even family members to action (Deber & Williams, 2003). In addition to identifying allies, you will need to identify and plan strategy around your opposition. When midwives or midwife lobbyists visit with legislators, the first thing asked is who is likely to oppose the bill. Who are the enemies of this bill? Legislators want to know this information up front. The politically savvy midwives will have identified these people ahead of time and will have attempted to meet and work with them prior to any attempts to move the legislation. This should be part of the time line: an internal environmental analysis and strategy for moving the legislation.

Introduce the Legislation: The First Step

The first step for a bill to become law is to have the legislation introduced. The ACNM needs to identify friendly legislators to author and introduce the bill. If the ACNM has members from *both sides of the aisle* (bipartisan members), the ACNM will have a greater chance of success. When legislation is introduced in the House, it is handed to the clerk of the House or placed in the hopper (Project Vote-Smart, 2004). The hopper is a box on the House clerk's desk where members can place bills and resolutions prior to their introduction. In the Senate, members must acquire the attention of the presiding officer to introduce a bill during the morning hour. The morning hour is the time set aside at the beginning of each legislative day. Each of these mechanisms sends the bill to the clerk of the Senate or the House. The clerk will give the bill a number and a title. A House bill is labeled with HR and a Senate bill is given an S, then the assigned number follows both. The bill is also labeled with the sponsor's name and sent to the Government Printing Office.

Moving the Bill Through Committee

From here, the Speaker of the House or the presiding officer in the Senate assigns the bill to the appropriate committee (**Figure 7–1**). For health care issues, the bills will usually go to an authorization committee and an appropriations committee. Often the House or Senate parliamentarian makes the actual referral decision. The committee may reject the bill or table the bill. If the bill is tabled it is never discussed in the committee again. Bills are scheduled on the calendar and hearings may be held to listen to the facts about the bill. At this time, the bill can be voted on or changed. The session during which revisions and additions are made to bills is called a *mark-up session*. If the committee does not act on a bill it essentially kills the bill. Conversely, if most of the committee votes in favor of the bill it is sent back to the House or Senate for debate. If substantial amendments are made, the committee can order a *clean bill,* which includes all of the amendments. This clean document becomes a new bill with a new number. The House or Senate must approve, change, or reject the committee amendments before each conducts a final vote. Most bills never make it out of the committee. Each year thousands of bills are sent to committees and only several hundred of these actually make it out of committee. The rest of the bills die in committee. This is the reason it is essential to have a person on the committee, and if possible the committee chair, as sponsors of the bill. Bill sponsors are more likely to be invested in moving the legislation through the committee and on to the whole chamber.

Bill Returns to the Full Chambers

The Speaker of the House and the Majority Leader in the Senate hold a great deal of power. They decide which bills will reach the floor and when. They will schedule the bills on one of the four House Calendars. In the Senate, the Majority Leader schedules the legislation on the Legislative Calendar. If a majority of Senators agree, the bill can be brought to the floor at any time.

Figure 7–1 How a Bill Becomes Law

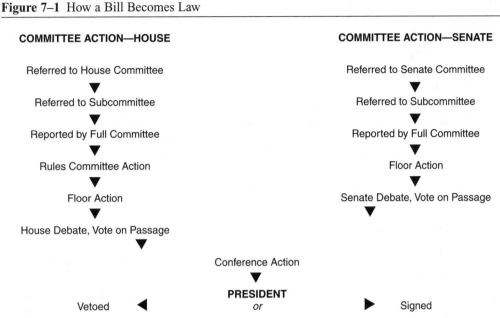

Once a bill makes it to the floor it is debated. The debate is guided by the bill's sponsoring committee and equal time is given to the proponents and opponents of the bill. In the House, once a vote is called there must be a quorum of 218 members present. If a quorum is not present, the House will adjourn until the Sergeant of Arms can round up the necessary quorum. In the Senate, debate is unlimited until a cloture is called. A cloture is a motion in the Senate to limit debate. It takes 60 member votes to invoke cloture. If cloture is called, each senator has only one hour of debate time. Senators can try to defeat a bill by doing something called filibustering. Filibustering occurs when a senator or several senators give long speeches in an effort to delay work in the Senate. Some politicians or Washington insiders describe a filibuster as *talking it to death*. This is often done by the minority party to avoid a vote. A cloture will end a filibuster.

After a vote occurs and the bill is passed, it is sent to the other chamber for consideration. If the bill passes both the House and the Senate, it goes to the president for his signature. If the House and Senate pass similar bills but not the same bill, they are sent to the Conference Committee. The Conference Committee is made up of members from each house who meet to iron out the differences in the bill. If the committee can compromise, it prepares a report called the conference report and submits it to each chamber. The conference report needs to be approved by both chambers of Congress.

The Bill Becomes Law

Finally, a bill becomes law when the president signs it. If the president does not sign the bill and Congress is still in session 10 days later, it becomes a law without the president's signature. Conversely, if Congress does not remain in session and the president does not sign the bill, it is called a pocket veto and does not become law. The president can also veto a bill and send it back to Congress. If a bill is vetoed the president must put his reasons for the veto in writing. To override a veto, a two-thirds majority of those present must vote in favor of the override. Once the bill becomes law by either a signature or an override, it is assigned an official number (Fact Monster, 2005; Project Vote-Smart, 2004).

Once a bill becomes law, it is the responsibility of a federal agency to see that rules are written and the law is enforced and followed. For issues concerning midwifery, the bill will be directed to one of several different federal agencies. The bill may be directed to DHHS, the Centers for Medicare and Medicaid Services (CMS), the Maternal and Child Health Bureau (MCHB), the Health Resources and Services Administration (HRSA), the Department of Justice (DOJ), the Department of Education (DOE), or the Federal Trade Commission (FTC).

Politics at the State Level

At the state level, the process of how a bill becomes a law is similar to the federal government in most states. There is some variation from state to state. To find out how the process works in your state, look for the state government Web site or request a Blue Book from a state assembly representative or state senator. The Blue Book in each state contains information about each state's history, symbols, legislator biographies, how a bill becomes a law, and many other state facts. The Blue Book is free and is an invaluable source of information for state politics.

The Politically Active Midwife

In 1986, then ACNM President Susan Yates announced to the graduating class at the Frontier School of Midwifery and Family Nursing that each midwife needs to practice business and politics, including the art and science, of nursing and midwifery. She proposed that the most effective way to establish nurse–midwifery in the political arena is to be visible on issues important to midwives and women's health (Gesse, 1991). Nurse–midwives has been a politically active group since the earliest days of women's suffrage. For example, early graduates of the Maternity Center Association's nurse–midwifery program became consultants in maternal–infant health in many state and federal agencies. As a result, early nurse–midwifery services were included in numerous federal projects (Gesse, 1991). The need for midwives to be politically active is just as great now.

There are many ways for midwives to become politically active. You can influence policy individually or jointly by developing plans, contacting legislators, attending town hall meetings, writing letters to the editor, calling in on radio talk shows and developing relationships with legislators and Congressional health legislative staff (Wakefield, 2004). Gesse (1991) studied nurse–midwives in order to determine the amount and type of political activity in which midwives participated. She found it was women's issues that motivated midwives to take political action. In 2005, midwives are still interested in women's issues, but need to be concerned about reimbursement and practice issues as well. Our very livelihoods depend on political activity.

Start a Resource File

To become politically active, the first thing you will need to do is to educate yourself about the current status of midwifery nationally and in your state. Put together a file of documents that are essential to midwifery practice. Examples of items in file should include are a copy of your State Practice Act, federal regulations, Medicare and Medicaid regulations, and requirements for direct access and third-party reimbursement (see Table 7–1). Each midwife will refer to this file frequently, so make sure to keep the file updated (Foster, 1998).

Exercise the Right to Vote

The easiest behavior to incorporate in becoming politically active is to exercise your right to vote. It is the right of every American to vote (Cooney, 2004). Midwives, regardless of party affiliation, need to participate in the electoral process. The vote is anonymous; no one knows who you vote for, but legislators will know you voted. Interestingly, legislators pay close attention to which (and how many) of their constituents show up to the polls and vote. Legislators actually buy the voting lists. When you contact their office, they may check the voting lists to make sure you vote. If you do not get out and vote, legislators do not respond to you in the same manner. Legislators respect voters, so get out and vote.

Midwife the Process

Policy development, moving issues, and righting the wrongs of previous legislation usually takes time. It is important for midwives to be patient and persistent. It may take several years to move the ACNM political agenda. It is easy to become frustrated with the slow progress, but without your continued involvement and persistence, change will never occur. Midwives are known for their patience and persistence during long labors as we midwife our clients. "Midwifing" legislation often involves much the same process. You can use your skills to midwife legislators and the political agenda.

Adopt Your Legislator

Midwives need to develop long-term relationships with elected officials. Think about developing the relationships as if you are adopting your legislators. Legislators and their staff respond better if you have developed relationships over time (Foster, 2002). Visit your legislators in both their local and national offices. Try to meet with each of your elected officials at least once per year. Read the local newspapers and watch for notices of town hall meetings. Attending town hall meetings is a great way to get midwifery issues heard and to remind those in office we exist. Remember, when you meet your legislators, you need to dress for success. Business attire in Washington, D.C., tends to be more formal than in other settings. When visiting in Washington, D.C., you should wear a suit. When visiting at the local office it is also important to dress professionally.

Midwives need to frequently remind those in the legislative offices about who we are, what we do, and for whom we care. When you visit offices, bring information along that helps to explain midwifery and your present position. Do not forget to take along business cards. It is important to be able to leave a business card when you visit each office. During the visit you will need to remind them of the educational requirements, certification, and licensing requirements for CNMs/CMs. You need to talk about the women and families you serve and the scope of your practice. Gather good stories about your practice that you can share with staff. In addition, you need to educate the staffers in each office about midwives being with women, not just with pregnant women. Staffers are often young and have a frequent turnover. Legislative aides frequently are the ones advising the legislators about health care issues. Therefore, we need to invest time and energy in the staffers.

Be creative. Consider giving an annual legislative or leadership award from your chapter to public officials who have demonstrated they are friends of midwives (Schmoozing, 1997). Invite your legislators to work. During the warmest part of summer, legislators return home to their constituents and are often available to make visits to midwifery clinical sites. Women's issues are currently popular with legislators. Inviting your legislator to work is a great way to build a relationship with the legislator (Cooney, 2004). In fact, during the 2004 elections, the candidates worked hard to attract women's votes. Legislators love mothers, babies, and crowds, so invite both. Do not forget to include the press. Positive press will help build your practice and will help to build your relationship with the legislator. It is easy to find your legislators. Go to the ACNM Web site, www.midwife.org. On the ACNM site, scroll down to Legislation & Health Policy, click on it, and select *Speak Out for Midwifery*. From there it is easy to access your legislators' names, offices, and addresses. When you call the office, ask for the scheduler and be persistent.

Prior to visiting with your legislator, and while on the *Speak Out for Midwifery* site, check on the legislators' voting records. Note the votes that were important to you and remember to thank the legislator for votes that you also supported. During the visit make sure you get a chance to talk about the current important issue impacting practice and the midwifery profession (Cooney, 2004).

Another great way to develop relationships with your legislator is to volunteer your time. Choose the candidate or legislator you would like to work for and call their campaign manager or campaign office. Volunteer to make telephone calls at the phone banks or to do literature drops door to door. Spending only a few hours volunteering on a campaign can help to build a lasting relationship with the legislator. Better yet, recruit other midwives and other individuals to also help with the campaign. In addition to volunteering to work on the campaign, donate money. A campaign cannot be successful without funds. Giving donations is another great way for midwives to be noticed. Remember to donate to the Midwives PAC, as well as candidates of your choice, because your donations are used to help build relationships with your legislators.

Your local ACNM chapter may want to consider starting either a PAC or a conduit, or begin organizational fund raising. A conduit or other organizational fund raising differs from a PAC in that donors give a certain amount of money and when it is time to donate, the person running the conduit will call and ask if it is alright to donate to a particular candidate. The names of the donors and the organization are listed on the conduit donation.

Spreading the Message

Do not forget to include consumers in your legislative work. Many birth centers and midwifery practices place patient educational materials on midwifery issues in the waiting rooms. Other practices have newsletters or some other mechanisms they can use to educate and enlist the support of consumers. When you are pursuing a legislative issue you may want to have your clients write letters of support. This could be as easy as leaving paper, stamped envelopes, addresses, and bullet talking points in the waiting area. This is a good way for your clients to use their time while waiting to be seen by you. Whenever possible, enlist your clients to write letters or to testify on behalf of midwifery. Politicians respond better to constituents than to midwives who they may perceive as having a vested interest in the legislation (Schmoozing, 1997).

Make your message short, easy, and to the point. Along with developing a time line to help move the legislation, it is important to write bullets or talking points to get the message across. Educate yourself, fellow midwives, and supporters. Arm yourself with information. Keep a paper trail as you work to move legislation. Elected officials and their staffers keep track of contacts they receive. In fact, they count pro and con contacts. If they are not receiving written communication and telephone calls, legislators assume the issue is not important for their constituents.

Originally, it was important to send handwritten letters through the U.S. Postal Service. However, since September 11, 2001, and the anthrax scare in Washington, D.C., letters by postal mail are no longer the preferred manner of communication. Instead, your handwritten letters can easily be faxed to the Congressional offices. Handwritten letters hold more weight than e-mails or telephone calls. Sending e-mails are also more accepted since September 11th, but are not viewed as well as letters. There are several tips for writing an effective letter (see **Table 7–2**). First, identify yourself as a constituent and begin with a clear statement describing the intent of the letter. Write the letter as an individual and include your occupation. Discuss only one issue per letter; be brief and to the point. It helps to make the issue local for the legislator. To do this, give them examples or stories from your practice, which is located in their district. Explain why the issue is important to women, mothers and their babies, and communities, all of whom are constituents. And finally, ask for the specific actions you want and ask for his or her position on the issue. As you develop a relationship with the legislative office, check to see what the office's preferred method of communication would be.

Table 7–2 Tips for Writing an Effective Letter

Identify yourself as a constituent.
Begin with a clear statement describing the intent of the letter.
Write the letter as an individual and include your occupation.
Discuss only one issue per letter; be brief and to the point.
Make the issue local for the legislator.
Explain why the issue is important to women, mothers and their babies, and communities.
Ask for the specific actions you want and ask for his or her position on the issue.

Telephone calls are not generally as effective as letters. If there is a rapid turnaround time, make telephone calls. In the case of telephone calls, legislative offices often keep track of how many pro calls and how many con calls have been made. However, telephone calls do not hold much weight. If you need to get your message out fast it would be best to make multiple contacts via multiple mediums and don't get discouraged.

After you have met with or contacted your elected official, make sure you send a follow-up thank you note for their time. Also thank them for their vote if they voted favorably (for or against) your issue. When they respond by mail write another thank you. Every correspondence the office receives from midwives will help keep midwifery issues on the forefront. And finally, remember there is power in numbers. Midwives need to present a unified front. Not only is it important for us to present a unified approach, it is important to network and to identify midwife allies. For example, there are many more nurse practitioners (NPs) than midwives in the United States. If we can enlist the support of other groups such as NPs, our legislative agenda is more likely to be moved forward.

One more important way to get out a message about women's health issues and midwifery is to formally testify before committees or at hearings. Providing testimony allows you to speak to multiple influential legislators at the same time. It also gives you a chance to make a prepared, well-thought-out, and researched statement in public. Speaking in a public forum also gives you a chance to get media exposure, which may serve to bolster your cause. When providing public testimony, you should focus on your personal, real-life experiences and how these experiences relate to the issue under consideration. For example, you may have experience with patients who rely on Medicaid or Medicare. Your voice at a hearing describing personal stories would be particularly effective. See **Boxes 7–1** and **7–2** for two examples of testimony.

Case Example

Recently, CNMs in the state of Wisconsin were able to move legislation removing supervisory language in only 2 years. In addition to removing the supervisory language, the new statutory language linked the scope of practice for nurse–midwives to the *Standards for the Practice of Nurse Midwifery*. Tying the scope of practice for nurse–midwives to this document, which is revised and updated regularly, allows for the evolution of nurse–midwifery practice as it occurs over time without requiring additional legislative change to the practice act. This successful legislative campaign began with the identification of the problem. CNMs in Wisconsin could not have admitting privileges in hospitals because they were not viewed as independent providers due to the supervisory language in the Nurse Practice Act. They also recognized that the scope of practice as described in the old act was no longer consistent with the present-day practice of nurse–midwives. They knew the only way to change their status was to change the portion of the practice act about midwifery. The nurse–midwives set up a legislative committee and invited the ACNM state senior policy analyst to come to Wisconsin to help get the process started. The policy analyst spent an entire weekend reviewing the issues with a number of midwives. Because many Wisconsin midwives were involved in the legislative process, there was a great investment in the outcome. The most important items accomplished that weekend were developing a time line and establishing talking points. The time line contained the strategy to move the legislation.

Meanwhile, two of the CNMs were working with a group of advanced practice nurses and the Wisconsin Nurses Association. This relationship was instrumental in serving to enlist this group of nurses as allies. The nursing groups were initially opposed to the CNMs opening the practice act. They were worried that other changes would be slipped into the practice act when it was opened for the midwives. The more the CNMs worked with the nurses, the more support they received from the nursing groups who ultimately became allies in the process.

One of the recommendations from the ACNM policy analyst was to hire a lobbyist. The midwives did not have to look very far. One of the members of the legislative committee is married to a lobbyist. He had previously worked with the Republican governor and had many relationships with Republican legislators. At the time, Wisconsin had a Republican governor, a Republican assembly, and a Democratic senate. Many of the CNMs in the state are Democrats, so having a lobbyist with these kinds of connections was key. Hiring a lobbyist is a great use of chapter moneys. However, lobbyists are not inexpensive. Money was raised through fundraising and an increase in chapter dues. The lobbyist got right to work and found a Republican sponsor in the assembly who also chaired the committee in which the bill was likely to be heard. While the lobbyist was working on the Republicans, one of the CNM committee members found a sponsor in the Senate. This senator is an advanced practice nurse who was eager to help move the legislation through the Senate. Both sponsors chaired the appropriate committees so they were able to see the legislation through both committees and then back to the senate and the assembly. This bipartisan approach led to the establishment of friends and supporters on both sides of the aisle.

During the months that followed, midwives met with all of the members of the committees in which the bill would be heard. At every meeting with legislators, the midwives were asked to identify proponents and opponents of the legislation. This meant they had to look for the groups that might oppose eliminating the supervisory language and expanding the scope of practice. First, they sought out friendly obstetricians who were also active members of the American College of Obstetrics and Gynecology (ACOG). These ACOG representatives took the legislation back to their members and gained full support from the Wisconsin Chapter of ACOG. Interestingly, it was the Wisconsin Medical Society and the Family Practice Physician Group who presented opposition. Members of the local chapter of ACNM met with these two groups to iron out the differences in order to gain their support of the legislation. One of the points the physician groups objected to was the use of statutory language describing nurse–midwives as primary care providers. To remedy this, one of the family practice physicians attempted to write her own definition of nurse–midwifery practice. Needless to say, this was unacceptable to the midwives, who were ultimately allowed to write the definition themselves. Through a series of meetings, a compromise was met so that all the groups involved were satisfied. This was an important step that alleviated opposition to the bill after it had been introduced.

Another issue was malpractice insurance. The physicians argued that if we were to become independent providers, we needed to carry the same malpractice insurance required of all independent practitioners in the state. In addition, the Wisconsin Association of Trial Lawyers indicated that they would use their control in the senate to kill the bill if we did not accept the requirement for medical malpractice insurance. Because of the potential problems this could create for the CNMs attending home birth, the legislative committee

Box 7–1 Testimony

5-17-05

To: Chairman Reynolds
        Members of the Senate Committee on Labor and Election Process Reform

From: Kathryn Osborne on behalf of the Wisconsin Chapter of the American College of
        Nurse–Midwives.

Chairman Reynolds, committee members, thank you for the opportunity to provide comments on Senate Bill 155. My name is Kathryn Osborne. I am licensed by the State of Wisconsin as a Registered Nurse, an Advanced Practice Nurse Prescriber and a Certified Nurse–Midwife. I am here today, on behalf of the Wisconsin Chapter of the American College of Nurse–Midwives (ACNM), to testify against Senate Bill 155. As women's health care providers, the Wisconsin Chapter of ACNM opposes any legislation that restricts a woman's access to health care. We believe that there are several mandates in SB 155 that will restrict access to health care and services.

I would like to start by clarifying that as advocates of self determination and individual choice, we understand that there are certain activities that some individuals would prefer not to participate in because of their "creed." That being said, we also understand that current law *already* addresses employment discrimination based on "creed." As you are aware, current law protects the religious conviction of individual employees, as long as making accommodations for that employee does not pose undue hardship on the employer. The employers we speak of here are health care providers. They are in the business of (and are professionally responsible for) providing safe, legal health care to members of a community. If the religious conviction of employees and/or potential employees interferes with the business's ability to provide safe, legal health care services then employers must be afforded the opportunity to hire individuals who will be able deliver such services. Statutorily requiring employers to maintain, or hire employees to the degree that they are not able to provide services that are recognized as safe and legal in this country, has the potential of rendering them incapable of conducting business. SB 155 requires employers to honor religious conviction to that degree.

The ability to fill a prescription is a critical element in the provision of health care. The mandates of SB 155 place the decision to proceed with a plan of care, established by a woman and her health care provider, in the hands of a pharmacist who for reasons of "creed" may refuse to fill the prescription. This is most likely to become an issue of restricted services in the rural areas of the state—areas where there may only be one pharmacist, one hospital, or one physician. Imagine for one minute, a young woman in Hayward, Wisconsin, who, following a sexual assault, is not able to get her prescription for emergency contraception filled because the only pharmacist in town refuses to fill it based on his "creed." Shall we further violate her by asking her to drive 25 miles to Spooner? And then she discovers that the pharmacist in Spooner refuses to fill it as well. After hours in an emergency room, following a violent assault, she now has to get back in her car and drive on to Rice Lake. This hardly seems like accessible health care, and it is certainly much more than a "minor inconvenience" as has been suggested by the proponents of this bill.

The effects of this bill will also be felt in our inner cities. I know that you are all aware of the high rates of teen pregnancy. My practice in Milwaukee provides evidence that teen pregnancy is a very real problem in the state of Wisconsin. Nationally, in addition to thousands of unplanned teen pregnancies, over 50% of all pregnancies in this country are unplanned. Access to safe and legal contraception is the only way to reduce this number and subsequently improve the overall health status of women. I have seen the lists created by several organizations that *incorrectly* include hormonal contraceptives (birth control pills and Depo Provera) as abortive agents—drugs that under the provision of SB 155 pharmacists would be allowed to refuse to dispense. Keeping this in mind, imagine the crisis we will experience if the two most common forms of contraception for inner city women are rendered unavailable because Wisconsin statute allows pharmacists to refuse to fill a prescription for hormonal contraception. How likely will it be for my client, who is dependent upon public transportation, to travel from pharmacy to pharmacy (with multiple bus connections) until she finds a pharmacist who will fill the prescription that will prevent one more teen pregnancy? Pharmacists are not and should not be asked to review contraceptive options, make recommendations, or provide counseling on the use of multiple forms of contraception. They are simply asked to do what they are educated and licensed to do—fill the prescription that was deemed most appropriate by the woman and her health care provider.

I would like to advocate for public policy that improves access to health care and moves us away from high rates of unplanned pregnancy, especially for young teens. This bill has the potential to do just the opposite by limiting access to health care for women of all ages and economic status, in all parts of the state. Health care needs of the patient, not the personal beliefs of pharmacists, should be the driving force in the provision of health care and the creation of health policy.

Thank you for your consideration of our concerns.

Respectfully submitted,

Kathryn Osborne, MSN, CNM
Wisconsin Chapter of the American College of Nurse–Midwives

took this issue back to the chapter. The chapter did not want to include statutory language that would be problematic for the CNMs attending home births. Following a lengthy discussion, the group reached the consensus that removing the supervisory language was the priority and that they would accept the professional and statutory obligation to carry the malpractice insurance.

The next events to take place were the public hearings in the senate and assembly committees that were considering the bill. Several CNMs gave testimony and many more gave the committee members written statements. The bills were heard in both committees without opposition. The lobbyist offered guidance and coaching along the way. His help was invaluable as the legislation continued to move forward.

Following passage in both committees, the bill was sent to the full assembly and senate for consideration. Prior to the introduction of the bill to both houses, members of local ACNM chapter visited the office of almost every senator and representative in the capitol. This important step afforded the midwives an opportunity to educate legislators about midwifery and answer any questions that might stand in the way of full legislative support of the bill. The bill passed unanimously in both the assembly and the senate. The collegial

Box 7–2 Testimony

5-25-05

To: Chairperson Owens
        Members of the Assembly Family Law Committee

From: Kathryn Osborne on behalf of the Wisconsin Chapter of the American College of
        Nurse–Midwives.

Madam Chair, committee members, thank you for the opportunity to provide comments on Assembly Bill 343. My name is Kathryn Osborne. I am licensed by the State of Wisconsin as a Registered Nurse, an Advanced Practice Nurse Prescriber and a Certified Nurse–Midwife. I am here today, on behalf of the Wisconsin Chapter of the American College of Nurse–Midwives (ACNM), to testify against Assembly Bill 343. As women's health care providers, the Wisconsin Chapter of ACNM opposes any legislation that restricts a woman's access to health care. We believe that the mandates of AB 343 severely restrict the access of UW students to health care that is recognized in this country as safe and legal.

Upon review of AB 343, it is clear that the intent of this bill is to limit a fundamental right of women in the year 2005—the right to plan when, and with whom they will bear children. Oral contraceptives have been available as a means to control fertility since 1960. Rendering them unavailable to women who attend the University of Wisconsin represents a giant leap backward. At a time when the university is trying to attract the best, and brightest, and most forward thinking students in the nation, it seems illogical to put in place a policy that identifies the University of Wisconsin as an institution that has moved back in time—almost half a century—with regard to meeting the health care needs of its student body.

Oral contraceptives, including emergency contraception, are among the most effective and widely used contraceptive methods in the United States. Their primary mode of action is the inhibition of ovulation. If taken properly, oral contraceptives are approximately 98% effective (Varney, 1997). When used within 72 hours of unprotected intercourse (or following contraceptive failure such as condom breakage), emergency contraception (Plan B) can be 85% successful at preventing unplanned pregnancy (Lakha, F. & Glasier, A., 2004). Passage of AB 343 would make these effective methods of contraception unavailable for UW students. It is highly unlikely that anything that goes on in this legislative session will change the sexual activity of UW students. The actions here can, however, greatly reduce the ability of UW students to act responsibly with regard to their fertility and controlling unplanned pregnancy.

The early studies of oral contraceptives, prior to their availability to the general public, were conducted in the 1950s among the women in Southeastern Kentucky. As is true today, the women of Appalachia embraced the idea of preventing pregnancy. They knew that limiting the size of their families was paramount if they had any hope of moving out of poverty. The federal government knew about the importance of family planning as it relates to reducing rates of poverty when it passed the Family Planning Services and Population Research Act of 1970 (Rooks, 1997). Just like those women in Southeastern Kentucky, students at the University of Wisconsin know that an unplanned pregnancy may have the effect of rendering them unable to finish school and subsequently earn a livable wage. I'm certain that the authors of this bill do not intend to contribute to the increasing drop-out rates from our nationally recognized university system.

In addition to reducing rates of poverty, decreasing the rate of unplanned pregnancy greatly reduces maternal morbidity and mortality. The United States has an embarrassingly high rate of maternal mortality (we rank somewhere around 21st in the world). At the present time, the risks associated with pregnancy far outweigh the risks of oral contraceptives, including emergency contraception. Additionally, we know that the rates of pregnancy termination rise in the absence of access to reliable contraception. Because illegal abortion is a major contributor to maternal mortality whenever there is poor access to contraception and legal abortion, the availability of these has played an important role in reducing high rates of maternal mortality (Rooks, 1997). At a time when access to legal abortion services is under attack, we cannot afford to reduce the availability of contraceptive services.

Please remember that passage of AB 343 will do nothing to change the sexual activity of UW students. It will only serve to impair their ability to prevent unplanned and unwanted pregnancies.

Thank you for your consideration of our concerns.

Respectfully submitted,

Kathryn Osborne, MSN, CNM
Wisconsin Chapter of the American College of Nurse–Midwives

relationship between the governor and the ACNM lobbyist also proved to be beneficial, and with the support of the assembly and the senate, there was no concern about the governor signing the bill. The day the governor signed the bill was a wonderful day in April. The bill was signed in the hometown of our lead Republican assembly sponsor. The press was invited, and it was a great day for midwifery.

Summary

As has been demonstrated throughout this chapter, the practice of midwifery is in fact inherently political. Midwives can and, through hard work, do, affect health care policies and the future of the midwifery profession. Laws impacting women's health consumers and providers are commonplace and ever changing. Politically active midwives can work to change and refine laws to benefit midwifery practice and improve the lives of women and their families throughout the world. Political action and activity need to be incorporated into the life and practice of all midwives.

Table 7–3 For Your Professional Files

State practice act
Federal regulations governing practice
Medicare and Medicaid regulations
Requirements for direct access and third-party reimbursement
ACNM Legislative Handbook

References

Ament, L. (2004). Generation of health care policy: Using evidence to implement change for a nurse–midwifery practice. *Policy, Politics, and Nursing Practice, 5*(1), 34–40.

American College of Nurse–Midwives. (2003). *State and federal policy agenda 2005–2006.* Retrieved May 26, 2005, from http://www.midwife.org/legis/agenda.cfm

American College of Nurse–Midwives. (2004). *State fact sheets.* Retrieved May 24, 2005, from http://www.midwife.org/legislative.cfm?id=186

American College of Nurse–Midwives. (2005). *Division of women's health policy and leadership.* Retrieved May 24, 2005, from http://www.midwife.org/about.cfm?id-58

Bodenheimer, T., & Grumbach, K. (1998). *Understanding health policy: A clinical approach* (2nd ed.). New York: McGraw-Hill.

Boufford, J., & Lee, P. (2002). Health policy making: The role of the federal government. In M. Danis, C. Clancy, & L. Churchill (Eds.), *Ethical dimensions of health policy* (pp. 157–183). New York: Oxford University Press.

Capps, L. (1998). Vital signs: Nurses' voices needed in the halls of Congress. *American Journal of Nursing, 98*(9), 80.

Cooney, P. (2004). Four easy steps to becoming more politically active. *Quickening, 35*(5), 9.

Deber, R., & Williams, P. (2003). Government, politics, and stakeholders in the United States and Canada. In P. Leatt & J. Mapa (Eds.), *Government relations in the health care industry* (pp. 3–21). Westport, CT: Praeger.

Emanuel, E. (2002). Patient v. population: Resolving the ethical dilemmas posed by treating patients as members of populations. In M. Danis, C. Clancy, & L. Churchill (Eds.), *Ethical dimensions of health policy* (pp. 227–245). New York: Oxford University Press.

Emanuel, E.J., & Emanuel, L.L. (1996). What is accountability in health care? *Annals of Internal Medicine, 124,* 229–239.

Epstein, A. (1996). Performance reports on quality, prototypes, problems, and prospects. *New England Journal of Medicine, 333,* 57–61.

Fact Monster. (2005). *How a bill becomes a law.* Retrieved May 26, 2005, from http://www.factmonster.com/ipka/A0770454.html

Federation of State Medical Boards of the United States, Inc. *Assessing scope of practice in health care delivery: Critical questions in assuring public access and safety.* Retrieved May 29, 2006, from http://www.fsmb.org/pdf/2005_grpol_scope_of_practice.pdf

Foster, B. (1998). *Schmoozing: How to be politically effective.* A primer from the American College of Nurse–Midwives. Retrieved May 26, 2005, from http://www.midwife.org/legis/display.cfm?id=201

Gesse, T. (1991). Political participation behaviors of nurse–midwives. *Journal of Nurse-Midwifery, 36*(3), 184–191.

Hartley, H. (2002). The system of alignments challenging physician professional dominance: An elaborated theory of countervailing powers. *Sociology of Health and Illness, 24*(2), 178–207.

Hartley, H. (2003). Impact of health policy at state and local levels: The case of certified nurse-midwifery. *Nursing and Health Policy Review, 2*(1), 25–34.

Kingdon, J. (1995). *Agendas, alternatives and public policies* (2nd ed.). New York: Harper Collins.

Kingdon, J. (2002). The reality of public policy making. In M. Davis, C. Clony, & S. Churchill (Eds.), *Ethical dimensions of health policy* (pp. 97–116). New York: Oxford University Press.

Leatt, P., & Mapa, J. (Eds.). (2003). *Government, politics, and stakeholders in the United States and Canada.* Westport, CT: Praeger.

Leavitt, J. (1986). *Brought to bed: Childbearing in Amreica, 1750 to 1950.* New York: Oxford University Press.

Longest, B. (2003). Strategic management and public policy. In P. Leatt & J. Mapa (Eds.), *Government, politics, and stakeholders in the United States and Canada* (pp. 23–47). Westport, CT: Praeger.

Mechanic, D., & Reinhard, S. (2002). Contributions of nurses to health policy: Challenges and opportunities. *Nursing and Health Policy Review, 1*(1), 7–15.

Milio, N. (1984). The realities of policymaking: Can nurses have an impact? *Journal of Nursing Administration, 14*(3), 18–23.

Oberlander, J., & Brown, L. (2002). Health policy and state initiatives. In M. Danis, C. Clancy, & L. Churchill (Eds.), *Ethical dimensions of health policy* (pp. 184–201). New York: Oxford University Press.

Project Vote-Smart. (2004). *Government 101: How a bill becomes law.* Retrieved May 26, 2005, from http://www.vote-smart.org/resource_govt101_02.php

Reed, A. (1997). Strategies for influencing state policy. A tip sheet for ACNM Legislative Contacts, p. 7.

Rodwin, J. (1994). Consumer protection and managed care: The need for organized consumers. *Health Affairs*, 15, 110–123.

Robinson, J. (1994). *The corporate practice of medicine:* Competition and innovation in health care. Berkeley, CA: University of California Press.

Shannon, T. (Ed.). (2004). *Health care policy.* Oxford, England: Rowman & Littlefield.

Wakefield, M. (2004). 2004: A federal and state health odyssey. *Nursing Economics, 22*(1), 47–48.

Wong, S. (1999). Reimbursement to advanced practice nurses (APNs) through Medicare. *Image: Journal of Nursing Scholarship, 31*(2), 167–173.

World Health Organization. (2000). *The world health report 2000—Health systems: Improving performance.* Retrieved July 3, 2006, from http://www.who.int/whr/2000/en/index.html

CHAPTER 8

Midwifery Scope of Practice

William F. McCool, CNM, PhD, FACNM and
Marion McCartney CNM, BSN, FACNM

Learning Objectives

1. Discuss the *Standards for the Practice of Midwifery*, how they were developed, and how they have evolved over time.
2. Describe guidelines for practice: purpose, use, and development.
3. Identify additional factors that define scope of practice.
4. Understand the historical background for the development of the *Core Competencies for Basic Midwifery Practice*.

Paramount to the practice of any health care provider is an awareness of the individual professional's scope of practice. The defining of this scope occurs on several levels, including the professional, governmental, and individual. Understanding and adhering to one's scope of practice is an important element in the protection of recipients of health care practices, as well as in the safeguarding of health care professionals themselves. A person with a broken bone does not seek care from a psychologist any more than an individual suffering with depression hopes to benefit from being cared for by an orthopedic surgeon. The prevention of such inappropriate and potentially dangerous scenarios is the very reason why defining one's scope of practice is vital to the well-being of individuals seeking health care, and is addressed accordingly by professional organizations, governmental legislators and regulators, educational programs, and individual health care facilities and practices. In midwifery education, students learn from the start of their training that safety is vital to offering quality midwifery care, and understanding one's scope of practice is a large part of achieving this.

Definition

How is scope of practice defined? In any health care profession in the United States, this is manifested through input on several different levels. These include:

- A professional organization's delineation of what is thought to be the area of health care in which its members should practice, and the extent to which this should occur. For example, in the midwifery profession, health care practices are limited to working with women and newborns, and do not include such practices as being the lead clinician performing a cesarean section or hysterectomy.
- A legislative body's passing practice laws establishing mechanisms by which to regulate health care practices in order to offer protection for the citizens of the region the legislator oversees. In the United States, this most typically occurs at the level of state governments, which license health care practitioners and define the regulations by which they may practice. Because this is state-regulated, the scope of practice can be different from one state to the next.
- Federal agencies presenting guidelines for the offering of care based on:
  - Federally funded scientific research that has examined the efficacy of health care practices, leading to the presentation of evidence about the maintaining or abandoning of practices based on their safety and cost. This research has originated or been funded by such research agencies as the National Institutes of Health (NIH) and various federal health services agencies.
  - Evaluations of health care costs as they apply to federal programs, such as Medicare and Medicaid, that help pay for the health care of many Americans and while doing so, indirectly establish guidelines for reimbursement from third-party payers/private insurers. The Health Care Financing Administration (HCFA), which administers the Medicare and Medicaid programs, has done much to define scope of practice in health care because of its reviews of individual practices and decisions about whether or not to fund them.
- Third-party payers, or health care insurance agencies, deciding for cost reasons which practitioners will be reimbursed for which procedures. In midwifery, this often has led historically to curtailment of practice because of the unwillingness of an insurer to reimburse midwives for services that they have been trained to offer (e.g., gynecological procedures). Thus, even though a midwife's training and experience may encompass a routine procedure that falls well within the individual's scope of practice, such as insertion of an intrauterine device, the inability for the midwife to be reimbursed for this service can result in an unnecessarily limited scope of practice.
- Individual health care facilities, such as hospitals, ambulatory clinics, and private health care practices, establishing practice guidelines by which individual professionals working within these institutions must conduct their offering of health care. These guidelines have been known by a variety of names, including "practice protocols" or "clinical practice guidelines," and are usually established and routinely reviewed by a committee composed of clinicians familiar with the health care practices being defined, or as in the case of individual private practices, by the affected clinicians themselves. In terms of written documentation, clinical practice guidelines are the most accessible means of defining an individual practitioner's scope of practice.
- Litigation proceedings resulting in decisions that set precedents for how care needs to be offered, even when that care may not be supported with evidence from scientific research. As an example, this level of influence on the scope of health care practice in

obstetrics can be seen with the persistent use of routine continual fetal monitoring during normal labors, despite evidence that shows this practice can result in increased morbidity (Thacker, Stroup, & Chang, 2001). Concern by practitioners of not being viewed as vigilant enough in the offering of care, should any litigation occur, can contribute to the use of unfavorable practices such as continual fetal monitoring.

- Practitioners themselves deciding on an individual basis which practices they are comfortable performing within the scope of what they have learned. Many midwives recognize this contribution to one's scope of practice as "the circle of safety" (Burst, 2000) learned while in midwifery school, and it involves such matters as each clinician's own ethics, personal beliefs, level of confidence in practice, and physical well-being or limitations. For example, a midwife may personally be opposed to abortion, and thus would decide not to be involved in offering care that required such a procedure.

Scope of Practice for CNMs and CMs in the United States

For certified nurse–midwives (CNMs) and certified midwives (CMs) in the United States, defining scope of practice can begin by seeking information from the American College of Nurse–Midwives (ACNM). The Department of Professional Services at the ACNM is often asked questions regarding the scope of practice of midwives, such as:

> *"What is the scope of practice of a midwife?"*
>
> *"Is it within the scope of practice for a midwife to _____?"*

In answering questions such as these, two essential ACNM documents, the *Core Competencies for Basic Midwifery Practice* and *Standards for the Practice of Midwifery*, provide the foundation for defining the CNMs/CMs' scope of practice in the United States. (These two documents, as well as additional resources that can be useful in responding to these questions, are listed in the References at the end of this chapter.)

Core Competencies

A key element in recognizing and understanding one's scope of practice is to become aware of the basic knowledge inherent to one's profession. In order for safe health care to be offered, each practitioner must first learn the key elements of their particular craft and be able to apply them in a helpful manner. Likewise, the general public must have confidence that the health care practitioners with whom they are working have the basic knowledge and training that are intrinsic to the care being offered. In the midwifery profession overseen in the United States by the ACNM, the skills required to safely begin practicing as a CNM/CM are described in the *Core Competencies for Basic Midwifery Practice*. First created in 1978, this document was developed to describe the fundamental knowledge, skills, and behaviors expected of a new practitioner who graduates from an ACNM accredited school (Avery, 2005). The focus, as highlighted in the title, has been on delineating those elements of offering midwifery care that are needed to begin *basic* midwifery practice.

Historical Background

Although the notion of a profession expressing the basic knowledge practitioners should have with regard to clinical practice arose mostly in the latter half of the 20th century, educational programs in the health care fields have long established basic knowledge that graduates should possess, and this has been reflected in the presentation of curricula. In medicine, formal medical colleges in the United States began with the founding of the College of Philadelphia in 1765 by, among others, Benjamin Franklin. Early medical schools depended on apprenticeship training in the clinical arena (Papa & Harasym, 1999), but began students' education with several months of classroom instruction. Specific topics that were covered were determined primarily by lecture notes of the faculty, and included anatomy, physiology, surgery, and obstetrics-gynecology (Papa & Harasym, 1999). The extent of what was taught varied considerably from one school to the next, and was dependent on the faculty present at each institution.

By the mid-19th century, medical textbooks began to be published and used in medical education. They did much to bring some standardization to health care education and practice, since different institutions and their faculty were now often teaching from the same text of knowledge, and becoming less dependent on individuals' notes (Papa & Harasym, 1999). However, medical education in the United States remained highly variable and inconsistent, and led to reforms in the latter part of the 19th century meant to, among other goals, bring greater standardization to the knowledge graduates of medical schools should have. It was at this time that most allopathic* medical schools moved into university settings, placed greater emphasis on a discipline-specific (rather than generalist) approach to learning, and began to lengthen the amount of time required to be educated as a physician (Papa & Harasym, 1999). Also relevant to the later notion of core competencies was the push at this time to move away from the practice of students memorizing notes and facts, and instead having them become independent thinkers who could critically analyze a situation, rather than simply view it based solely on prior knowledge (Papa & Harasym, 1999). Thus, the curriculum, like later competencies, would not be a listing of facts or practices to be learned, but instead general concepts requiring attention as part of one's education. To simply present lists of specific information to be memorized would eventually have become daunting as medical knowledge increased, and would have allowed for a limited amount of analytical thinking.

As the 19th century came to a close, allopathic schools of medicine were utilizing increasingly similar curricula, and beginning to graduate similar practitioners of medicine. However, allopaths were far from being the only clinicians offering health care in the United States. In addition to nursing, which became formalized as a health care profession in the mid-1800s, there existed midwives, homeopaths, botanists, and a number of differ-

---

* *Allopathy* refers to the practice of conventional, or "regular," medicine that is most commonly practiced today by medical doctors (MDs). Although some medical historians disagree with the use of this term to describe the medical model, it historically has linked modern physicians with their predecessors who came to approach health care delivery as a system dependent on tradition and the use of scientific method to dictate practice. In this chapter, *allopathy* will be used to describe the practice of physicians following the medical model of care.

ent practitioners who offered a variety of remedies and lifestyle activities to help improve health. The practice of health care was highly individualized, with clinical practice varying considerably from one geographic region to the next, one culture to the next, one philosophical belief system to the next, and one educational background to the next. And even within the diverse philosophies and beliefs of health care, actual clinical practice varied considerably from one individual clinician to the next (Wertz & Wertz, 1989).

Early in the 20th century, this lack of consistency of practice, and the guidelines by which to do so, began to change. The allopathic physicians, or "regular doctors," were almost exclusively composed of individual men from the wealthier classes of the time. Their styles of learning and practice, which had at one time been as erratic as that of other disciplines, was increasingly becoming influenced by a rational, scientific form of disease prevention and health care that originated in Europe with the acceptance of germ theory. Wealthy allopaths training in German medical schools returned to the United States in the late 19th and early 20th centuries to promote the growth of expanded medical education with curricula that integrated clinical education with basic laboratory science (Ehrenreich & English, 1973).

Although the training and care of "regular doctors" was undergoing an unprecedented focus on a standardized form of education and practice, the United States was in the midst of social change brought on by the Industrial Revolution. Financial empires were being built by such entrepreneurs as Vanderbilt, Carnegie, and Rockefeller. The amount of wealth amassed by these individuals was staggering, and led to a number of social changes in the United States, including the growth of organized philanthropy. "Foundations" backed by such prominent capitalists as Carnegie and Rockefeller set about altering the social and cultural landscape of the country to suit the belief systems of the wealthy who supported these benevolent organizations (Friedman & McGarvie, 2003). One of the top priorities of these early foundations was to reform the seemingly chaotic nature of health care in the United States. A standardized, respectable practice of medicine was sought, and this coincided with the promotion of the European style of scientific training that was becoming more popular with allopaths in the United States.

At the start of the 20th century, large amounts of foundation money were put forward to help support medical education. The question was, however, which schools following which curricula should receive the industrialists' funds. To answer this, the Carnegie Corporation sent an employee, Abraham Flexner, on a national tour of health care schools that existed at that time. In 1910, the Flexner Report was released, and in it the author argued that philanthropists should only support the allopathic route to health care practice, originally promoted in the United States at Johns Hopkins University, because Flexner believed this form of academic medical education was the most beneficial to ill people. To critics, Flexner's choice was a forgone conclusion, because the practitioners of allopathy were from the same social class as the philanthropists, and like their benefactors, were almost exclusively white and male (Ehrenreich & English, 1973).

Among a number of changes brought about by the Flexner Report, including the near elimination of nonallopathic forms of health care practices (discussed later in the chapter under "Standards of Practice"), was the call for standardization of medical education according to the principles of allopathy. The move by medical schools in the latter half of the

19th century toward a consistent core of education across all training institutions received a significant boost from this 1910 report. Americans became increasingly able to identify that allopathically trained physicians were practicing according to a standardized approach to health care, no matter what school or region of the country they came from. Although several additional major changes in medical education were made during the 20th century, including the introduction of organ systems–based curricula in the 1950s and problem-based curricula in the 1970s (Papa & Harasym, 1999), the basic notion of a standardized basis for all medical education continues to be a major result of the Flexner Report.

Long before the release of the Flexner Report, the profession of nursing also had begun addressing the issue of standardized education. The era of modern nursing began in the United States during the Civil War of 1861–1865 (Kalisch & Kalisch, 2003). Pressed into service by the needs of the thousands of wounded and sick from the war, women in the North both volunteered and were paid to assist in the care of soldiers as they were brought off battlefields to hospitals. Initially trained by surgeons who ran the hospitals, the nurses were beholden in most institutions to strict rules of work and behavior established by the male surgeons. However, there was no formal standardization of training, which varied from one hospital to the next. The situation was even less formalized in the South, where societal prejudices against women working in such roles as nursing limited the number of volunteers willing to endure the lack of welcome they received at most hospitals (Kalisch & Kalisch, 2003).

Following the Civil War, individuals trained as nurses pushed for the establishment of formal schools of nursing in the United States. Although there had been some training pro-grams of nurses and midwives in the late 18th and early 19th centuries, such as New York Hospital and the Philadelphia Lying-In Charity, the first formal training schools for nurses did not open until the 1870s. These early professional nursing schools had established cur-ricula, often based on the work and educating of nurses in England by Florence Nightingale. However, classes were initially taught informally by physicians, and nursing textbooks did not become readily available until the last years of the 19th century. Early curricula for nursing students was focused more on behavior and dress than on theory and practice (Kalisch & Kalisch, 2003).

With the growth of hospitals and the increasing role for nurses in offering health care came a recognition by superintendents of nursing training schools of the need to better de-fine the profession and to standardize what nursing students learn. Toward this end, the American Society of Superintendents of Training Schools for Nursing, later named the National League of Nursing, was founded in 1893 (Fondiller, 1999). Among the goals es-tablished by this organization, primary was the establishment and maintenance of a uni-versal standard for educating nurses.

In part because nursing became a complementary function of medicine, allowing physi-cians to diagnose and prescribe while nurses carried out the actual implementation of care, the nursing profession grew considerably throughout the 20th century, along with hospi-tals and the practice of modern medicine itself (Ehrenreich & English, 1973). Along with that growth came a desire among nursing leaders to maintain standardization of nursing education and practice, which has been promoted by the use of nursing textbooks, standard examinations upon graduation, and ongoing incorporation of nursing research into the cur-ricula of nursing schools.

Midwifery's Core Competencies

Although midwifery had been present in the United States long before its founding as a nation, the profession was almost exclusively learned empirically, with little or no formal education available to the women practicing as midwives. What formal education was available regarding women's health was open only to wealthy males who were training in European-styled medical schools (Ehrenreich & English, 1973). And as stated previously, until the 20th century there was limited standardization in what was being taught regarding obstetric and gynecological care, or medical care in general.

At the start of the 20th century, the work of midwives faced a pivotal challenge from the medical establishment. The status of women in general, including midwives' image as health care providers, reached an all-time low at the turn of the century (Swenson, 1968). Social forces during the Victorian era and the Industrial Revolution rendered women exploitable in the workforce and at home, yet powerless in social and political circles. Within this climate, midwives were increasingly labeled as ignorant and incompetent, and their practice of helping women deliver at home became viewed as unsafe when compared to hospital deliveries in the presence of physicians and nurses, even though morbidity and mortality statistics were similar in both arenas (Varney et al., 2004). Because most midwives were of poorer, uneducated classes, even if there was a desire to define and standardize midwifery care at this time, there was no manner in which midwives could communicate and unite at a level needed to accomplish such a task.

The abysmal status of women's health care, especially with regard to pregnancy and birth, began to receive the attention of the public health community and local and federal governments in the first two decades of the 20th century. The Children's Bureau was established by the federal government in 1912, and conducted studies that confirmed the dire status of maternal–child health in the United States. Despite efforts by the medical community, such as the Flexner Report described previously, to place blame for poor health statistics on health care groups other than the allopaths, advocates for improved maternity care lobbied for the formal education of traditional midwives, rather than their banishment. This led to the founding of such midwifery educational endeavors as the Bellevue School of Midwifery in New York City and the midwifery course at the Preston Retreat Hospital in Philadelphia (Varney et al., 2004). However, exactly what was taught at those institutions depended on the knowledge of the faculty involved, and as with medical schools at the time, did not conform to any defined national standards.

The increasing need for quality maternity care led to the introduction of nurse–midwifery into the country in the mid-1920s. Mary Breckinridge from Kentucky brought British-trained nurse–midwives to her home state to help improve health care for women in rural Appalachia. Meanwhile, in New York City, the Manhattan Midwifery School in 1925 and the Lobenstine Midwifery School in 1932 were opened to train graduate nurses in how to become midwives. The latter was created by the Maternity Center Association in New York with the goal of improving maternal–child care in the city, and was formally known as "The School of the Association for the Promotion and Standardization of Midwifery." This was the first public recognition of any need to standardize what midwifery care was, and grew in part from the positive results Breckinridge and the British-trained midwives were demonstrating in Kentucky with improving mothers' and babies' health (Varney et al., 2004).

A formal curriculum based on British nurse–midwifery training was established at the Lobenstine Midwifery School, and emphasized the particulars of antenatal, intrapartal, and postpartal care. Meanwhile, Breckinridge in Kentucky had been continuing her dependence on British-trained midwives for the running of the Frontier Nursing Service (FNS). With the advent of the Second World War, those loyal to Britain wanted to contribute to the war effort in Europe and left Kentucky. This led to the need for FNS in 1939 to establish a school in Kentucky, named the Frontier Graduate School of Midwifery. As with the Lobenstine Midwifery School in New York, the Frontier School had a curriculum based on the British nurse–midwifery educational system (Varney et al., 2004). Serendipitously, this meant that nurse–midwifery training in different regions of the United States was similar in its content and approach, thus moving toward a standardized description of what a formally trained midwife was and what skills she had learned. The roots of future core competencies were being established.

Nurse–midwifery as a profession began to grow, and in the 1940s and 1950s, seven additional nurse–midwifery education programs were opened. The expansion in numbers of graduate nurse–midwives led to the founding in 1955 of a national organization, the American College of Nurse–Midwifery (ACNM, which was later renamed the American College of Nurse–Midwives), to represent the interests of nurse–midwives in the United States. Included among the longstanding objectives of the organization have been the study, development, and evaluation of *standards* for midwifery care of women and infants and for midwifery education. This desire to standardize care and education led to such developments as official ACNM reviews of educational programs beginning in 1966 and the requirement of nurse–midwifery graduates to take a national certification examination, starting in 1971 (Carrington & Burst, 2005).

As the number of midwifery educational programs grew in the 1960s and early 1970s, so too did the variety of curricula being used by these programs. A task force established by the ACNM in 1973 reported on this diversity in curricula, and subsequent discussions by nurse–midwifery educators and leaders eventually led to a recommendation that a set of core competencies be developed that would be expected of all nurse–midwifery graduates in the United States. Created by the ACNM's Education Committee (1979), the *Core Competencies in Nurse–Midwifery: Expected Outcomes of Nurse–Midwifery Education* were approved in 1978 by the Board of Directors of the ACNM (Avery, 2005). For the first time in the history of midwifery in the United States, it was officially documented what skills and knowledge any clinician graduating from a nurse–midwifery program needed to have in order to safely practice. Since then the *Core Competencies* have been revised a total of four times (in 1985, 1992, 1997, and 2002) to reflect both historical developments and changes in the health care system (Avery, 2005). The curriculum in all ACNM Division of Accreditation (DOA) accredited education programs is based on the *Core Competencies*. They remain to this day a blueprint for the extent of knowledge and skills required for a beginning practitioner graduating from a nurse–midwifery program in the United States.

Realizing that practice would evolve and that individual and institutional differences would influence decisions regarding expanding practice beyond the *Core Competencies,* the ACNM developed *Guidelines for the Incorporation of New Procedures into Midwifery*

Practice in the early 1970s. In 2003, these guidelines were incorporated into the *Standards for the Practice of Midwifery* as Standard VIII (see below). They provide a mechanism for evaluating the need for a particular procedure, establishing a process for education, and evaluating and maintaining competency. The actual procedure for expanding one's scope of practice, such as learning to be a first assistant at surgery, to use a vacuum extractor, or to perform colposcopies, is described in the ACNM document entitled "Expanded Midwifery Practice" (available at the ACNM website, http://www.acnm.org).

Standards of Practice

Essential to the safe practice of any health care clinicians, including midwives, are the standards by which they practice. Standards help to define the safe parameters by which individual practitioners are able to offer care, and play a major role in maintaining the safety of clients who receive this care. Clinical knowledge is vital for one to practice safely. Also vital is knowing when and how to apply that knowledge. Being cognizant of the standards of practice for one's profession does much to assist the clinician in providing safe and helpful care.

Standards of practice vary from one profession to the next, and depend on educational background and historical limits of practice. Yet, no matter what the profession, it has become an established tradition in modern health care delivery that all educated and licensed practitioners be held to a set of standards that are created, and periodically updated, to help guide the clinician in offering safe and effective care. These standards are usually established by the professional organization that represents a particular clinical profession, and in the case of CNMs and CMs in the United States, the *Standards for Practice* have been established by the ACNM (American College of Nurse-Midwives [ACNM], 2003).

Historical Background

As stated previously, prior to the 20th century the practice of health care in the United States was highly individualized, with great variety in clinical practices. A number of loosely organized styles or philosophies of practice did exist (e.g., midwifery, allopathy, homeopathy, and botany), but even within these groups, the concept of "standards of practice" did not exist in any formal sense, and there was little scientific or consistent basis on which such standards could be formed (Ehrenreich & English, 1973; Papa & Harasym, 1999).

By the start of the 20th century, matters began to change. The increasing use by allopaths of a scientific approach to understanding diseases and their cures led to greater consistency in how "regular doctors" were practicing. Meanwhile, the growth of philanthropic foundations during the Industrial Revolution (discussed previously) resulted in the search for standardized, respectable practices of medicine, which were identified by Flexner in 1910 as those institutions supporting allopathic medicine. It was not long before the effects of the Flexner Report were felt throughout the health care fields. With little to no financial backing, practitioners of disciplines other than allopathy soon struggled to maintain acceptable forms of education and practice (Ehrenreich & English, 1973).

Midwifery, which was an almost exclusively female practice that lacked any form of professional organization, faced an even more difficult task of survival than more organized groups such as homeopaths and botanists. Matters worsened when allopaths began to use their increasing wealth and status to introduce and support legislation that would ban health care practice by anyone other than graduates of their own educational institutions. The phrase "practicing medicine without a license" soon entered legal and social communities throughout the United States, forcing practitioners of a variety of previously accepted modalities, including midwifery, to practice incognito, or to abandon their profession altogether (Ehrenreich & English, 1973).

Although devastating in its effect on all but practitioners of allopathy, the Flexner Report did bring about a practice that continues today among most health care professions—the use of established standards of practice. For the first time in American health care, individuals claiming to be physicians were expected to be educated in a certain discipline (in this case, allopathy), and to practice according to principles established by experienced clinicians and educators in that discipline. Some of the first sets of standards were established in 1919, not by physician groups, but by hospitals in the United States. However, the drive for these standards was led at that time by the American College of Surgeons (Bowman, 1920) and stood to benefit those professionals, namely allopathic physicians, whose philosophy of care was the basis of practice in most American hospitals. Eventually, individual physicians' groups followed suit and established standards of practice for the medical specialties that they represented. The American College of Obstetricians and Gynecologists (ACOG) was established in 1951, and in 1959 issued its first edition of *The Manual of Standards in Obstetric-Gynecologic Practice* (Mengert, 1977).

Interestingly, the nursing profession was cognizant of the need for standards of care even prior to the release of the Flexner Report, but linked these standards to the actual licensing of nurses by individual states. The first practice act in the United States was established in North Carolina in 1903 (Robertson & Sanders, 2005), and set the standards by which nurses in that state were to practice. Within 20 years, all states had their own individual practice acts, with many actually defining exactly what a nurse could or could not do (Robertson & Sanders, 2005). Eventually, national nursing organizations began to set standards for nursing subspecialties, producing more general national guidelines for particular types of nursing care. The Nurses Association of the American College of Obstetricians and Gynecologists (NAACOG), founded in 1969 and later renamed the Association of Women's Health, Obstetric and Neonatal Nurses (AWHONN), released its first edition of the *Manual of Standards of Practice* in 1974 (Wohlert, 1979).

Midwifery's Standards of Practice

The survival of midwifery in the United States following the damage to the profession initiated by the Flexner Report was in large part due to the establishment of nurse–midwifery care in the 1920s, both in Kentucky and New York City. From the outset, nurse–midwives sought to offer care that was based on formal education and training similar to that found in the profession of midwifery in England. Early in its existence as a profession, nurse–midwifery in the United States was guided by such groups as the Frontier Nursing

Service and the Association for the Promotion and Standardization of Midwifery in New York (Dawley & Burst, 2005). Eventually, a group of nurse–midwives brought together in 1944 by Hattie Hemschemeyer, director of the midwifery education program at the Maternity Center Association in New York, expressed the need for a national midwifery organization that would, among other things, "develop and maintain standards for nurse–midwifery practice and supervision" (Dawley, 2005). This initiative led to the founding that year of an autonomous section for nurse–midwifery in the National Organization of Public Health Nurses (NOPHN).

The dissolution of NOPHN in 1952 left nurse–midwives without an inclusive national organization, and led to a call from Sister Theophane Shoemaker, a Medical Mission Sister and nurse–midwife, and Hattie Hemschemeyer for nurse–midwives to meet in Chicago in 1954 to reopen discussions about the formation of a national nurse–midwifery organization. Members of a newly established Committee on Organization, whose work soon led to the formation in 1955 of the ACNM, drafted several statements, including those that addressed standards for both the practice and education of nurse–midwives. By 1966, the organization more formally addressed standards of practice by publishing a document entitled *Functions, Standards, and Qualifications for the Practice of Nurse–Midwifery*. To accompany these guidelines, in 1969 the ACNM also published *Standards for a Nurse–Midwifery Service* to help identify safe and effective practice characteristics for running a midwifery service (Dawley & Burst, 2005).

The *Functions, Standards, and Qualifications for the Practice of Nurse–Midwifery* document was revised in 1975 and again in 1983. Eventually, the document's name was changed to the *Standards for the Practice of Nurse–Midwifery,* which was updated in 1987 and 1993. In 2003, the document was revised again, and has since been called *Standards for the Practice of Midwifery* (ACNM, 2003). Currently, there are eight general standards described, and just as *Core Competencies* are meant to establish what midwives need to know at the time of graduation, the *Standards for Practice* are meant to guide midwives in practice throughout their professional careers. They contribute significantly to each midwife's recognition of her scope of practice.

Additional Factors Defining Scope of Practice

Although the *Core Competencies* and the *Standards for Practice* have perhaps the greatest overall influence on defining a midwife's scope of practice, several additional factors play a role. These include:

1. *State laws and regulations:* Although the practice of midwifery by CNMs is legal in all 50 states, the extent to which a midwife can practice varies from one state to the next, and can obviously change with time as laws and regulations are altered or created. Typically, a state law defines in general terms who can practice health care and is therefore eligible for a license to do so, and then specific guidelines are determined by a regulatory board that consists mostly of experts within the health care field being regulated. Unfortunately for midwives, few states actually have boards of midwifery, and in most states midwives' practice is regulated by boards of nursing or medicine. State laws and regulations that define the scope of practice

of a midwife are addressed in two ACNM publications available from the ACNM Resource Catalog: *Nurse–Midwifery Today: A Handbook of State Laws and Regulations* (ACNM, 2002), and *Direct Entry Midwifery: A Summary of State Laws and Regulations* (ACNM, 2001). Some state laws explicitly reference the ACNM standards, thereby permitting advanced practice procedures consistent with the guidelines.

2. *Federal agencies:* The federal government plays a significant role in defining scope of practice through:

   a. Federally funded scientific research and training programs, primarily through the Department of Health and Human Services (DHHS), which reports on the latest medical research findings and helps fund educational programs and clinical care sites. By suggesting treatment regimens for particular illnesses (e.g., "Sexually Transmitted Diseases Treatment Guidelines" published regularly by the Centers for Disease Control and Prevention [CDC]) or funding federal health clinics in underserved areas, DHHS is able to define, and possibly limit, the practice of health care practitioners.

   b. Federal programs, such as Medicare and Medicaid, that help pay for the health care of many Americans. In establishing guidelines and spending limits for reimbursement of clinicians and institutions for care delivered, the federal government, through the Health Care Financing Administration (HCFA), can put limits on the amount and type of care that can be offered. For example, the federal Medicaid program will not pay for abortion care, thus putting financial limitations on those practitioners, including midwives, who would be able to offer that form of care. The federal government also plays a large role in the reimbursement practices of third-party payers/private insurers, who often use federally funded health care as a benchmark for the practices they will fund, and for the amount of funding they will offer.

3. *Third-party payers:* Health care insurance agencies, which are private companies requiring profits for solvency, will often make decisions about what services to pay for based on a number of factors, including cost and the recommendations of medical personnel within the companies. The decisions of payment made by insurance companies can alter individual practitioners' scopes of practice, limiting choices of care to certain procedures, or even certain personnel. For example, historically, midwives have been excluded from some insurers as practitioners eligible for payment for reasons that often go unexplained (Goldsmith, 2004). Actions such as these point to the need for midwives to be professionally involved in such matters as sitting on advisory boards for insurers, keeping abreast of insurance industry policies, and lobbying for change when policies restrict the care that can be offered to women.

4. *Health care facilities:* Hospitals, ambulatory clinics, and private health care practices usually maintain or require *clinical practice guidelines*, or *practice protocols,* which set parameters by which clinicians within the facility are required to practice. In addition, the *Standards for the Practice of Midwifery* (ACNM, 2003) are

clear about the need for developing practice guidelines. Specifically, Standard V states that "midwifery care is based upon knowledge, skills, and judgments which are reflected in written practice guidelines." Some guidelines can be quite detailed, such as guidelines often found at family planning clinics (e.g., Planned Parenthood), whereas others are developed using general suggestions that allow for more flexibility in management and decision making.

No matter what the type of clinical guidelines, it has become increasingly vital for all practitioners to work under a formal set of parameters, with many publications currently available to serve as prototypes for establishing guidelines. Though the ACNM publishes a number of clinical bulletins, clinical practice statements, and handbooks that can assist midwives in the development of clinical practice guidelines, the ACNM does not publish specific clinical practice guidelines. Rather, individual midwives and/or practices establish specific guidelines to describe the parameters for midwifery management, physician management, and collaborative management that are appropriate for the individual clinician and practice setting. Practice guidelines usually are established for each specialty area, which include but are not limited to antepartum, intrapartum, postpartum/newborn, and gynecology/family planning.

The ACNM is often asked for guidelines regarding client selection and management (e.g., At what gestational age may a midwife care for a patient? or Must a client with twins [or diabetes or any number of conditions] be collaboratively managed or referred?) Such decisions—and the development of guidelines that address such decisions—are best made by the individual midwifery practice. In defining their scope of practice and the populations served, individual midwives will consider many factors, including:

- The clinical setting in which care is provided
- The skills and expertise of the individual midwife or midwives
- The skills and expertise of the consultant physician(s)
- Legal parameters under which they practice

It should be noted that in addition to the recommendations or requirements of many health care institutions and organizations such as the ACNM, regulators, accreditors, and insurance companies will not approve of a clinical practice that is without written guidelines for practitioners.

5. *Litigation:* Outcomes or findings from legal cases that involve health care offered by a practitioner can do much toward defining scope of practice. This defining can occur on a legal, professional, or personal level. Legally, a decision of a case can set legal precedent, or can lead to a change in legislation. Professionally, after having been named in a legal case or decision, a practitioner may be unable to obtain malpractice insurance, thus severely limiting or ending one's scope of practice. Being involved in a litigation case, especially as a defendant, can lead to a practitioner altering the way in which health care is delivered, no matter what the outcome of the case being heard (Guidera & McCool, 2003). Thus, one's practice,

including the scope of it, can change dramatically as a result of involvement in lit-igation. What can be particularly frustrating to a clinician is that the outcome may not necessarily be related to scientific evidence, but depend more on opinion and emotion. Yet the effect of the outcome is the same—a less-than-optimal level of practice.

6. *Individual practitioner's philosophy, ethics, experiences, and personality:* Health care clinicians bring to their practices individual philosophies and beliefs about how they perceive their scopes of practice. Even when the notion of an individual philosophy of care is not recognized or acknowledged, it is clear that clinicians' practices are influenced by their thoughts, experiences, morals, ethics, and confi-dence in their skills, along with what they have learned in formal education. So, for example, clinicians who are opposed to abortion will not include termination care in their scopes of practice. It is important, however, to note that all clinicians are expected to offer emergency care when necessary, no matter what their personal philosophy or beliefs.

Summary

It is clear that "scope of practice" is not simply defined or described, yet it is vital to the practice of midwifery and all health care delivery. Although it seems obvious that no cli-nician would practice in an unfamiliar field of care, it is important to formally recognize just what one's knowledge and skills are, especially for the benefit of the individuals who will be receiving the care offered. Although identifying one's scope of practice is not a sim-ple task, parameters by which to do so have been discussed in this chapter. For CNMs and CMs in the United States, these parameters can be identified through the ACNM's *Core Competencies* and *Standards for Practice*; governmental laws and agencies; third-party payers/insurers; practice guidelines established by institutions, organizations, or individual practitioners; litigation outcomes; and individual philosophies, ethics, experiences, and personalities. It is vital to midwives offering safe and beneficial care that the time is taken to define one's scope of practice and then to actually practice accordingly.

Acknowledgments

The authors would like to thank Sara Scott, SNM, from the University of Pennsylvania Midwifery Graduate Program, for her assistance in preparing this chapter.

Table 8–1 For Your Professional Files

Core Competencies for Basic Midwifery Practice (ACNM, 2002)
Direct Entry Midwifery: A Summary of State Laws and Regulations (ACNM, 2001)
Nurse-Midwifery Today: A Handbook of State Laws and Regulations (ACNM, 2002)
Standards for the Practice of Midwifery (ACNM, 2003)

References

American College of Nurse–Midwives. (2001). *Direct entry midwifery: A summary of state laws and regulations.* Retrieved September 30, 2005, from http://www.midwife.org

American College of Nurse–Midwives. (2002). *Nurse–midwifery today: A handbook of state laws and regulations.* Retrieved September 30, 2005, from http://www.midwife.org/legis/print.cfm?id=209

American College of Nurse–Midwives. (2003). *Standards for the practice of midwifery.* Retrieved September 30, 2005, from http://www.midwife.org/prof/display.cfm?id=138

American College of Nurse–Midwives. Education Committee. (1979). Core competencies in nurse–midwifery: Expected outcomes of nurse–midwifery education. *Journal of Nurse-Midwifery 24,* 32–36.

Avery, M. D. (2005). The history and evolution of the core competencies for basic midwifery practice. *Journal of Midwifery and Women's Health, 50,* 102–107.

Bowman, J. G. (1920). Hospital standardization series: General hospitals of 100 or more beds, report for 1919. *Bulletin of the American College of Surgeons, 4,* 3–36.

Burst, H. V. (2000). The circle of safety: A tool for clinical preceptors. *Journal of Midwifery and Women's Health, 45*(5), 408–410.

Carrington, B. W., & Burst, H. V. (2005). The American College of Nurse–Midwives' dream becomes reality: The Division of Accreditation. *Journal of Midwifery and Women's Health, 50,* 146–153.

Dawley, K. (2005). Doubling back over roads once traveled: Creating a national organization for nurse–midwifery. *Journal of Midwifery and Women's Health, 50,* 71–80.

Dawley, K., & Burst, H. V. (2005). The American College of Nurse Midwives and its antecedents: A historical time line. *Journal of Midwifery and Women's Health, 50,* 16–22.

Ehrenreich, B., & English, D. (1973). *Witches, midwives, and nurses—a history of women healers.* New York: Feminist Press.

Fondiller, S. H. (1999). One hundred years ago: Nursing education at the dawn of the 20th century. *Nursing and Health Care Perspectives, 20,* 286–288.

Friedman, L., & McGarvie, M. (Eds.). (2003). *Charity, philanthropy, and civility in American history.* New York: Cambridge University Press.

Goldsmith, J. (2004). Nurse–midwives encounter new roadblocks. *American Journal of Nursing, 104*(2), 25–26.

Guidera, M., & McCool, W. (2003, June). *When bad things happen to good midwives: Recovering from poor outcomes in midwifery practice, implications for practice and education.* Paper presented at the 48th Annual Meeting of the American College of Nurse–Midwives, Palm Desert, CA.

Kalisch, P., & Kalisch, B. (2003). *American nursing: A history* (4th ed.). Philadelphia, PA: Lippincott Williams & Wilkins.

King, T. (2000). Clinical boundaries: What parameters determine a midwife's scope of practice? *Journal of Midwifery and Women's Health, 45*(6), 448–449.

Mengert, W. (1977). *History of the American College of Obstetricians and Gynecologists: 1950–1970.* Chicago: American College of Obstetricians and Gynecologists.

Papa, F. J., & Harasym, P. H. (1999). Medical curriculum reform in North America, 1765 to the present: A cognitive science perspective. *Academic Medicine, 74,* 154–164.

Roberts, J., & Sedler, K. D. (1997). The core competencies for basic midwifery practice: Critical ACNM document revised. *Journal of Nurse Midwifery 42,* 371–372.

Robertson, L., & Sanders, S. (2005). *Ohio standards of safe nursing practice.* Retrieved September 30, 2005, from http://www.nursingceu.com/courses/65/index_nceu.html

Swenson, N. (1968). The role of the nurse–Midwife on the health team as viewed by the family. *Bulletin of the American College of Nurse–Midwifery, 13,* 128–132.

Thacker, S., Stroup, D., & Chang, M. (2001). Continuous electronic heart rate monitoring for fetal assessment during labor. *Cochrane Database of Systematic Reviews, 2,* CD000063.

Varney, H., Kriebs, J., & Gegor, C. (2004). *Varney's midwifery* (4th ed.). Sudbury, MA: Jones and Bartlett.

Wertz, R., & Wertz, D. (1989). *Lying in: A history of childbirth in America* (2nd ed.). New Haven, CT: Yale University Press.

Wohlert, H. (1979). NAACOG—The first 10 years. *JOGN Nursing, 8,* 9–22.

CHAPTER 9

Practice Structure

Lynette Ament, RN, CNM, PhD, FACNM

Learning Objectives

1. Discuss various practice models.
2. Discuss advantages and disadvantages of various practice settings.
3. Evaluate strategies for seeking a position.
4. Review the components of an effective résumé.
5. Discuss effecting interview skills.
6. Identify key elements in marketing midwifery practice.
7. Identify the use of data sets in demonstrating your worth.

Whether you begin to seek your first midwifery position or your twenty-first, the first essential step is to do a self-inventory (Zaumeyer, 2003) (see **Table 9–1**). Begin by asking yourself some basic questions, such as what are your short- and long-term goals? Include both your personal and professional goals. In your answer to these questions consider what quality of life you seek. Does a large city with an active night life appeal to you? Can you envision yourself in a rural, close-knit community? Or is there somewhere in-between that would best provide what you are searching for? Can you see yourself in one setting over the short term and a different setting for somewhere to settle in?

Next, examine your philosophy of midwifery. What are the essential elements that compose your view of what midwifery means to you? Is it a specific type of care, such as a small practice where you follow your own clients from first visit through birth and beyond, or is it the type of care that is provided? This question may tie in very closely with your desired quality of life. Although you may envision a practice where you can provide constant continuity, a lifestyle that requires being on call 24 hours a day, 7 days a week may not be one you can support. You might be on the other end of the spectrum, where scheduled shifts within a practice that espouses minimal interventions and family-centered care works best for you. Anywhere in between you will find a practice that rotates call on a scheduled basis.

Table 9–1 Self-Inventory Guide

Personal and Professional Goals
  Short-term goals
  Long-term goals
Quality of Life
  Rural
  Urban
  Hours worked
Midwifery Philosophy
  Continuity of care vs. care provided
Strengths
  Clinical
  Administrative
Needs
  Economic
  Clinical

Adapted from Zaumeyer (2003).

The last step in the self-inventory is to identify your strengths and needs. What are your clinical abilities? Are you a new graduate with mentoring needs or are you a seasoned clinician who can manage more complicated diagnoses? Do you have administrative skills? This does not necessarily mean that you will seek out a position as a practice director, but it may mean that you are capable of accepting leadership responsibilities within the organization, such as chairing the quality assurance committee. Last, do you have needs for economic security that must be met?

The job market may not always allow for you to realize all of your goals in one position, but most likely there will be one position that will fulfill a majority of your needs. Although it is true that this position may not be where you will spend the next 20 years, by carefully examining your needs, strengths, and limits it will more surely assist you in finding satisfaction in the position.

Practice Settings

There are many options available to you in regards to practice settings (see **Table 9–2**). The options range from a large institutional setting to a small private practice. The range of midwifery services also varies, from full-scope practice to only prenatal care or gynecological care. The ACNM (American College of Nurse-Midwives [ACNM], 1997) position statement on practice settings states, "Every family has a right to a safe, satisfying childbirth experience, with respect for cultural variations, human dignity and the rights as consumers to freedom of choice and self-determination. The certified nurse–midwife and certified midwife may practice in a variety of settings including hospital, home and birth center. In any practice setting, provision for the safety of mother and baby is a primary concern."

There are many midwifery practices in institutional settings. Midwives practice in tertiary care facilities in practices owned by the institution itself, managed care entities, med-

---

Table 9–2 Practice Settings

Institution
   Hospital
      Tertiary care center
      University teaching hospital
      Community hospital
      Birth center
   Clinic
Home
Free-standing birth center
Family planning clinic
Private practice
University health service
Federally qualified community health center

---

ical schools, private or public midwifery practices, and midwifery faculty practices. Midwives also practice in small community hospitals. Typically, these settings offer full-scope midwifery care.

Certified nurse–midwives attended 7.6% of all births in 2003. Approximately 1% of CNM-attended births in the United States occur in the home setting (Centers for Disease Control and Prevention [CDC], 2005). There are several resources available to midwives wishing to learn more about home births or to establish a home birth practice (ACNM, 2003). Another 1.9% of CNM-attended births occur in freestanding birth centers (CDC, 2005). In the 2003 ACNM annual survey, 6.4% of members indicated they attend births in birth centers, and 3.7% indicated they attend births in the home (Schuiling, Sipe, & Fullerton, 2005). Besides freestanding birth centers, birth centers also exist within hospitals. The National Birth Center Study (Rooks et al., 1989) demonstrated that birth centers are safe alternatives to hospital deliveries for healthy women. For more information about birth centers, refer to the National Association of Childbearing Centers (NACC) at www.birthcenters.org.

Some midwives choose not to practice full scope midwifery and work in clinic or office settings. More CNMs/CMs are working in federally qualified community health centers, which may or may not offer full scope care. Private practices, university health centers, and family planning clinics are also settings that may offer only outpatient opportunities. The 2003 ACNM membership survey indicates that the majority of members (27.6%) are employed in hospitals/medical centers, 24.9% are employed in a physician group practice, 6.2% are employed in midwifery practices, and 4.7% are employed in community health centers (Schuiling et al., 2005).

Practice Models

Just as there are a variety of midwifery practice settings, there are a variety of practice models. Some midwives decide that they would like the autonomy of owning their own practice; others decide that an employment arrangement works best for them. There are successful, privately owned midwifery practices. Practices may be either solo-owned, owned with other midwives, or owned with other providers. Advantages of owning your own practice include autonomy of practice, such as deciding how many patients you will see and for how long (Buppert, 2004). You can also have greater control over quality issues, including who you employ. Disadvantages and barriers also exist when owning your practice. You will be responsible for all financial aspects of the practice, from establishing managed care contracts to paying for rent, supplies, and employees. You are also responsible for building and marketing the practice so that you have patients to see. Both the advantages and disadvantages have trade-offs; for example, managed care payments may not allow you the luxury of spending 2 hours with a new patient if you need reimbursement to cover expenditures.

Many midwives choose to enter into an employee/employer relationship. Some advantages to this model are obvious: You will receive an agreed upon income and do not have to oversee day-to-day business operations. Disadvantages may include less practice autonomy and control over work schedule. Hospitals, clinics, universities, and private practices are examples of employee/employer models.

Practice models involve more than just employment arrangements. You may choose to work in a practice with only midwives. Other types of practice models include faculty practices, midwife/physician models, midwife/nurse practitioner models, and interdisciplinary practices, such as in community health centers. **Table 9–3** compares and contrasts various practice models.

Physician arrangements are also a consideration when seeking a position. If you choose to work in an employee/employer model then typically the arrangement has already been established. The *2002 Joint Statement of Practice Relations between Obstetrician-Gynecologists and Certified Nurse–Midwives/Certified Midwives* states that "in those circumstances in which obstetrician-gynecologists and certified nurse–midwives/certified midwives collaborate in the care of women, the quality of those practices is enhanced by a working relationship characterized by mutual respect and trust as well as professional responsibility and accountability. When obstetrician-gynecologists and certified nurse–midwives/certified midwives col-

Table 9–3 Practice Models

Practice Model	Benefits	Disadvantages

Self-ownership	Autonomy of practice
	Quality control
	Employee control
		Obtaining managed care
		  contracts
		Financial responsibilities—rent
		  and payroll

Employee/employer	Consistent income Predetermined work hours	Less control over work schedule Lack of autonomy in practice
Midwife-owned practice	Philosophy of care Peer support	Managed care issues Need to find physician collaborator
Physician-owned practice	Physician collaboration Interdisciplinary care	Medical model of care Lack of autonomy in practice Isolation from midwifery colleagues
Community health center	Interdisciplinary care Care to vulnerable populations	Salary not as competitive as other markets May or may not be full scope

laborate, they should concur on a clear mechanism for consultation, collaboration and refer-ral based on the individual needs of each patient" (ACNM & American College of Obste-tricians and Gynecologists [ACOG], 2002). You should also be familiar with the practice act requirements for the state in which you choose to practice; you may be required to have physi-cian supervision and/or practice guidelines on file with the state.

Physician collaboration can be arranged through the employee/employer relationship and varies based on the arrangement. The physician may be the employer or the employee. Midwives also arrange for collaborative services with physicians on a contractual basis. Physicians may request a prearranged monetary reimbursement in return for a certain number of hours of service, and/or they may request third-party payer reimbursement for services provided.

Seeking a Position

There are many factors to consider when seeking and applying for a midwifery position. Once you have done a self-assessment of your goals and needs and have become knowl-edgeable about the state regulatory environment where you may be looking, you are ready to begin examining positions. There are multiple ways to seek a position. First, you could look for advertised openings. Venues for this include eMidwife, ads in *Quickening* and the *Journal of Midwifery & Women's Health*, professional recruiters, and newspaper and In-ternet ads. You may also find available positions through your local ACNM chapter or via networking. Many midwives seek positions in practices that have no advertised openings. If possible, before sending a cover letter and résumé, do your homework.

Examine the mission, vision, and philosophy of the organization and/or the practice. Many organizations and practices have web sites and this information may be accessible that way. It may appeal to you to work for a practice whose mission is to serve vulnerable populations. Other midwives may be attracted to the triad of missions of a teaching insti-tution: teaching, practice, and research. Other components of the organization that are es-sential for you to know about include the model of care delivery (for example, will you see the same patients as their primary care provider, or do all patients see all providers?), clin-ical programs offered (for example, are nutritional services, social services, or a diabetes clinic offered?), patient populations, and physician collaborative arrangements. If you are seeking a full-scope practice, knowing about the birth setting is essential, and the same questions should be asked of the birth setting. In addition, examine the community. What are the community resources available to the population that is served? What are the com-munity needs? Chapter 3 outlines data to be gathered in a community assessment; care-fully examine the data you collect.

Preparing Your Résumé

Your résumé is a reflection of your professional achievements, educational background, per-sonal accomplishments, and career goals. It is also a reflection of your overall profession-alism and your ability to market yourself. A résumé and cover letter may be your first contact with the prospective employer. Your résumé must be eye-catching and set you apart from other applicants.

First, a brief review about the difference between a résumé and a curriculum vitae. A résumé is a brief synopsis of education, professional experience, community service, and career goals. It may include your professional achievements, such as awards and honors. A curriculum vitae is a more detailed description of your presentations, publications, courses taught, and community service activities. A résumé should be no longer than one to two pages; a curriculum vitae may be several pages in length. A résumé is used to apply for a clinical position. A curriculum vitae is usually used to apply for academic or research positions, professional awards, or management positions.

Most résumés are written in reverse chronological order; that is, each category outlines achievements by year. The typical order of a résumé is as follows:

- Demographics
- Objective
- Education
- Certifications
- Experience
- Honors/awards
- Professional memberships
- Community service activities

Your objective should be brief and coincide with the position advertised. If you are forwarding your résumé to an employer without an advertised position, leave the objective broad rather than specific. For example, "to obtain a full-scope nurse–midwifery position" is broader than "to obtain a position in infertility care." Under experience, provide a short description of your overall responsibilities and include any special or leadership responsibilities. If you have established yourself in practice, you may wish to include three to four bullets under employment positions that list key accomplishments per position. Remember to use action verbs when describing these accomplishments, such as *implemented*, *developed*, and *established*.

If you are a new graduate or have held positions outside of midwifery, include those as appropriate. If you are a new graduate and worked as a nursing assistant in postpartum care or in another type of health agency, list it. If you are a new graduate and have just changed careers, include your most recent employment positions and bullet your salient accomplishments. If you are an experienced clinician and have held positions outside of midwifery but in health care or a related field, list them. The same holds true for the education category. If you are a new graduate you may list your clinical rotations and types of experiences under groupings by either course or rotation. If you list by course, remember to list the course name with the course number. You can include such information as type of setting (rural, urban, community hospital, birth center) and practice model (midwifery-owned practice, community health center). **Box 9–1** is an example of an effective résumé.

Cover Letter

Your cover letter that will accompany your résumé is also an important marketing tool. It must be concise yet capture the essence of your strengths and potential contributions to the

Box 9–1   Effective Résumé

Lynette Ament, CNM
123 Main Street
Rural, New Hampshire 54321
(123) 456-7890
Email: lynette.ament@internet.com

OBJECTIVE	To obtain a full scope nurse–midwifery position		
EDUCATION	PhD	University of Wisconsin–Milwaukee (Nursing; Minor Public Administration)	1996
	Certificate	University of Illinois–Chicago (Nurse–Midwifery)	1993
	MSN	Loyola University (Perinatal Nursing)	1987
	BSN	Loyola University	1982

CERTIFICATIONS

1993	CNM	ACNM Certification Council (#06480)

EXPERIENCE

2001–2004	Certified Nurse–Midwife, University of New Haven Women's Clinic, West Haven, CT
1998–2004	Certified Nurse–Midwife, per diem staff, Planned Parenthood of CT
1996–1997	Certified Nurse–Midwife, Associates for Women's Health, S.C., Waukegan, IL • 1st nurse–midwife in private practice in Lake County • 1st nurse–midwife with hospital privileges in Lake County
1994–1997	Certified Nurse–Midwife, Family Planning Division, Lake County Health Department, IL
1993–1997	Certified Nurse–Midwife, Clinical Instructor, University of Wisconsin–Madison Medical College, Sinai Samaritan Medical Center
1982–1995	Staff Nurse, Lake Forest Hospital, Ante-, Intra-, & Postpartum Care. Chairperson, OB Primary Care Committee, Lake Forest, IL

HONORS

2004	Fellow, American College of Nurse–Midwives
2003	DHHS Primary Care Policy Fellowship
2002	Kitty Ernst Award, American College of Nurse–Midwives
1990	Sigma Theta Tau International, Alpha Beta Chapter

ACTIVITIES

	American College of Nurse–Midwives
2000–2006	Chair, Policy Development and Evaluation Section
1995–2000	Political and Economic Affairs Committee
1995–2000	Professional Liability Committee
2004–Current	New Hampshire Board of Nursing, APRN Liaison Committee

REFERENCES	Available upon request

prospective practice. Your letter should begin by addressing a specific person, not "to whom it may concern." Do your homework and find out who that person is. If it is an advertised midwifery position send your cover letter and résumé to the listed contact. If you are sending your résumé and cover letter to a practice in an area where you would like to obtain a position, address it to the midwifery practice director (if there is one) or the practice director. Make sure you have the spelling and credentials correct. For example, if the person's credentials are ND, DNSc, or PhD address them as Dr., not Ms. or Mr.

The first paragraph should state the purpose of your letter; for example, you are writing to apply for a certain position or explore employment opportunities within the practice. If you are responding to an ad or someone personally referred you to the practice, state so in this paragraph. The next one to two paragraphs should highlight your strengths and experiences to demonstrate your qualifications for the position you are seeking. If you have experience with vulnerable populations, community health centers, are fluent in a foreign language, or have done volunteer work with similar populations state so here. Last, close your letter with a succinct paragraph that states that your résumé is enclosed for their review, and that you are available for an in-person interview (give dates if you will be traveling to the area) or telephone conversation. Avoid beginning every sentence with "I" and limit the letter to one page.

Proofread both your letter and résumé for grammar and spelling. Print both your résumé and cover letter on business-type stationery. Send both in a typed envelope. Whether or not you are responding to a specific ad, follow up your mailing with a telephone call.

Interviewing

Once you have captured the attention of a potential employer you will have the opportunity to demonstrate in person what you have to offer. Interviews are a time for you to be interviewed and for you to interview the practice. Both the employer and the employee should use this time to assess whether the position is a good fit for a positive working relationship. If distance is a factor, some potential employers may prefer a phone interview for screening purposes. A phone interview is just as important as an in-person interview, so be attentive when responding and asking questions. If this practice has not utilized a midwife before, you must demonstrate not only your worth to the organization, but also the contributions midwifery will bring to the practice.

Prior to the interview, review your short-term and long-term professional goals. Compare these with the philosophy and mission of the practice. If you must travel overnight for the interview, typically the practice will cover travel expenses. Plan to dress for success. Although practitioners in the office may have a casual dress code, wear a suit. Limit jewelry and unique expressions, such as hair color, style, or body art. Bring a notepad if you wish to have a list of your questions or write notes.

In preparing for your interview, ask about the format. Will you be interviewing with just one person; if so, who is that person (both name and role)? If you will be meeting with others, ask for a schedule in advance so that you know their names and roles within the practice. These interviews may occur on a one-on-one basis or in a group setting, or both. You may meet midwives, physicians, business managers, and hospital administrators. If this is a full-scope practice, be sure that you will have the opportunity to visit the birth site.

Basic principles to remember for your interview include being yourself, that is, relaxed and able to portray yourself in a manner that your prospective employer will be able to assess who you are. Be positive—do not offer negative comments about your educational experience or prior job experiences. In midwifery, it is most likely that someone you are interviewing with knows your educational program, employer, or someone else who knows them. Maintaining a positive attitude is also a positive reflection of your enthusiasm about midwifery and the position. Answer the questions in full sentences; instead of a "yes" or "no" answer, elaborate on your response.

Fair employment laws prevent your prospective employer or any of the practice's employees from asking you about your religion, age, marital status, or other personal questions. Interview etiquette for you also includes not asking about salary or compensation until the prospective employer brings up the topic.

Go to the interview prepared for questions. Typical questions that you will be asked include:

- What attracts you to the practice?
- How many (#s of clinical experiences) have you done?
- Why did you/are you leaving your current position? (Remember to be positive, such as looking for growth or new practice opportunities.)
- What are your strengths and needs?
- Describe a challenging clinical situation.
- What can you bring to the practice?
- Describe a challenging physician situation.
- How many patients do you usually see in a practice day?

Go to the interview prepared to ask questions. Ask for a copy of the position description, including position expectations. Questions you should consider asking include:

- What are you looking for in an ideal candidate?
- What is an average work week like?
- What is the average volume for the practice?
- What are the productivity requirements?
- What are your cesarean section, episiotomy, and epidural rates?
- What types of quality assurance and peer review projects do you have?
- What office accommodations are available?
- What types of mentoring are available to new midwives?
- What is the reporting structure here?
- Will I have nonclinical responsibilities?
- What types of resources are available (books, continuing education, grand rounds, etc.)?

If it is a full scope practice, include questions such as:

- What is the birth environment like for midwives?
- What category are the hospital privileges?
- What are typical call/shift hours versus clinical hours?

Once you have returned home from the interview, always remember to send handwritten thank you notes. You should write an individual note to each person you interviewed with, and if an administrative assistant was responsible for scheduling your interview and/or travel arrangements, remember to also send that person a thank you. Timeliness is important, so complete this task as soon as possible.

The next task to do after returning home is completing a postinterview evaluation. Take some time to evaluate what you have learned and compare it to your expectations and desires. **Table 9–4** is a rating tool to help you assess whether this practice will be a good fit for you.

Contract Negotiations

Congratulations! You have successfully navigated the résumé, cover letter, and interview and have just been offered the position. If you are interested in the position, and before the negotiations begin, let the practice director know you are interested in pursuing this opportunity. If you are no longer interested in the position, also let the practice know; do not wait until you are offered the position to decline it. And then remember, unless the director offers you something that is openly stated as non-negotiable, negotiate. There are several resources available about the art of negotiation; the purpose of this section is not to teach you about the art of negotiation, but to provide you with items that should be considered when negotiating a contract.

Salary is typically the first item discussed. If possible, investigate the mean and range of salaries for midwives nationally and/or in that region. ACNM collects this data and periodically prints it in the *Journal of Midwifery & Women's Health*. In 2003, 20.5% of ACNM members earned between $60,000 and $69,000 and 17.5% earned between $70,000 and $79,000 (Schuiling et al., 2005). Salary typically is offered as a straight salary, an hourly rate, or salary plus productivity. If it is not clear with the offer, clarify what the terms of salary will be. There are potentially five possible payment arrangements: salaried employee, salary plus profits, portion of profits only, partner/owner, or independent contractor (Matyac, Fitchitt, & Dearing, 1996).

Table 9–4 Postinterview Evaluation

Rate your responses to the following questions:

1 = acceptable   2 = unsure   3 = unacceptable

Practice philosophy	1	2	3
Patient volume	1	2	3
Patient demographics	1	2	3
Patient outcomes	1	2	3
Productivity requirements	1	2	3
Clinical hours	1	2	3
Practice partners	1	2	3
Support staff	1	2	3
Practice facilities	1	2	3
Birth facilities	1	2	3
Nonclinical responsibilities	1	2	3
Availability of resources	1	2	3
Orientation	1	2	3

If your salary will include some form of compensation for productivity, clarify what the definition of productivity is. Compensation for productivity is typically monetary payment in addition to your base salary for the volume of work that you produce. If your productivity compensation will be by numbers of births or procedures performed, carefully evaluate whether this will impact your or the practice's quality of care. Will you or your partner(s) be more willing to begin oxytocin stimulation or induction so the birth will occur during your call period? Will you or your partner(s) be more willing to perform other procedures? Productivity is also measured by new patients brought into the practice. If you are responsible for attracting new patients, what marketing resources are available to you? Another form of productivity pay is pay-for-performance. This is an incentive begun by managed care organizations to pay providers for quality care, that is, for meeting benchmarks in care for your cohort of patients. For midwives, this could be achieving a predetermined benchmark of the percentage of your patients who receive first trimester care, or certain laboratory tests, such as mammograms and pap smears. Some bonuses come in the form of an overall productive practice and are equally divided among practice members.

Verify the number of hours per week that you will be expected to work, both in the office and on call/shifts. If this is not in writing, ask that it be included in the contract. Will you be expected to cover sick and vacation time for other members of your practice? Is office salary a different compensation rate than call time? Is there overtime and/or holiday compensation?

The next item for negotiation is benefits. Although some benefits are not negotiable, such as retirement plan, life insurance, disability insurance, health care, dental, and optical care, some items are negotiable. What is the amount of paid vacation that you will receive? Does this increase with time of service? Do you get paid sick time, and if so, how much? What paid holidays will you receive, and how does the practice rotate holidays among the providers? If you have already scheduled vacation or other time away that begins after you would begin employment, negotiate that right now with your new employer.

Clarify what your professional liability coverage will be and, once covered, ask for a copy of the policy face sheet. Will you be covered under the organization's policy or as a rider to a physician? Know what the limits of the policy are and whether you have a claims made or occurrence policy. Ask if the practice will cover a tail for you if you leave. For more information about professional liability coverage, refer to Chapter 6.

There are several expenses that you will incur by virtue of being a health care professional. Some of these expenses include association memberships, subscriptions to professional journals and data search engines, licensing fees, DEA registration fees, and continuing education costs. Depending on the size and type of your practice, most practices will offer compensation for some or all of these expenses.

There will typically be business expenses in association with being a member of a practice. If you are relocating, will these expenses be reimbursed? If part of your position requires call of any kind, does the practice reimburse for pager and/or cell phone services? Is mileage for call provided?

If there is an employee handbook, ask to receive a copy. Know how your work performance will be evaluated, how often, and by whom. You may have a 3- or 6-month conditional appointment. If this is the case, during that time your employer may not need a justifiable reason to terminate you. Knowing the criteria from which you will be evaluated will help you set your own performance benchmarks.

If this is a private practice, it is not atypical to have a restrictive covenant. Restrictive covenants protect the practice against the potential loss of clients if you leave the practice and patients follow you. Restrictive covenants are enforceable in many states, and midwives have been successfully sued for breach of a restrictive covenant. If you voluntarily or involuntarily leave the practice, a restrictive covenant in your contract may prevent you from practicing within a certain mile radius of this current practice, prevent you from practicing at certain hospitals, and delineate a specified number of years for this restriction. The best negotiation is to get a restrictive covenant removed from your contract. If it will not be removed, only you can determine if this is a part of the contract that you can accept.

Another important item to review in an employment contract is the termination of contract conditions. What are the conditions under which you could be terminated? It has been known to happen in some midwifery practices that the employer decides he or she no longer needs or has the resources to afford nurse–midwifery services, typically because the practice volume cannot support the existing numbers of providers, and the midwives are terminated with little to no notice and no compensation package. Ensure that your contract specifies that if you are terminated because your position is terminated, that you will be given adequate notice (typically 2–4 weeks) and adequate compensation (many professionals negotiate 6 months or greater).

Before you finalize your employment contract, seek consultation with a lawyer. The legal fees you may incur at this juncture of contract negotiations are well worth the money spent if you choose not to use these services and the covenants of the contract are not honored. If your employer refuses to offer you a contract, you must decide if you can live with unknown and/or uncertain terms. That is, your hours, compensation, benefits, and even your job can be changed or terminated at any time. If you do not have a contract and you and your employer have a disagreement about services, you can be terminated. This can occur and it has happened to many midwives in the past. **Table 9–5** provides a list of items to consider in contract negotiations.

Starting Your Own Practice

Starting your own practice is a labor-intensive endeavor and, if successful, can be very rewarding, both professionally and economically. It is not an endeavor a midwife should enter lightly; it requires significant planning and foresight. There are several publications and organizations available to help you begin your practice. The ACNM document, *Guidelines for Establishing a Nurse–Midwifery Practice*, is an excellent resource.

Several types of ownership are possible, and each has distinct legal and tax implications. In a sole proprietor, you and the business are one and the same. Any expenses, debts, or legal liability belong to you (Buppert, 2004). Partnerships involve the establishment of a business relationship with two or more individuals. In this type of a relationship, each partner is equally responsible for debts, legal liability, profits, decision making, and overall administration of the business. The main advantage of a limited liability company (LLC) is

Table 9–5 Contract Negotiations

1. *Type of Position: salary, hourly?*
2. *Benefits*
   a. Salary
   b. Health, dental, optical insurance
   c. Paid vacation (#)
   d. Paid sick leave (#)
   e. Paid holidays (#)
   f. Life insurance, retirement annuity
3. *Other Professional Benefits*
   a. Tuition reimbursement
   b. Expense account/continuing education costs and paid time off
   c. Professional membership dues
   d. Professional journal subscriptions
   e. Professional licenses
   f. Pager/cell phone
   g. Mileage
   h. Bonuses
      i. Productivity by volume or
      ii. Productivity by effectiveness
   i. Malpractice insurance
      i. Amount of coverage
      ii. Personal policy or rider
      iii. Tail
4. *Other*
   a. Work hours: office, call, administrative time, committee or other responsibilities
   b. Paid for overtime?
   c. Scheduling of appointments: how many per day, time per visit
   d. Productivity data
   e. Length of orientation
   f. Employee handbook

Contract
1. Position description
2. Work hours/expectations
3. How evaluated? When? By whom?
4. Salary (and benefits)
5. Duration of contract
6. Amendment and modification agreement
7. Restrictive clause?
8. Termination of contract conditions
   a. Of the person
   b. Of the position
   c. Length of notice
   d. Compensation

income and losses pass through the individuals similar to a partnership, but some of the legal liability (not professional liability) protection is similar to a corporation. A corporation is a business with its own identity separate from any individuals who own it. Corporations may disburse income on a pro-rated basis comparable to the amount of individual investment(s), have legal limits on individual liability (not including professional liability), and profits are taxed. In some states, members of different professions with different licenses are not allowed to form a corporation; thus, in some states you are not allowed to be a partner in a corporation owned by a physician, and vice versa.

One important element in examining the feasibility of starting your own practice is the development of a business plan. **Table 9–6** provides an outline of elements to consider when writing a business plan. The process of developing a business plan will clarify your ability to be a risk taker, articulate your clinical expertise, determine your basic management skills, and determine your basic financial skills. A business plan is the blueprint for the development of your practice; it solidifies your ideas into an organized format, clarifies the role of others, makes you think about aspects you might not have considered, and serves as a benchmark for actual performance. A business plan will help you to quantify resources, evaluate finances, and prioritize objectives.

The cover page contains demographic information: business name, contact information, and name of principle owners. The executive summary is typically one to two pages in length and contains your statement of purpose and a summary of your proposal. When

---

Table 9–6 Business Planning

Benefits of a Business Plan
- Makes you think about many aspects you might not have considered
- Helps to solidify ideas into an organized format
- Clarifies the role of others: collaborating physicians, other health professionals
- Serves as a benchmark for actual performance

Business Plans Help You To
- Quantify resources
- Evaluate finances
- Prioritize objectives

Elements of a Business Plan
- Cover page
- Executive summary
- Practice organization
- Market analysis
- Market plan
- Regulatory issues
- Facility and space requirements
- Equipment requirements
- Accounting, taxes
- Financial data
- Time lines

addressing practice organization, components to consider include the type or form of the business (solo or group, organizational chart), the size of the business (who and how many will staff the practice, position descriptions, and whether or not services such as credentialing and billing will be outsourced), and the services that will be provided. A good market analysis should include your market size (can your practice grow?), a description of who your clients will be, competition in the area, and trends of similar businesses in the area. Your marketing plan will include your marketing philosophy and how you plan to market your practice. The operating plan section details specific regulatory, facility, space, and equipment issues, including accounting needs and professional liability coverage. The start-up budget, available capital, operating budget, breakeven analysis, and sensitivity analysis are included in the financial data section. Last, a good business plan will provide a time line for acquiring the physical plant, hiring staff, and opening. Supporting documents may include your résumé and references and a collaborating physician agreement.

There is a tremendous amount of details to address in starting any business, including a midwifery practice. There are several significant start-up costs, such as utilities, office equipment (computer, printer, fax, copier, credit card processor), office cleaning, signage, medical equipment (for each exam room and overall), office supplies (pens, paper, medical records), and business licenses. Poor planning, poor market analysis, poor budgeting, and inadequate inventory are all characteristics of failure. The first step in starting a practice is to know your strengths and know when to ask for help.

Instead of completing the formal process of securing your own business, you may consider becoming an independent contractor. An independent contractor is responsible for his or her own taxes, insurance, health benefits, equipment, and sometimes office space (Buppert, 2004). Some midwives who work as independent contractors contract with another health care provider for usage of space, supplies, and personnel to see midwifery patients; they reimburse that provider for such services and then keep the remainder as profit.

Marketing Your Practice

Whether you own your own practice or not, you need to be savvy in marketing both your practice and your profession. Marketing can also be viewed as public relations. Buppert (2004, p. 418) identified the process of public relations: 1) develop the message; 2) determine the target(s) for the message; 3) identify the best way to deliver the message; 4) disseminate the message; and 5) evaluate the success of your efforts. The message should be consistent with your goal: promoting CNMs/CMs as primary care providers for women across the life span. In midwifery the message is simple: All women deserve a midwife! The targets for your message are the women in your community and beyond.

Midwives provide high-quality, cost-effective care. Become familiar with the national data that support this statement and your own practice data; data will speak much better than generalized statements about outcomes. Marketing midwives will educate consumers, generate practice income, and create new midwifery job opportunities (Hamric, Spross, & Hanson, 2000). In addition to generalized marketing of midwifery, in order to market your practice you will need to know more about your market area. Refer to the data you collected in the Chapter 3 end of chapter exercise. The findings from this exercise will give you information on the average age of women in your community, its birth rate, and the socioeconomic status of the women. If looking specifically at growing your practice, you will know whether and how your practice can grow, including the payer mix in the area. Also look at your competition. What is the number of other practices in the area? How many of them are midwifery practices? Have there ever been midwifery practices in your area and what is their history?

There are many venues in which to market your practice. These venues include newspaper and other print ads, brochures and fliers, and yellow page listings. Carry business cards with you wherever you go and make sure you always give them to your current patients. Personal testimonials are excellent marketing tools; if you have a positive outcome or heart-touching story, call your local radio station, television station, and newspaper to tell them the story. You can also write the story yourself and submit it to the local newspaper(s). Other marketing strategies midwives have used include writing a weekly women's health or childbearing column in their local newspaper(s).

Learn where women go for support or information groups in your community. Look for a local young mother's organization, a LaLeche League group, or a book club. Ask for the opportunity to speak to these groups on a topic that would be of interest to them. Seek out professional opportunities in your community and/or volunteer activities. Does the community have a health-related advisory committee, or are there professional boards that you could join on topics of interest to you, such as a local nursing advisory board? Begin to network and build your community.

Knowing Your Impact

Sometimes the survival of your practice depends on the data you generate. This could mean the survival of not only your individual position, but also of the midwifery practice. The midwifery role is more vulnerable than many other roles in a health care practice and may be the first to be eliminated when the budget is reviewed. As an employee, CNMs/CMs may not be provided with the financial data demonstrating their contribution to the practice/institution (Ament, 2000; Matyac et al., 1996). Several resources are available for data collection. The ACNM data set series consists of data sets for five clinical areas: antepartum, intrapartum, postpartum, newborn, and primary care. There are also software programs available for purchase to help you organize and evaluate your data.

There are several pieces of information you will want to evaluate with your data set. Documenting not only the amount of care you provide, but also the quality of care you provide will demonstrate growth in your practice, positive patient satisfaction, midwifery outcomes, and economic value. Do not wait until you are asked for the data to share it. Share your data on a regular basis with your partner(s), your employer, your managed care organizations, and your consumers. If you meet or exceed local and/or national benchmarks, publicize the information on your brochures, with the media, and so on. Being proactive in your use of data will eliminate the need to be reactive and will assist in preventing unexpected changes in your employment.

Practice Directors

Every practice with a midwife should have a midwifery practice director. There are several resources and supports available for practice directors. The midwifery Service Directors Network (SDN) is an organization (separate from ACNM) that provides a network for administrators of midwifery practices. The Midwifery Business Institute is an annual conference that covers a broad array of topics for current and future practice directors.

Summary

Given the nursing shortage, the professional liability crisis, and the growing costs of health care, it may be difficult to predict the rate of growth of midwifery practices over the next decade. In looking towards what the future holds for the practice climate of advanced practice nursing, Aiken (2003) examines a myth that can be extrapolated to midwifery: The increase in advanced practice nurses (midwives) will saturate demand and result in employment difficulties. There will always be women who need midwives, and we have not yet achieved a critical mass of midwives to care for all women. When we reach that critical mass and after the celebrations are over, we will look towards new and innovative midwifery practice settings and models.

Chapter Exercise

To prepare for your first new midwifery position or your next job search, you need to develop a professional portfolio. The portfolio is intended to promote your professional development and achievements. It is also designed to facilitate your participation in assessing and evaluating your practice needs. A portfolio is a means to preserve your work, fostering the importance of building on previous work. The development of a portfolio begins during your educational experiences. Upon graduation from your midwifery program, your portfolio is tangible evidence of knowledge acquired throughout your program.

It is a part of your professional responsibility to maintain and continue a portfolio. Purchase a binder or folder in which to assemble your material, and then prepare a table of contents and/or use dividers. Assemble the following items for your portfolio and update it on a regular basis:

Professional Portfolio Template

1. **Résumé**
2. **Academic Summary**
   a. Final Statistics
   b. Summary of Clinical Sites
      Under each clinical site, provide:
      - Name of site and dates of assignment
      - Type of experience (antepartum, gyn, pc, intrapartum, full-scope)

- Brief summary of site: sociodemographics of clients, type of midwifery service, service setting
3. **Abstract of Scholarly Work(s)**
4. **Copy of Final Summary from Academic Program**
5. **Credentialing Materials**
   a. Diploma from midwifery program
   b. ACC/AMCB certificate
   c. CNM/CM license
   d. RN license (where applicable)
   e. DEA and state prescriptive authority license
   f. Copy of CEU certificates

Table 9–7 For Your Professional Files

ACNM Essential Documents Package
ACNM Handbook: Home Birth Practice (2004)
ACNM Handbook: Minding Your Own Business: Business Plans for Midwifery Practices (2000)
ACNM Handbook: Marketing & Public Relations: A Complete Resource Guide (2000)
ACNM Guidelines for Establishing a Midwifery Practice
ACNM QuickInfo
   Administration of Midwifery Practices
   Birth Centers
   Career Development
   Data Collection
   Home Birth
   Marketing Your Practice
   Productivity & Compensation
   Quality & Effectiveness
ACNM Position Statement on Practice Settings

References and Bibliography

Aiken, L. H. (2003). Workforce policy perspectives on advance practice nursing. In M. Mezey, D. McGivern, & E. Sullivan-Marx (Eds.), *Nurse practitioners: Evolution of advanced practice* (4th ed., pp. 431–442). New York: Springer.

Ament, L. (2000). Certified nurse–midwives' knowledge of reimbursement issues. *Journal of Midwifery & Women's Health, 45*(2), 157–160.

American College of Nurse–Midwives. (1997). *Statement on practice settings.* Washington, DC: Author.

American College of Nurse–Midwives. (2003). Home Birth. *QuickInfo.* Washington, DC: Author.

American College of Nurse-Midwives & American College of Obstetricians and Gynecologists. (2002). *2002 joint statement of practice relations between obstetrician-gynecologists and certified nurse–midwives/certified midwives.* Washington, DC: Author.

Buppert, C. (2004). *Nurse practitioner's business practice and legal guide* (2nd ed.). Sudbury, MA: Jones and Bartlett.

Centers for Disease Control and Prevention. (2005, September 8). Births: Final data for 2003. *National Vital Statistics Reports, 54*(2).

Hamric, A. B., Spross, J. A., & Hanson, C. M. (2000). *Advanced nursing practice: An integrative approach* (2nd ed.). Philadelphia: W. B. Saunders.

Matyac, H. G., Fitchitt, B. L., & Dearing, R. H. (1996). Compensation models of certified nurse–midwives in clinical practice. *Journal of Perinatal amd Neonatal Nursing, 10*(1), 36–45.

Mezey, M., McGivern, D., & Sullivan-Marx E. (Eds.). (2003). *Nurse practitioners: Evolution of advanced practice* (4th ed.). New York: Springer.

Rooks, J. P., Weatherby, N. L., Ernst, E. K., Stapleton, S., Rosen, D., & Rosenfield, A. (1989). Outcomes of care in birth centers: The National Birth Center Study. *New England Journal of Medicine, 321,* 1804–1811.

Schuiling, K. D., Sipe, T. A., & Fullerton, J. (2005). Findings form the analysis of the American College of Nurse–Midwives membership surveys: 2000–2003. *Journal of Midwifery & Women's Health, 50*(1), 8–15.

Zaumeyer, C. R. (2003). *How to start an independent practice: The nurse practitioner's guide to success.* Philadelphia: F. A. Davis.

CHAPTER 10

Credentialing

Lisa Summers, CNM, DrPH

Learning Objectives

1. Define "credentialing," "privileging," and "appointment."
2. Discuss the role of JCAHO in the process of obtaining clinical privileges in a health care institution.
3. Define "LIP" and discuss what determines whether a midwife is an LIP.
4. Describe the major differences between credentialing via the human resources route versus the medical staff route.
5. List the important steps in the process of obtaining clinical privileges in a health care institution.

This chapter provides an overview of two administrative procedures that must be mastered in order for a midwife to practice: clinical privileges and credentialing. The American College of Nurse–Midwives (ACNM) handbook, *Clinical Privileges and Credentialing*, third edition, covers this topic in depth and provides checklists and practical advice that are indispensable for midwives facing their first application for privileges to provide care in a hospital or other health care setting as well as for those wishing to deal more effectively with the credentialing process. The handbook contains appendices with useful reference materials and sample documents that should serve as a supplement to this chapter.

This chapter is organized into three sections. The first provides important background information regarding key organizations, terminology, and the impact of state laws and regulations. The second addresses the processes for obtaining clinical privileges in a hospital. The last section addresses the credentialing process in the managed care arena.

The ACNM has also worked to develop resources for hospital administrators, credentials committees, and others involved in the process of credentialing midwives. An article containing background information about the education, licensure, and scope of practice of midwives appeared in *Synergy*, the official publication of the National Association of Medical Staff Services, and is also available on the ACNM Web site, www.midwife.org. A resource packet specifically for credentials committees and medical staff offices entitled *Clinical Privileges for Midwives* is available for purchase through the ACNM Resource Catalog and Shop ACNM.com.

Key Organizations

The Joint Commission on Accreditation of Health Care Organizations (JCAHO)

The Joint Commission is a private not-for-profit accrediting body responsible for the promulgation of standards that, when met by hospitals and health care organizations, make them eligible for Medicare and other forms of third-party reimbursement. The stated goal of the organization is to improve that quality of care for patients. JCAHO is one of only two accrediting agencies whose approval process is required in order for a health care organization to receive reimbursement for services provided to Medicare and Medicaid clients. This status gives JCAHO the unique opportunity to influence government health care policies.

Established in 1951 as the Joint Commission on the Accreditation of Hospitals, the organization was an outgrowth of early efforts to set minimal essential standards for hospitals. JCAHO is now a joint venture of the American Medical Association, the American Hospital Association, the American College of Surgeons, the American College of Physicians, and the American Dental Association. JCAHO originally conducted only hospital accreditation, but has expanded to other settings including psychiatric facilities, long-term care facilities, substance abuse programs, community mental health programs, home care agencies, and health care networks. In 1989, the term *hospitals* was changed to *health care organizations* to reflect this expanding sphere of influence.

The decision-making body of the Joint Commission is a 28-member Board of Commissioners (BOC), with 21 commissioners representing the 5 member organizations. One position is designated for a nurse-at-large who is also appointed by the BOC. The ACNM is a member of the JCAHO Liaison Forum and, over the years, a number of nurse–midwives have served on JCAHO task forces and expert panels.

JCAHO MEDICAL STAFF STANDARDS

Originally written for physicians only, in 1983 the JCAHO adopted medical staff standards that recognized that the medical staff might include licensed individuals other than physicians and dentists. However, requirements for "prompt medical evaluation by a qualified physician" limited the utility of that recognition. Each subsequent revision to the medical staff standards has had an impact on the ability of midwives to obtain clinical privileges that allow them to practice to the full extent of their education and licensure. Although most of the changes have been positive and JCAHO denies all allegations that it wishes to use JCAHO standards to limit access to hospital privileges for those who are not physicians, the standards still offer access and protections to physicians that are not available to midwives.

The National Committee for Quality Assurance (NCQA)

Though not as central to the credentialing process as JCAHO, it is important that midwives have some understanding of the NCQA and its Health Plan Employer Data and Information Set (HEDIS) program, addressed in detail in Chapter 12. Many health plans will request HEDIS data in the credentialing process.

Terminology

Terms such as *credentialing*, *clinical privileges*, *clinical practice privileges*, *hospital privileges*, and *hospital practice privileges* are often used interchangeably in the health care field. As a practical matter, the clinician is expected to present his or her credentials to support an application for clinical privileges, such as qualifications and licensure. "Clinical privileges" include various subcategories of specific privileges (for example, admitting, discharge privileges, or performance of specialized procedures). Privileges to admit and discharge clients are the hallmark of practice autonomy, as well as a JCAHO-specified requirement for medical staff membership.

Credentialing vs. Privileging vs. Appointment

Credentialing is the first step in the process that leads to *privileging*, and that may lead to *appointment* to membership on the medical staff. The credentialing process includes a series of activities designed to collect relevant data that serve as the basis for decisions regarding granting of privileges and, possibly, appointment to membership on the medical staff.

Credentials review is the process of obtaining, verifying, and assessing the qualifications of an applicant to provide patient care, treatment, and services in or for a health care organization.

The *privileging process* typically entails processing the application, evaluating the applicant's information, and making recommendations to the governing board for applicant-specific delineated privileges, notifying the applicant, monitoring the use of privileges, and an on-going system for monitoring quality of care.

The purpose of verifying credentials data is to ensure that:

- The individual requesting privileges is the same individual identified in the credentialing documents.
- The applicant has attained the credentials as stated.
- The credentials are current.
- There are no challenges to the credentials.

Midwives must be familiar with the Medical Staff chapter of the JCAHO *Hospital Accreditation Standards (HAS)*. These standards are published annually and are typically available in the medical staff office, the medical records department, or the nursing administration office of a hospital or other health care institution. JCAHO's definition of licensed independent practitioners (LIPs), addressed in more detail in the following section, is of critical importance. More information about JCAHO is available on its Web site, www.jcaho.org.

Licensed Independent Practitioners (LIPs)

With the publication of the 2004 *HAS*, JCAHO revised slightly the definition of an LIP. An LIP is "any individual who is permitted by law *and by the organization* to provide care, treatment, and services, *without direction or supervision*." The language in italics (added) explains why it has become so important that midwives encourage legislators, regulatory boards, and hospital bylaws committees to avoid the use of "direction and supervision" in laws and regulations that address the practice of midwifery. JCAHO underscores the importance of state laws and hospital bylaws by noting, "The Joint Commission does not determine if a practitioner is an LIP. State law and hospital policy determine whether a practitioner can practice independently" (Joint Commission on Accreditation of Healthcare Organizations [JCAHO], 2004, p. 291).

The Impact of State Laws and Regulations

It is important that every midwifery practice and/or midwife be thoroughly familiar with the state laws and regulations that impact the practice of midwifery. It is even more critical to ensure that certified nurse–midwives and certified midwives meet the JCAHO definition of a licensed independent practitioner. A summary of the state laws as they relate to the practice of CNMs and CMs is available in the ACNM handbook, *Clinical Privileges and Credentialing*.

Although most states do not address hospital privileges for CNMs/CMs, eight states and the District of Columbia have enacted statutes that either permit hospitals to grant clinical practice privileges to CNMs or APNs or prohibit hospitals from discriminating against CNMs or APNs with respect to granting clinical practice privileges and/or membership in the hospital's medical staff. Legislative activity is always evolving with the potential for more states to enact statutes on clinical privileges for CNMs/CMs. It is important to monitor state legislative activity.

For more information on states that address hospital privileges for CNMs, the ACNM publication, *Nurse–Midwifery Today: A Handbook of State Laws and Regulations*, is available on the ACNM web site.

Obtaining Clinical Privileges in a Hospital or Health Care Organization

Credentialing is the first step in the process that must be followed to obtain clinical privileges to practice in a hospital or other health care organization. "The credentialing process includes a series of activities designed to collect relevant data that serve as the basis for decisions regarding appointment to membership on the medical staff, as well as privileges recommended and the delineation of privileges recommended by the medical staff" (JCAHO, 2004, p. 307). Credentialing for managed care contracts is addressed later in this chapter.

Two Routes to Obtaining Clinical Privileges

Privileges to practice in a hospital can be obtained via one of two mechanisms outlined in either:

- Human resources (HR) department policies and procedures and JCAHO HR standards (JCAHO, 2004, pp. 261–270) or
- Medical staff bylaws and JCAHO's *HAS* Medical Staff chapter (JCAHO, 2004, pp. 291–326).

Credentialing via the HR route reflects the fact that the individual is an employee of the institution and typically does not allow participation in medical staff committees. Be aware of the due process accorded to employees via this route. (For further information about due process, refer to "Denial of Privileges.") The HR route is used for LIPs and non-LIPs employed by the institution (this could be a hospital or a related organization, such as a health science center). The JCAHO *Hospital Accreditation Standards (HAS)* contains a chapter regarding credentialing via this route. HR policies outline an evaluation process for initial training and ongoing competency as well as a job description with clinical responsibilities outlined.

The medical staff route is always used for physicians and dentists and may include other LIPs as well. Members of the medical staff are also allowed membership in a number of important policy-setting committees. The remainder of this chapter focuses on the process of obtaining clinical privileges as a member of the medical staff.

Denial of Privileges

Historically, many believed that if a practitioner was denied hospital privileges, this fact must be reported to the National Practitioner Data Bank (NPDB). In the past, ACNM has cautioned members to withdraw their applications if they had reason to believe the hospital would deny privileges just because they were a midwife. In fact, the NPDB understands that practitioners may be denied privileges for administrative reasons that are not a reflection on their competence/conduct. Denial of privileges for administrative reasons, meaning your competence and/or conduct was not evaluated, is not a NPDB reportable event.

Categories of Medical Staff Membership

Although all members of the medical staff have clinical privileges, not all health care providers with clinical privileges are members of the medical staff. The "medical staff" often has various categories of membership. There are no universally accepted standard definitions or terms used to describe those categories of medical staff membership.

Typically there are "full medical staff" or simply "medical staff" and then one or more categories that may be called associate to medical staff, allied health professional, special assistant, or specialized professional personnel. The range of privileges, influence, and due process protection offered in these other categories frequently falls far short of those guaranteed to physicians and dentists. For example, if you are not a member of the medical staff you may not have the right to vote on department policies; there may be no guarantee of due process if accused of substandard performance; and there may be no recourse when an application for privileges receives no action. Full medical staff privileges are considered the gold standard. If midwives are included in any other category, they should be fully aware of the implications of such a differentiation.

Under JCAHO standards and most hospital bylaws, medical staff members can admit or discharge patients, have the right to vote or hold office, and have the right to due process if their membership or clinical privileges are subjected to disciplinary procedures. Under former JCAHO standards (and arguably under the 1996 version), anyone who meets the definition of "licensed independent practitioner" is eligible to hold admitting and discharge privileges and to become a member of the medical staff.

Documentation

The process of obtaining privileges requires the accumulation and dissemination of a large quantity of information. It is critical to follow all of the directions, provide complete and legible information, and document each step of the process.

A record of every communication sent or received, no matter how informal or unimportant it may seem at the time, may solve many problems in the future. Retain originals and at least one copy of any document related to the application. A personal journal with a chronological accounting of every detail in the process may also be helpful

If a midwife is applying for privileges in a setting where midwives are well integrated into the system, she or he may wonder why so much caution and detail we needed. It is important to remember that credentialing requires a trail of paperwork that documents all of your past experience. In addition, a future job may bring with it the challenge of being the first midwife to apply for privileges. Getting paperwork organized from day one is a very good investment in the future. The ACNM (2005) *Clinical Privileges and Credentialing Handbook* contains more detail on this process, including a list of items to document.

Key Players

The process of obtaining clinical privileges involves contact with many different individuals and groups—the medical community, the nursing staff, the health care agency, hospital or clinic administration, other midwives, and the public. The process may be influenced by numerous factors, some of which may seem to have little, if any, relationship to the actual practice of midwifery. Each person draws upon his or her own understanding, experiences, and prejudices when interacting with a midwife both as a health care professional and as an applicant for privileges.

For example, a prior bad experience with an entirely different category of "nonphysician health care provider" may influence the willingness of one or more members of the medical staff to even consider the idea of a midwifery application. Similarly, members of the nursing staff may be supportive, but they might also feel threatened by a midwife's status as an independent practitioner. The local community may rally in favor of midwifery with petitions or other strong demonstrations of support for midwives or it may simply be indifferent.

The ACNM (2005) *Clinical Privileges and Credentialing Handbook* contains a list of individuals most likely to be encountered in the application process, from the chief executive officer to staff nurses to the board of trustees. It is important to understand the role of each of these key players and have a plan for communicating effectively with them.

Particularly critical are chief of staff or president of the medical staff (typically elected by the medical staff members) and the credentials committee. The credentials committee investigates and provides an initial approval or rejection of applications for privileges. The credentials committee (or administrative personnel assigned to it) reviews applications, checks references, and often conducts one or more interviews with applicants. It is not unusual to find that one application may suffice for several institutions. In this case, it is more difficult to get to know the individuals involved.

A number of community groups also play an important role in the process. The client/patient base—current clients and patients of the midwife and/or of the collaborating physician as well as potential clients (many of whom may be currently clients of competitors)—may contain individuals who can inform and persuade key players in the institution. Special interest groups, such as women's groups, family planning organizations, community health centers, health care activists, the state and local nursing associations, childbirth educators, and other midwives may play a role. Even local schools, civic associations, and local government officials may have an interest in seeing midwives on staff at the hospital. Finally, the media, including newspapers, magazines, newsletters, scientific journals, radio and TV broadcast stations, and local cable television, may play a role in educating key players about midwifery, creating a demand for midwifery services, and occasionally, shedding light on a difficult situation.

The Privileging Process

There are many steps to the privileging process that are outlined in detail in the ACNM (2005) *Clinical Privileges and Credentialing Handbook*. A highly abbreviated list is included here.

Preapplication Preparations

- Obtain a copy of all state regulations that govern admitting privileges to hospitals.
- Obtain a copy of and carefully review the medical staff or network bylaws.

Determine if nonphysician health professionals are not mentioned in the bylaws or if midwives are delegated to some non-MD category that precludes admitting privileges and/or medical staff membership.

If a bylaws change or amendment is needed, determine whether you want to work for this change prior to or after you obtain clinical privileges. Changing the bylaws, if you have support from within the system, can delay getting privileges, since this process may take 6 to 12 months. If there is resistance to including midwives in the bylaws, the process may take much longer and will require a careful strategy. On the other hand, limited privileges may make it impossible to build a financially viable business.

- Obtain a copy of OB department bylaws.
- Obtain an application for privileges.
- Carefully review the application so that you can prepare to meet all of the requirements.
- Organize midwifery practice documents.

Your professional files should include the documents listed in **Table 10–1.**

Locate a Current Edition of JCAHO's Hospital Accreditation Standards

JCAHO's Web site provides information about its publications. You may wish to purchase this publication or check for it in the medical library or medical staff office. The JCAHO Web site has some information about current updates.

Finalize Plans with Consultant/Collaborating Physician

Identify the physician with whom you will have a collaborative relationship. Meet with the collaborating physician to develop a plan of action. Discuss key players and steps of the privileging process. Identify any areas of concern to either party.

Establish Peer Support

Involve the local midwifery community in your plans.

Establish Credibility

Find out how key players perceive midwives and midwifery and address any misconceptions. When building support, go beyond the midwifery/obstetric community and make use of various contacts.

Submitting the Application

Complete and submit the application in accordance with previously developed strategy. Notify your midwifery education program (and other educational/academic references) to submit a transcript and alert other references and former employers either to submit letters of reference or to expect to be contacted by the hospital for such references, whichever route is required by the application process. Former employers and all institutions where you may have practiced or possessed clinical privileges may also be contacted by the credentials committee, and they may also access the National Practitioner Data Bank (see

Chapter 6) and the state boards in all states where you have been licensed as an RN or otherwise authorized to practice as a midwife. There is typically an application fee.

Interview

A personal interview may be part of the application process. View this as an important opportunity to provide information to key players who may be unfamiliar with midwifery practice. Be aware of the importance of presenting a professional appearance.

Midwives, particularly those undergoing this process for the first time, often feel that they are being examined particularly carefully. The volume of paperwork required can begin to feel oppressive. Keep in mind, however, that the application process is a detailed and extensive one *for all providers*. Before challenging any requirements as unreasonable, find out if those requirements are imposed upon physicians and other providers.

Temporary Privileges

Although increasingly rare, physician applicants for privileges and medical staff membership are sometimes granted temporary privileges that they may exercise with appropriate restrictions or probationary status while the application is processed. If the bylaws permit temporary privileges for non-MDs, a midwife may consider requesting them from whatever office has the authority to grant them to physicians. If temporary privileges are denied, the issue can be dealt with at that time, or alternatively, continue to keep records regarding this denial to use in the future as needed, while continuing to focus on the permanent application.

Delineation of Privileges

The "delineation of privileges" is a list of all possible functions and procedures considered appropriate by the department, typically provided on a preprinted form. Some OB departments use the same form for all practitioners credentialed to provide obstetric care; others develop separate forms for each practitioner. A sample delineation of privileges form specifically for midwives is included in the Appendix of the ACNM *Clinical Privileges and Credentialing Handbook*.

The practitioner typically is asked to identify the procedures he or she is qualified to perform from the list provided (e.g., admission history and physical, a full spectrum of intra- and postpartum care, and specific procedures such as provider performed microscopy, episiotomies, vacuum extractions, repair of third or fourth degree lacerations, etc.). The delineation of privileges may also indicate whether or not a midwife may write or give verbal orders to the nursing staff and whether the physical presence or co-signature of a collaborating physician is required in connection with any procedure or order.

The sample form developed by the ACNM makes a clear distinction between standard privileges (the clinical skills and judgments described in the ACNM *Core Competencies for Basic Midwifery Care*), and expanded practice privileges (clinical skills, procedures, or components of practice that may be acquired beyond basic midwifery education). If you request privileges for expanded practice procedures (e.g., first assisting at surgery, use of a vacuum extraction device, circumcision), you should expect to produce documentation that you have received appropriate training in the procedure consistent with the ACNM *Standards for the Practice of Midwifery*.

When clinical privileges are granted, it is important to review the approved delineation of privileges list carefully to determine if the privileges that were requested have been granted or limited. The delineation of privileges should conform as closely as possible to one's practice guidelines. The actual scope of practice within the hospital should conform to both documents, as well as to departmental rules and regulations.

Probation or Preceptor Period

When the application is approved, notification should be received in writing. Once initial privileges are granted, it is not unusual to be required to serve some probationary or preceptor period. This is usually specified in the bylaws or in departmental rules and regulations. ACNM takes the position that such probation should be no different, either in duration or nature, than for a newly privileged physician in the same department with similar privileges.

Renewal of Privileges

JCAHO medical staff standards (MS.4.20) specify that privileges do not exceed a period of 2 years. Consequently, hospitals require privileges to be renewed on a regularly scheduled basis, such as every 1 or 2 years. Rules governing the process are included within the medical staff bylaws and, according to ACNM's position, should be no different for midwives than for physicians.

The growing emphasis on monitoring the quality of care is reflected in the process for renewal of privileges. The process for renewal of privileges is not a "rubber stamp" for those already credentialed. Rather, it involves the same steps as those outlined for granting initial privileges *and* requires the medical staff to evaluate a practitioner's performance. JCAHO specifies that the evaluation of a practitioner's ability to perform certain procedures includes a review of nine separate criteria, including involvement in a professional liability action, practitioner-specific mortality and morbidity data, and peer recommendations. "Each reappraisal includes information concerning professional performance, including clinical and technical skills and information from hospital performance improvement activities, when such data are available" (JCAHO, 2004, MS.4.40.4).

If you plan to expand your practice to include procedures such as vacuum extraction or circumcision, it is imperative that you:

- Receive appropriate training (be wary of the "see one, do one, teach one" culture).
- Document that training.
- Ensure that your delineation of privileges form is updated to reflect an expanded scope of practice.

You can expect that medical staff will monitor an expanded practice in accordance with JCAHO's 2004 *HAS* MS4.40.5, which clearly states: "Practitioners do not practice outside the scope of their privileges." For more information on relevant ACNM guidelines and standards, see "Expanded Midwifery Practice" in the ACNM QuickInfo series, available on the ACNM Web site. Refer to Chapter 8 for more information on expanded scope of practice.

Other Responsibilities

Along with the rights of medical staff membership come a host of responsibilities, including dues payment and attendance at staff meetings.

Denial of Privileges, Downgrading of Privileges, and the Appeals Process

Unfortunately, applications for clinical privileges are not always approved. The ACNM handbook devotes an entire chapter to advice for the midwife in two distinct but related situations: 1) the midwife whose application for clinical privileges has been denied, and 2) the midwife who has obtained clinical privileges but is experiencing a downgrading or limitation of those privileges. In both of these situations, it is common for midwives to wonder if the actions of the institution constitute restraint of trade or anticompetitive practices. Refer to Chapter 6 for a discussion of antitrust and restraint of trade issues.

Problems with Clinical Privileges

Although the majority of applications and renewals go smoothly, especially for the midwife who is prepared and follows the directions, a variety of problems can develop. For a thorough analysis on topics such as denial of privileges, downgrading of privileges, due process, and restraint of trade see the ACNM (2005) *Clinical Privileges and Credentialing Handbook.*

The reasons that the ACNM does not publish specific guidelines regarding client selection and management are the same reasons that a credentials committee or hospital OB department might wish to avoid such specific guidelines. Clinical practice guidelines are best developed by an individual midwifery practice in collaboration with their consulting physicians. In defining their scope of practice and the populations served, individual midwives will consider many factors, including:

- The clinical setting in which care is provided
- The skills and expertise of the individual midwife or midwives
- The skills and expertise of the consultant physician(s)

When an institution faces questions such as, "At what gestational age may a midwife care for a patient?" or "Must a client with twins (or diabetes or any number of conditions) be collaboratively managed or referred?" the answer may rightly be different when applied to different midwifery practices within the institution. One practice in which highly experienced midwives collaborate closely with perinatologists may co-manage a particular client that another midwifery practice would refer. Individual clinical practice guidelines, written by midwives in consultation with their consulting physicians, can provide the "designated mechanism" required by JCAHO.

The preceding information should prove helpful to ACNM members who experience attempts to downgrade clinical privileges. Members are also invited to discuss their specific situation with the professional services staff. Consultation with an attorney may be important, particularly if there is evidence of anticompetitive behavior.

Credentialing for Managed Care Organizations

Just as hospitals wish to verify a clinician's credentials as a part of the privileging process, managed care organizations (MCOs), as well as professional liability insurance carriers, also want similar background information on all clinical providers prior to writing a contract. Managed care credentialing is somewhat different from hospital credentialing. Hospitals are held to JACHO standards whereas most managed care organizations are held to the standards and guidelines of the National Committee on Quality Assurance (NCQA) when credentialing providers as well as federal and state laws and regulations that pertain to credentialing providers. NCQA, the accrediting agency for managed care organizations, has set similar guidelines for credentialing all practitioners (see Chapter 12, pp. 255–256). Midwives will find that much of the information required by MCOs is the same as for hospital credentialing.

In order to increase the chances of success when dealing with an MCO, learn about the organization before you begin the process. Each state insurance agency has a list of all health insurance companies licensed to practice in the state. Obtain information from the individual companies to find out who is on the board of directors, the number of members covered, and the annual report (see **Box 10–1**). The ACNM *Clinical Privileges and Credentialing Handbook* includes a list of the key players and critical information typically needed.

In the past, the *Standards for the Accreditation of MCOs*, published annually by NCQA, addressed only credentialing of physicians. The current *Standards for Credentialing and Recredentialing*, however, speak to *practitioners*. There is no language that would create problems for MCOs that want to credential midwives.

Like the general public, individuals in MCOs often have little factual information on midwives. Prepare a packet of information to send to your contact at the MCO contracts department. You may also want to include a packet to the medical director, and the directors of the public relations and sales departments. These people are interested in saving

---

Box 10–1   Obtaining Information about MCOs

Use any of the Internet search engines and enter the name of the MCO and "credentialing." You are likely to find a section of their Web site specifically for health care professionals. It will address the credentialing and renewal process and will often include clinical guidelines, CE information, referral systems, and a host of other information.

money, attracting new members, and keeping them satisfied, so it is helpful to show them that midwives do exactly those things! Do not assume that these people have any information about midwives. It is important to look very similar to physicians when approaching new MCOs, so this information should be polished and professional.

When asked what midwives should do to get the attention of MCOs, one medical director who experienced the benefits of contracting with CNMs said, "Brag more!" Be friendly, don't whine or complain, invite them to your office, feed them, and schmooze. If you are told that the MCO cannot contract with you because it does not have a credentialing form for midwives, offer to revise and fill out a physician form that can then be used to create the new midwifery form, which will save time and money and speed the process along for you. Remember, the average length of time to obtain a managed care contract is 4 to 6 months or longer, so begin the process at the earliest opportunity.

For more information on strategies, see Chapter 9 of the *ACNM Marketing and Public Relations Handbook* (ACNM, 2000).

This section on contracting is a very brief overview of a very complex subject. For additional information on contracts, consult the ACNM handbook *Guidance for CNMs in Managed Care Contracting* and the National Association of Childbearing Centers video, *How to Review a Managed Care Contract*, available through www.BirthCenters.org or call 215-234-8068.

Summary

Midwives have important and unique contributions to make to the health care of women and families, especially in this increasingly complex and changing health care environment. The process and issues surrounding clinical privileging are similarly complex and evolving. However, obtaining clinical privileges is critical to providing care, and is therefore central to midwifery practice. We hope that this chapter and ACNM documents will offer assistance in this challenging pursuit as CNMs and CMs continue to expand and grow in their role of providing responsive care to communities.

Be aware that individuals and organizations other than the ACNM have published materials and provided advice regarding credentialing midwives. Such advice has not always been in the best interest of midwives. Recent versions of these materials have incorporated more language from the ACNM, and the fairly strong language regarding physician supervision has been toned down. Midwives should, however, be familiar with the advice and information being provided to the credentials committees in their institutions. If you have questions regarding specific resources, please feel free to contact the ACNM Department of Professional Services.

Key Points:

- The process of obtaining clinical privileges in a health care institution can be time-consuming and requires meticulous attention to detail.
- Hospital Accreditation Standards published by JCAHO provide a critical framework for the process, though the specific mechanisms by which midwives are credentialed

will be defined in the institution's bylaws and precisely carried out by medical staff professionals in that institution.

Chapter Exercises

1. Choose a local health care institution, perhaps one where you plan to seek clinical privileges, and learn about its credentialing process for midwives. You are likely to obtain some basic information from its Web site. Next, talk with local midwives to learn how they are credentialed, what contacts they have in the medical staff office, and if there are current issues being explored (e.g., a change in the category for midwives or a change in the delineation of privileges). Obtain a copy of the bylaws and other relevant information. *If appropriate*, arrange to visit the medical staff office. If you intend to be the first midwife to seek privileges in the institution, this will be a key step in the detailed process addressed in the ACNM *Clinical Privileges and Credentialing Handbook*.

2. Obtain the relevant information above from the midwives and write a report on the status of midwives in the institution according to bylaws (category, relationship to physicians, limitations on privileges, responsibilities, etc.) and evaluate how prepared you are to complete the application for privileges.

3. Find out when the state affiliate of the National Association of Medical Staff Services (NAMSS) holds its annual meeting. On the NAMSS Web site, www.namss.org, click on "links" and then "NAMSS affiliates" and look for its calendar or an announcement of the meeting. Work with your local ACNM chapter to exhibit at the meeting, or see if you can arrange for a presentation about midwifery. For a handout, make copies of the article on credentialing midwives that was published in *Synergy*, the NAMSS bi-monthly publication. The article can be downloaded from the ACNM Web site.

Table 10–1 For Your Professional Files

- National and state laws and regulations governing midwifery practice (including prescriptive authority)
- Practice guidelines and any relevant clinical agreements with a collaborating physician (state law may require such documents)
- Information regarding reimbursement policies of federal, state, and private insurers
- Pertinent medical practice laws and regulations
- Regulations in the state hospital code, and laws or regulations relating to admitting or other clinical privileges for midwives (or all non-MDs). The state department that regulates hospitals is a good source for these provisions, or an attorney may research them. Also, check for any state law provisions that govern the performance of the admission history and physical exams by midwives or other non-MDs.
- License(s): RN, CNM, DEA, APN.
- Professional liability policy(s) current and past.
- Education transcripts.
- Certification contact information for original source verification.
- Work history with references.
- Records from all other sites where privileges have been granted.
- Continuing education records.
- List of references and current contact information.
- Documentation regarding mastery of skills that are beyond the ACNM Core Competencies.

References

American College of Nurse–Midwives. (2005). *Clinical privileges and credentialing handbook* (2nd ed.). Silver Spring, MD: Author.

American College of Nurse–Midwives. (2000). *Marketing and public relations handbook.* Silver Spring, MD: Author.

Joint Commission on Accreditation of Healthcare Organizations. (2004). *Hospital accreditation standards.* Oakbrook Terrace, IL: JCR.

Summers, L., & Williams, D. (2003, May/June). Credentialing certified nurse–midwives and certified midwives. *Synergy*, 30–38.

CHAPTER 11

Managed Care and Payment

Joan Slager, CNM, MSN, CPC

Learning Objectives

1. Differentiate payment under government programs from payment under private programs.
2. Define the rules governing the various payment mechanisms.
3. Discuss the significance of reimbursement for professional services.
4. Understand federal and state statutes that govern reimbursement.
5. Define and identify the use of billing codes.
6. Identify the criteria for billing.

Payment for services rendered is a primary concern for all health care providers. In order to receive payment from *payers* such as insurance companies, managed care organizations, or government health care plans, you must learn to navigate the payment system and understand the rules associated with submitting claims and getting paid. This chapter will give you an introduction to some of the payers that you must become familiar with as well as provide an introduction to the basic concepts of billing and coding.

Government health plans include Medicare for the aged and disabled; Medicaid for people with low income; military health plans such as CHAMPUS and Tricare; Rural, Migrant and Community Health Centers; the Children's Health Insurance Program; and the Indian Health Service.

The Centers for Medicare and Medicaid Services (CMS) administers the Medicare program and partners with states to administer Medicaid and the State Children's Health Insurance Program (SCHIP). CMS also is responsible for the administrative simplification standards from the Health Insurance Portability and Accountability Act of 1996 (HIPAA), surveying and certifying health care facilities to assure quality of care, and setting quality standards for clinical laboratories. The CMS national headquarters is in Baltimore, Maryland. Ten regional offices work with contractors who administer the Medicare program and also work with the states to administer Medicaid, SCHIP, and HIPAA. The regional offices also survey and provide certification of health care providers.

CMS, formerly known as the Health Care Financing Administration (HCFA), revises, identifies, and implements the rules for compensation of services provided to enrollees in government programs. The CMS publishes changes to these rules in the *Federal Register*. The *Federal Register* is published weekly and contains information about proposed and adopted regulations or sections of the regulations. The document also contains comments, suggestions, and history regarding regulations. Most public libraries have copies of the *Federal Register* or it can be accessed on line at www.cms.gov.

Access to CNMs Under Federal Programs

In 1997, President Clinton created the Advisory Commission on Consumer Protection and Quality in the Health Care Industry and charged this committee with developing measures to assure quality and value and protect the health care consumer and workers in the health care system. From that charge, the Patients' Bill of Rights was developed. The right to choose was one of the components of the Patients' Bill of Rights. This gave women the right to choose qualified specialists such as obstetrician–gynecologists and nurse–midwives for their health care. Thus, all recipients of government health plans are allowed direct access to midwifery care without obtaining a referral or authorization from a primary care provider.

Medicare

Medicare is a social insurance program and is regulated by the federal government. The Medicare program was enacted in 1965 and is financed by payroll taxes from workers and their employers, beneficiary premium payments, and general federal revenues. Medicare provides health insurance to people age 65 or older, people under age 65 with disabilities, and people who have permanent kidney failure requiring dialysis or transplant.

Traditional fee-for-service Medicare has two parts. Part A covers inpatient hospital services, skilled nursing facility services, some home health services, and hospice care. Part B covers professional services, outpatient hospital services, some home health services, and medical equipment and supplies. Medicare contracts with insurance companies to pay for professional services under Part B. The traditional Medicare model is available everywhere in the United States.

In order to bill Medicare, you must apply for a unique provider identification number (UPIN). The UPIN is the mechanism developed by the Secretary of Health and Human Services to identify health care providers who furnish services for which payment may be made under the Social Security Act. A health care provider wishing to provide and bill for Medicare services must complete HCFA forms 855 and 855-R (obtained from CMS at www.cms.gov). The application is reviewed to assure the provider is not excluded from participating in any federal agency, is licensed to practice according to applicable federal and state laws, and is qualified to provide medical or health services. Professional services are billed on the CMS 1500 form (which can be obtained online from CMS) on which you include your UPIN number to indicate who provided the care or services.

Two important issues for midwives with respect to Medicare are the payment rate assigned to midwives and the *incident to* rules. Medicare evaluates physician payment for specific services annually. Currently, midwives billing for services rendered to Medicare recipients receive 65% of the physician reimbursement rate as payment. This amount is an arbitrary amount and is not the result of any data analysis or logic. Accepting such discounted payment for midwifery services makes it difficult for midwives to remain financially viable.

Medicare is often viewed as the "gold standard" for reimbursement for many commercial carriers. What this means is that commercial carriers may adopt the Medicare level of reimbursement for midwives in their plans when they contract with midwives for payment of services provided to their enrollees. Thus, even if you do not provide care for the elderly or disabled, it is important to monitor the Medicare rules and regulations.

Some midwives or their employers, due to the deeply discounted Medicare payment rate, bill services provided by midwives in the name of or incident to a physician. Payment is received at 100% of the physician rate when billing incident to a physician. Certain rules apply when billing for Medicare incident to a physician:

* The physician must see the patient for the initial visit.
* The physician must be involved in the ongoing care of the patient.
* The physician must address any new problems.
* The physician must be *physically present* in the office suite when the care is provided.

The physician does not need to be consulted during the visit nor does he or she need to co-sign any notes or document that a review of the patient's chart took place.

Many Medicare recipients are members of a *Medicare Managed Care* plan. In any managed care plan, the member is assigned a primary care provider who acts as a *gatekeeper* with regards to access to the health care system. A gatekeeper acts as the primary care provider. Participants in the plan must first see the primary care provider, who then approves or authorizes a referral to a specialist if the condition of the patient cannot be managed by the primary care provider. Managed care plans contract with health care providers who agree to care for members of the plan for a preset rate. Due to this contract arrangement, midwives may participate with these plans and receive payment outside of the traditional 65% of the physician rate. Medicare incident to rules may or may not apply.

Medicaid

Medicaid is a federal/state health plan that pays for medical care for individuals or families with low income. Medicaid, also established in 1965, is jointly funded by the federal and state governments. States have different federal matching rates to fund the services provided under their Medicaid programs. The portion of the Medicaid program that is paid for by the federal government is called the Federal Medical Assistance Percentage. It is determined annually for each state by a formula comparing the state's average per capita income level with the national average. The federal government matches at least half of the state's spending.

Although eligibility is determined by individual states, to be eligible for federal funds states are required to provide Medicaid coverage for individuals who receive federally assisted income maintenance payments. Medicaid coverage is usually for low income individuals or families, aged, blind, or disabled persons, and those defined as medically needy. Most states have "state-only" programs for people who do not qualify for Medicaid. Federal funding is not provided for state-only plans. You should refer to your state's Medicaid manual for a comprehensive list of eligible individuals.

States are also allowed flexibility with regards to the services covered by Medicaid; however, federal requirements are mandatory in order for states to receive federal matching funds. Mandated services include inpatient and outpatient hospital services, prenatal care, vaccines for children, family planning services and supplies, rural health clinic services, laboratory and x-ray services, physician services, nursing facility services for persons age 21 or older, home health care for persons eligible for skilled nursing services, pediatric and family nurse practitioner services, nurse–midwife services, and federally qualified health care services. Also included are early periodic screening, diagnostic, and treatment services for children under the age of 21.

Each state sets its own rules with respect to payment of midwives. This is due in part to a lack of uniformity of the description of scope of practice for midwives from state to state. You must research your individual state's rules and regulations that apply to the provision of care to Medicaid recipients. Medicaid may or may not adopt the Medicare incident to rules. As with Medicare, you must obtain a Medicaid provider number from the state regulatory board. You should note that the federal laws regarding billing for Medicaid services do not require physician direction or supervision of you unless supervision or direction is required according to the individual state's rules and regulations.

Most states have a Medicaid Managed Care structure. Payment under these plans requires a provider to enroll as a preferred provider; that provider may receive payment on a different fee structure than "straight" Medicaid. You should research Medicaid rules, regulations, and requirements for billing in the state in which you intend to practice (found in the state Medicaid manual). You must also research the documents within state agencies (Board of Nursing, Board of Public Health, Board of Medicine, Board of Midwifery) that may govern midwifery practice because Medicaid allows for billing that is within your scope of practice as defined by state law.

Despite the federal mandate that allows women to seek midwifery care, and in the presence of nurse–midwifery-supportive state rules and regulations, midwives may experience difficulty receiving payment from Medicaid for some services. In the state of Michigan, for example, midwives are reimbursed at 100% of physician reimbursement for maternity care and gynecological care if it is for family planning. Medicaid would not reimburse for some services such as non-stress testing or colposcopy. Additionally, midwives were prohibited from billing for some services that Medicaid reimbursed nurse practitioners within the same state for.

You should remember that since Medicaid is regulated by the state, changes to the Medicaid payment policies require regulatory changes—thus they do not require legislation. What this means is, in order to change Medicaid rules and regulations, midwives may meet with the regulatory body (Medicaid) and request or negotiate change. If the regulatory body resists change or refuses to reimburse midwives for services they are legally authorized to perform under state law, the regional CMS office may be contacted to investigate failure to comply with federal regulations.

Regulatory bodies do not like legislation that mandates changes in policy, so enlisting the aid of a state representative or senator who is prepared to introduce legislation regarding a change often opens doors to negotiation.

Military Plans

Military personnel and their families are covered by government health plans called Tricare (a military managed care plan) and the Civilian Health and Medical Program of the United States (CHAMPUS). Midwives may provide care to recipients of these programs provided the services are covered benefits of the program and the midwife is licensed as a registered nurse, educated in a program accredited by the American College of Nurse–Midwives (ACNM), and certified by the ACNM or the ACNM Certification Council (ACC). Under CHAMPUS, midwives are authorized as individual professional providers of care provided the services are authorized by CHAMPUS. Midwives may provide care independent of physician referrals and supervisors. Reimbursable services are defined according to the scope of practice as determined by the local licensing agency for the jurisdiction in which care is provided.

Payment for services under CHAMPUS mirrors the Medicare fee schedule; thus, the midwife receives 65% of the physician's fee schedule for services rendered to CHAMPUS recipients.

Third-Party Payers

Although patients covered by federal government health plans often comprise a large percentage of the midwife's case load, many midwives provide care to patients insured by private insurers or health plans. These plans are much more loosely regulated than government plans.

"Third-party payers" often refers to private insurance plans—health care plans purchased by employers or individuals. These plans vary widely in their covered benefits and reimbursement for services. When purchasing coverage with these plans, the employer or individual has the opportunity to select which services may be covered and what out of pocket expenses are the responsibility of the consumer of the services. Federal mandates with respect to accessing midwifery care do not apply for the majority of these plans. States can enact laws that mandate coverage for midwifery services, however.

Employers that purchase coverage from private insurers may receive a discount in premiums because they purchase insurance coverage for a group of people. The employees covered by these plans may have to pay for some of the services they receive. The plan may pay for 80–90% of costs while the subscriber bears the responsibility for paying for the remainder. The subscriber often must pay a co-pay for routine services such as office visits.

The co-pay is a set out-of-pocket expense born by the subscriber. The plan pays the balance of the visit.

Subscribers are also frequently required to pay initial expenses for services until a deductible has been met. The deductible is a set amount of out-of-pocket expense that is the responsibility of the subscriber. Once the deductible has been met, the plan's coverage arrangement is put into effect. This process resets and begins again at the end of the contract year with the plan. Usually most contract years end at the end of a calendar year.

Insurance companies often enroll health care providers in their plans as preferred providers. As long as the subscriber seeks care from a preferred provider, the subscriber is able to enjoy the maximum benefits allowed by the plan. This is known as in-network services. If the subscriber elects to obtain services from providers not enrolled with the plan, such services are deemed out of network and the subscriber may pay a larger co-pay or be responsible for a higher portion of the payment.

Managed Care Plans

In an effort to control health care costs, consumers and providers of care have experimented with alternatives to traditional fee-for-service health plans. Prepaid health plans that attempt to manage the costs of health care have been around for many years. According to Kongstvedt (2001), many factors influenced the growth of managed care, including a shift in physician practices from a single practitioner to a group model. With enactment of Medicare and Medicaid legislation in 1965, more hospitals became investor owned and corporate controlled. In the 1970s, membership in health maintenance organizations (HMOs) escalated as more businesses began contracting with HMOs to control the rising costs of providing employee insurance benefits.

Managed care organizations (MCOs) are commercial plans that are designed to provide for access to care and control of health care costs. Many organizational models of MCOs have been developed to manage care.

Health Maintenance Organizations

Members enrolled in these plans are assigned a primary care provider who is responsible for the primary care needs of enrollees in the plan. Referrals for specialty services require the authorization of the primary provider. Such plans also have drug formularies that list the prescription drugs covered by the plan. The primary care provider receives monthly payment according to a formula that includes the number of *covered lives* in the plan and the average services provided over a set period of time, such as a year. This payment system to providers is called "capitation." The key to cost savings with a HMO is efficiency in care delivery. The HMO consumer must utilize the plan's physicians, hospitals, laboratories, and so on.

Preferred Provider Organizations (PPO)

A preferred provider organization is a provider network that contracts directly with an employer to provide health care services to the employer's employees. Patients are given incentives to use the providers in the network who have agreed to follow the PPO's utilization policies to control costs. Patients may select services outside of the PPO, but will pay higher costs for the services.

Exclusive Provider Organization (EPO)

Subscribers to this type of health plan must utilize the services of the providers in the plan or must pay out of pocket for services.

Point of Service Plans

Similar to HMOs, participants in this type of health plan see a primary care provider who receives payment according to the plan's contracted agreements with providers. The participant may elect to receive care outside of the network of providers but will pay higher premiums or co-pays to do so.

Independent Practice Association (IPA) or Organization (IPO)

In this model, an HMO contracts with a physician organization, which in turn contracts with individual physicians. The physicians see the patients in the plan in their own offices as well as patients in other plans. The HMO reimburses the IPA on a capitated basis, but the IPA may reimburse the physicians on a fee-for-service or capitated basis.

All health care programs, whether they be a government program or a commercial insurance plan, have the same requirements. They will pay for services that are:

- A covered benefit of the plan
- Provided by a qualified health care provider
- Medically necessary
- Documented in the medical record
- Coded correctly (numerical codes applied to clinical services for billing purposes)

The Rules of Billing and Coding

Many entities govern payment of services. The federal government and some of its health care plans were discussed previously.

State rules and regulations govern payment with respect to midwives by describing the midwives' scope of practice, relationship with a physician, and prescriptive authority. Midwives must be licensed by the state in order to provide services and bill for them. Governing bodies vary from state to state. Midwifery rules and regulations may be found in a variety of organizations within a state's government including the Board of Nursing, Board of Public Health, Board of Midwifery, or Board of Medicine.

According to the American College of Nurse–Midwives, 38 states mandate third-party reimbursement for midwifery services (American College of Nurse–Midwives [ACNM], 2002b). This means insurance companies must reimburse midwives directly for contracted services. In order to receive payment for services, you must submit an application and become *credentialed* with the insurance company. The credentialing process verifies your education, professional work history, and malpractice history. Once credentialed, you can then *contract* with the insurance company for payment. An application is obtained from the payer and once approved you can begin submitting bills to the payer for services rendered. Credentialing is the process of confirming that a provider is qualified to provide services, whereas contracting is the process involving payment from a payer to a provider.

It is important for you to understand how your individual state defines midwifery scope of practice. You would not be allowed to bill services provided in that state that were outside of your scope of practice. For example, an individual state may determine that infant circumcision is a surgical procedure and not within the scope of practice of a midwife. Midwives in that state would be prohibited from billing and receiving payment for the performance of infant circumcision. Requirements for physician oversight may also affect billing practices. Some payers will require a copy of the collaborative practice agreement between a midwife and his or her consulting physician if physician supervision is required by state law. Prescriptive authority may indirectly affect billing practices because supplies such as intrauterine devices or injectable contraceptives may be considered pharmaceuticals by the state and therefore the midwife must have prescriptive authority to prescribe or dispense such supplies in order to receive payment for providing these supplies to patients.

Learning the rules and regulations associated with billing for medical services are paramount because you must translate clinical services into revenue if you are to survive in today's health care market. Even those employed by large institutions or managed care organizations must demonstrate a financial value to the organization. Care providers are expected to be productive and generate revenue that covers the cost of doing business as well as (in many cases) making a profit. There are also regulations regarding billing and coding that you must be familiar with in order for you to be in compliance with the law. Such regulations address documentation requirements and coding processes that only the clinician can perform because he or she is the one providing the service.

Some clinicians fail to appreciate the value of learning the billing and coding language. They feel hiring a professional coder or billing service is an alternative to learning the language themselves. There are several reasons why this will not work:

- The clinician is the one responsible for the bill.
- Mastery of coding will increase reimbursement.
- The clinician is the only person in the exam room, operating room, or delivery room with the patient.

As mentioned before, you must translate clinical services into actual revenue. This is accomplished by becoming fluent in a language spoken by insurance companies and other payers. As of October 2003, the Health Insurance Portability and Accountability Act (HIPAA) standardized this language by way of the Uniform Data Set.

The Health Insurance Portability and Accountability Act of 1996 is a part of insurance reform. Implementation of HIPAA is the responsibility of the Department of Health and Human Services, the Department of Labor, and the Department of the Treasury. CMS works with the states to comply with the small group and individual market provisions of

HIPAA. HIPAA rules are categorized into three sets of standards: Transaction Standards, Security Standards, and Privacy Standards. All three sets of standards combined improve efficiency and effectiveness of health care by encouraging the use of information systems.

Billing codes were standardized to support the electronic exchange of data. These transaction standards automated billing for health care in much the same way as ATMs automated banking and universal product codes (UPCs) automated retail. This type of coding also simplified data collection, data analysis, and reporting. All services with more than 10 employees must now bill government agencies electronically.

With automated billing and the exchange of information electronically, HIPAA also made provisions for protecting a patient's privacy; thus, privacy rules and regulations were also implemented as a precursor to the implementation of the coding set and electronic billing. The Privacy Standards impose boundaries on the use and disclosure of private health information (PHI). They require accountability and adherence to appropriate safeguards from health care providers and others in order to protect an individual's PHI.

The Privacy Standards propose "minimum necessary standards" limiting access to PHI to the work force on a need to know only basis as determined by role or job function. The standards also increase a consumer's control over their health information.

Coding

This section will discuss the coding language that is necessary for billing insurance companies and government health plans. It is not the intention of this chapter to provide comprehensive instruction for billing and coding midwifery services. You should seek formal billing and coding instruction to comply with billing regulations and to ensure maximum reimbursement for services rendered.

Current Procedural Terminology

Current Procedural Terminology (CPT) codes are developed by the American Medical Association and updated yearly. The CPT book that contains and describes these codes is divided into six sections:

- Evaluation and management
- Anesthesia
- Surgery
- Pathology and laboratory
- Radiology
- Medicine

There are over 7500 CPT codes. Midwives will usually use codes found in the "surgery" and "evaluation and management" sections of the CPT book. Obstetrical services and gynecological procedures are found in the surgery section (10021–69990) and ambulatory care and some hospital services are found in the evaluation and management section (99201–99499).

CPT codes describe services provided or procedures that are performed. They tell the payer what the clinician did and determine the level of payment. The CPT code book provides instructions for coding in each section and subsection.

Many CPT codes are *global* codes. Global codes are codes that bundle services that are commonly performed together into one code. An example of this is the CPT code 59400. This is a global obstetrical code that includes routine antepartum care, vaginal delivery, and postpartum care. All services routinely performed are included in this code. Services such as nonstress testing, ultrasounds, and nonroutine lab work are not included in the global obstetrical services. CPT prohibits *unbundling* of these codes unless instructed by the payer. For instance, in some states, Medicaid instructs health care providers to bill individual prenatal visits as evaluation and management visits and does not accept global antepartum codes. Individual payers determine the number of prenatal visits that are included in the global code. You should be familiar with the payers' rules because it may be possible to bill for additional visits that are not covered in the global services.

Additional prenatal visits for complications related to pregnancy such as preterm labor or pregnancy-induced hypertension may be billable services outside of the global charges if the total number of visits exceeds the contracted number of prenatal visits allowed by the insurance company. Additionally, if you perform services that are not related to the pregnancy, billing for these services is allowed separate from the global charges. A separate visit is not necessary, provided the antepartum charges are billed globally. In cases where the antepartum visits are billed individually, a separate visit to address the unrelated problem may be scheduled or a higher level of service may be billed, taking into account the amount of history, physical exam, and medical decision making that comprise the total visit.

You are cautioned to examine payer contracts to understand the rules that apply in such cases. Sometimes you may not receive payment for evaluation and management services billed during pregnancy unless a referral from the patient's primary care provider is obtained. Any services provided during pregnancy that are not considered by the payer to be routine care may need prior approval or authorization from the primary provider. For example, it is discovered at a routine visit that a pregnant patient is suffering from an upper respiratory infection. You may be equipped to diagnose and treat the illness, but if you are not considered a primary care provider or do not obtain authorization to treat the upper respiratory infection from the patient's primary provider, payment will be denied by the patient's insurance company.

Evaluation and Management Codes

Evaluation and management codes occupy the first section of the CPT book. This is because they are the most widely used codes in the book. The evaluation and management section of the CPT manual is used for coding services such as office visits, counseling, consultations, hospital rounds, emergency room visits, and outpatient observation services. Virtually every specialty uses evaluation and management codes. The codes represent traditional encounters with a health care provider for management of health-related problems.

In January of 1992, the Resource-Based Relative Value System (RBRVS) was phased into CPT. The RBRVS was developed in the 1980s at Harvard. It provided a formula for determining physician compensation for services and procedures using the amount of work involved, the cost of providing the service, and the liability associated with the service or procedure. Measurement of each of these factors became necessary in order to assign a relative value for each service.

Since a majority of patient encounters you will have are billed using evaluation and management (E&M) codes, and CMS requires documentation that supports the level of evaluation and management billed, a detailed discussion of those codes follows.

In nearly all E&M codes, three components of the encounter with the patient must be considered:

- History
- Physical examination
- Medical decision making

Performance and documentation of the elements of each of these components will determine the level of evaluation and management code that is submitted for payment. For outpatient encounters, five levels of service are available for use (99201–99205 and 99211–99215). Selection of a code also requires identifying *new patients* and *established patients* within a service.

A *new* patient is a patient who presents for care and has not received billable services from anyone of the same specialty within the same group for a period of 3 years. Billable services include lab work or other face-to-face services billed by the service. Phone calls and prescription renewals are not considered billable services.

> *Example:* A woman is a patient of an internist in a large multi-specialty group. She has an abnormal pap smear and is referred to the midwives for colposcopy and management as necessary. She is a *new* patient because the internist is not in the same specialty as the midwives.
>
> *Example:* A private practice physician joins a midwifery practice after working for 7 years in the community. She brings to the midwifery practice a number of patients. Some of these patients elect to see the midwives for their annual exams. They are *established* patients of the practice if they have seen the physician who is new to the group within the last 3 years.

Once it is determined whether the patient is new or established, a level of service can be assigned based on the amount of history, physical, and medical decision making involved in the visit.

HISTORY

To determine the level of history, four components of obtaining a history are used:

- Chief complaint (CC)
- History of the present illness (HPI)
- Review of systems (ROS)
- Past, family, and social history (PFSH)

All evaluation and management visits require the documentation of a chief complaint or reason for the visit.

A history of the present illness is documented describing elements of the chief complaint such as:

- Location
- Duration
- Severity
- Onset
- Alleviating factors
- Aggravating factors

A review of systems is a systematic inventory of systems or body areas that may also be affected by the chief complaint.

The final element of a patient's history includes the patient's past medical history, pertinent family history, and the patient's social history, which may include substance use such as tobacco, alcohol, or drugs. Marital status, education, contraceptive use, and sexual history are all components of a social history.

Depending on the components of the history taken during an evaluation and management service, a level of history is determined. Four levels of history are considered:

- Problem-focused history
- Expanded problem-focused history
- Detailed history
- Comprehensive history

Table 11–1 will assist you in determining the level of history for an evaluation and management visit.

To select a level of history, you must document the highest level where all criteria (CC, HPI, ROS, and PFSH) are met.

PHYSICAL EXAMINATION

Determining the level of physical examination depends on the amount of examination that is performed and documented. The levels of examination in evaluation and management coding are the same four categories as the levels of history:

- Problem-focused
- Expanded problem-focused
- Detailed
- Comprehensive

You have the option of using evaluation and management 1995 or 1997 guidelines for documenting the physical exam. The 1995 guidelines count the number of systems or body areas that are examined to determine the level of physical exam. The 1997 guidelines describe essential elements of a physical according to specialty areas. The GYN exam has several elements identified by bullets that are counted to determine the level of examination that is documented.

Table 11–1 Elements of Obtaining a History

History	Problem-Focused	Expanded Problem-Focused	Detailed	Comprehensive
CC	Yes	Yes	Yes	Yes
HPI elements	1–3	1–3	4	Extended
ROS	None	Pertinent + 1	2–9	>10
PFSH	None	None	Pertinent 1 of 3	Complete 2/3 est., 3/3 new

Table 11–2 will assist you in determining the level of physical examination for an evaluation and management visit.

Medical Decision Making

The final component that determines the level of an evaluation and management visit is the amount of medical decision making that is involved in the encounter. Medical decision making has four levels to consider:

- Straightforward
- Low
- Moderate
- High

Choosing the level of medical decision making depends on the consideration of three areas:

- The number of diagnoses or treatment options to consider
- The amount of data reviewed
- The risk of either the disease, the diagnostic modalities, or the treatment required

Table 11–3 will assist you in determining the level of medical decision making for an evaluation and management visit.

The level of medical decision making is chosen by determining which category is most representative of the patient's problem. To assign the appropriate E&M code for an office service, the midwife must consider the history, physical exam, and medical decision

Table 11–2 Elements of a Physical Exam

Exam	Problem-Focused	Expanded Problem-Focused	Detailed	Comprehensive
1995	Affected system	Affected + 2–4 symptomatic or related systems	Affected + 5–7 systems	Affected + 8–12 systems
1997	1–5 elements identified by a bullet	6 elements identified by a bullet	12 elements identified by a bullet	All elements identified by a bullet

Table 11–3 Elements of Medical Decision Making

Medical Decision Making	Straightforward	Low Complexity	Detailed	Comprehensive
Differential diagnoses	Minimal diagnoses or management options	Limited diagnoses or management options	Multiple diagnoses or management options	Extensive diagnoses or management options
Data reviewed	Minimal, none or low complexity	Limited data reviewed	Moderate data reviewed	Extensive data reviewed
Risk of complications, morbidity, or mortality	Minimal risk	Low risk	Moderate risk	High risk

making involved. **Tables 11–4** and **11–5** can be used to assist with this. For new patients, the highest level of service of all three categories is used to determine the proper code. Stated another way, the code selected can be no higher than the lowest category of history, physical, or medical decision making. For example, a new patient is evaluated for right lower quadrant pain. A detailed history, an expanded problem-focused exam, and medical decision making of high complexity are documented. A 99202 is billed since the exam is the lowest level documented.

If the same situation is applied to an established patient, the highest level of two of three categories is used to determine the level coded. Thus, a detailed history, expanded problem-focused exam, and medical decision making of high complexity would be coded as 99214. Two of three components (history and medical decision making) were at least at a level 4.

Not all encounters include a physical exam, or sometimes the bulk of the encounter is spent in educating or discussing test results or treatment plans with the patient and/or his or her family. The times or length of service in Tables 11–4 and 11–5 are used to determine the level of service billed when more than 50% of the visit involves counseling, education, or risk factor reduction. If this is the case, the level of service billed correlates to the face-to-face time spent with the patient. The length of the visit should be documented in the medical record. If the midwife does not intend to bill based on the length of the visit, or if less than 50% of the visit is spent providing education, counseling, or discussing risk factor reduction, the length of the visit does not need to be documented.

Table 11–4 New Patient Evaluation and Management Visits

	History	Exam	MDM	Time
99201	PF	PF	S	10 minutes
99202	EPF	EPF	S	20 minutes
99203	D	D	L	30 minutes
99204	C	C	M	45 minutes
99205	C	C	H	60 minutes

	History	*Exam*	*MDM*	*Time*
Table 11–5 Established Patient Evaluation and Management Visits				
99211				5 minutes
99212	PF	PF	S	10 minutes
99213	EPF	EPF	L	15 minutes
99214	D	D	M	25 minutes
99215	C	C	H	40 minutes

You are cautioned to use all three components of evaluation and management coding when determining the correct level of visit to code. Midwives have traditionally chosen the level of visit based on how difficult the encounter seems or the amount of time the visit took. This will often lead to undercoding or the selection of incorrect codes that are not supported by documentation in the medical record. Undercoding will result in a lower payment from the payer than what the provider is actually entitled based on the level of service actually provided. It is a well accepted adage that what is not documented is not done. In billing and coding what is not legible is not documented. Thorough documentation is required to support the level of evaluation and management visit billed.

Preventive Medicine Codes

Another type of evaluation and management visit codes commonly used by midwives are the *preventive medicine* codes. Preventive medicine codes are used for the annual well woman exam and include a comprehensive history, comprehensive physical exam, and routine health screening and risk factor reduction. The level of visit chosen depends on whether the patient is a new or established patient and on the patient's age.

Table 11–6 illustrates the preventive medicine codes that are used for well woman exams.

In addition to office visits, evaluation and management visits are also used for hospital services such as initial admissions, rounding, and discharge visits. They are also used for outpatient observation services such as triage visits and emergency room visits. Refer to a CPT code book for a full description of evaluation and management codes. CPT codes are revised annually, so a current edition of a CPT code book is essential.

Modifiers

It is easy to understand that not all patient encounters can be readily pigeon-holed into CPT codes. For this reason, modifiers, found in Appendix A of the CPT code book, can be added to codes to further define the code. Modifiers can indicate a prolonged or difficult procedure. They can be used to indicate bilateral procedures or discontinued procedures.

> *Example:* A 53-year-old established patient presents for her well woman annual exam. She also complains of a breast lump and nipple discharge. In addition to a comprehensive history, a comprehensive exam, and counseling and risk factor reduction appropriate for the woman's age,

Table 11–6 Well-Woman Exams

Age	New Patient	Est. Patient
12–17	99384	99394
18–39	99385	99395
40–64	99386	99396
>65	99387	99397

the midwife obtains a detailed history about the breast lump and discharge including when the symptoms first appeared. A thorough breast exam is documented including a description and location of the lump, color of discharge, and any other pertinent observations. A pap smear of the discharge is obtained, a mammogram is ordered, and a surgeon is consulted. The midwife bills for the preventive medicine visit (99396) and also bills an evaluation and management visit according to the level of history, exam, and medical decision making unique to the breast lump that was performed and documented (99213, for example). A 25 modifier is appended to the evaluation and management code (99213-25) to indicate a *separate and significant evaluation and management service* was performed on the same day as another service.

The 25 modifier allows reimbursement for two services performed on the same day. Some procedures have both a technical and a professional component.

> *Example:* A nonstress test is performed in the midwife's office on a patient who is post dates. The midwife bills for the nonstress test (59025). Similarly, a midwife is called to review the fetal monitor tracing of a woman who presented to labor and delivery reporting decreased fetal movement. The midwife reviews the tracing and determines the tracing is reactive. She documents the results and advises the woman to keep her next scheduled appointment. The midwife bills for a nonstress test with a modifier 26 to indicate she performed only the professional component of a nonstress test (59025-26).

The technical component of the nonstress test will be billed by the hospital. The 26 modifier reduces payment from the insurance company because only the professional component was performed by the midwife.

For a complete list of modifiers and their descriptions, see Appendix A of the CPT code book.

International Classification of Diseases, 9th Revision (ICD-9)

The International Classification of Diseases (ICD) coding system dates back to 17th century England. The codes, originally called the London Bills of Mortality, were used to collect information regarding the most frequent causes of death. In 1937, the codes were renamed the International List of Causes of Death and were primarily used for statistical purposes. The World Health Organization used these codes when tracking morbidity and mortality. In 1977, the U.S. National Center for Health Statistics took the statistical study a step farther and added clinical information to the codes. The result is the International Classification of Diseases, 9th Revision, Clinical Modification (ICD-9-CM).

The ICD-9-CM codes are maintained by the Coordination and Maintenance Committee, co-chaired by the National Center for Health Statistics and the Centers for Medicare and Medicaid Services. The committee meets twice yearly to discuss revisions of the codes. The changes, published in the *Federal Register*, become effective October 1 of each year. The newest version of ICD codes, ICD-10, is already in use for statistical purposes. The Clinical Modification of ICD-10 will be implemented soon.

For billing purposes, ICD-9-CM codes are used to establish the medical necessity for a service or procedure and determine if the clinician is paid. Failure to establish medical necessity for a service will result in denial of payment. Three or four ICD-9 codes can be paired with a CPT code to establish the medical necessity for a service or procedure.

ICD-9-CM is organized into three volumes:

- Volume 1, Tabular List
- Volume 2, Alphabetic Index to Diseases
- Volume 3, Procedural

To navigate the ICD-9-CM book, the condition, diagnosis, symptom, or complaint is located in the alphabetic index or Volume 1 of the book. Once the condition, diagnosis, symptom, or complaint is found, a corresponding number assists with locating a specific code in the tabular section or Volume 2, of the book. You should always pay attention to the symbols in the book that may direct you to a more specific code. Nonspecific codes may result in denied or downgraded payment. Most ICD-9-CM codes are three-digit numerical codes followed by a decimal and one or two other numbers. Very few ICD-9-CM codes are three-digit codes alone. Most coding requires use of the forth or fifth digit for specificity.

Most conditions complicating pregnancy require five-digit codes. The fifth digit is applied to describe when in the pregnancy the complication occurs. Failure to code to the highest level of specificity—using the fifth digit—may result in denial of payment.

> *Example:* A woman calls the office 4 days postpartum stating something is coming out of her vagina. She is evaluated in the office and retained fetal membranes are noted protruding from the cervical os. The membranes are removed with ring forceps and the woman is given a prescription for antibiotics and methergine. The office visit is coded as 99213 with a diagnosis of 667.14 (retained portion of placenta or membranes, without hemorrhage). The last digit (4) indicates that this is a postpartum condition or complication.

V CODES

Not all patients seek medical care for a symptom, diagnosis, condition, or complaint. Well patient visits, follow-up, or counseling visits are coded using V codes (V72.31—routine gynecological examination). V codes may also indicate a patient is at risk for a condition, but at the current time of service is well. V codes are listed in a separate section of the ICD-9-CM manual.

> *Example:* A woman presents with a vaginal discharge and cultures are obtained. A CPT code of 99212 is billed with 623.5 (vaginal discharge) as the diagnosis. Another woman presents for screening for sexually transmitted diseases. She denies any symptoms. A 99212 is billed for the office visit and V74.5 (special screening for venereal disease) is indicated as the medical reason for the visit.

> *Example:* A woman is scheduled for more frequent prenatal visits since she has demonstrated preterm labor contractions with cervical change. The diagnosis for these extra visits could be 644.0 (threatened premature labor). Conversely, another woman who has delivered a previous infant at 32 weeks is seen more frequently during a second pregnancy but has no symptoms of preterm labor. The diagnosis for the extra visits is V23.41 (pregnancy with history of preterm labor).

Alternative Billing Concept Codes

Alternative Billing Concept codes (ABC codes©) are five-character alphanumeric symbols that have been developed by a company called Alternative Links based in Albuquerque, New Mexico. These codes are for integrative health care products and services and are based on a wellness model rather than the disease model upon which CPT codes are based. Alternative Links maintains that ABC codes do not replace CPT codes, but rather complement them by coding for wellness services not covered by CPT.

The codes reflect care delivered by providers such as acupuncturists, massage therapists, midwives, nurses, and social workers. Alternative Link has also developed provider modifiers for the codes. The modifier indicates which type of provider is billing for a specific service. These modifiers would assist insurance companies in determining if a code should be reimbursed because the codes and the providers qualified to bill for them would be part of the insurance company's database. ABC codes are also HIPAA compliant.

For more information on ABC codes, access the Alternative Link Web site at www.alternativelink.com.

Billing

In previous sections of this chapter, the codes that translate clinical services into a language spoken by insurance companies and other payers have been discussed. Accurate coding is essential in order to receive payment for services and avoid fraudulent billing.

Beware that *coding* and *billing* are not synonymous. Although it is possible to find legitimate codes in the CPT book that describe services performed, billing rules may prohibit their use in certain situations. Some payers may require services be billed in a specific manner, or consider some codes to include several services. Often billing rules are implied rather than specifically stated in coding manuals. For example, codes that represent "repair of genital lacerations" can be found in the integument section of the CPT code book, but most payers would expect that a repair of a genital laceration incurred during a vaginal birth would be included in the global obstetrical charge. The prudent midwife should check with the payer involved if he or she is unsure how to apply codes in a specific clinical situation. If the situation is unusual, a letter of explanation or additional documentation describing the service may prevent delays or denial of payment.

It is always a wise investment to become familiar with the practice's billing manager. Professional coders and others responsible for billing for the practice may be unfamiliar with the practice of midwifery or with rules and regulations that may apply in certain situations with respect to midwives. Educating the billing staff and managers and enlisting them as advocates helps to assure that your services are billed for properly. Additionally, you can learn a great deal from professionals who have been formally educated in billing and coding.

You should also familiarize yourself with the contracts that pertain to your practice. You must be aware of specific billing rules and regulations that are unique to individual payers. You must know what services are considered covered benefits of individual plans and of any specific requirements for referrals, documentation, or billing incident to a physician when necessary.

Fraud

Fraudulent billing can take many forms and is punishable by fines and/or imprisonment. You may be found guilty of fraudulent billing if you billed for services fraudulently or knew of illegal billing practices that occurred on your behalf. In cases where improper billing occurred and was due to ignorance, health care providers have been ordered to pay back funds that may represent overpayment. Additionally, fines are imposed for fraudulent billing practices. Examples of fraudulent billing include upcoding—billing a higher level of service than was performed or that is supported by documentation; unbundling—billing separate codes for services usually represented by a global CPT code; undercoding—billing a lower level of service than that which was provided; or billing for services that are not medically necessary.

The Office of the Inspector General (OIG) is responsible for examining billing compliance and investigating fraud with respect to billing federal government programs. Each year the OIG publishes its work plan, which details areas of billing and coding that will fall under scrutiny for that year. It is not uncommon for incident to billing and billing by nonphysician providers to be on the work plan. Thus, you must remain up to date with billing rules and regulations. The Office of Inspector General Work Plan for the current year and previous years can be found at http://oig.hhs.gov/publications/workplan.html.

Health care providers convicted of billing fraudulently may lose their opportunity to participate in health plans. Those who have lost billing rights with Medicare and Medicaid are listed in the National Practitioner Data Bank (NPDB). The purpose of the NPDB is to allow state licensing agencies to examine the records of health care providers who have settled malpractice claims or been excluded from participating with Medicare and

Medicaid. For more information on the NPDB, access their Web site at http://www.npdb-hipdb.com.

Summary

The processes of billing, coding, and receiving payment for midwifery services are complex. You must become educated in these processes so as to remain financially viable and comply with the law. In review, payers pay for services that are:

- A covered benefit of the plan
- Provided by a qualified health care provider
- Medically necessary
- Documented in the medical record
- Coded correctly

Consistently and accurately meeting these requirements will help to assure timely payment for clinical services.

Chapter Exercise

One of the essential people you will need to get to know in your practice is the business manager or the person who will coordinate your payer credentialing and process your claims for payment. In order to both function and survive in practice you will need to be able to access critical data about your practice, in addition to understanding the billing rules and regulations. Each office operation varies slightly, so make an appointment with your business manager and/or practice billing coordinator and spend one-half day with her or him.

Answer the following questions:

- Who manages the practice data?
- Can you retrieve data on your volume of patients by diagnosis, managed care entity, and billables generated?
- What are the relative value units (RVUs) for each provider and how do they compare?
- Does the practice compare data between and among providers?
- What is the process in the practice for credentialing providers?
- Does the practice bill under your provider number, a practice number, or incident to?
- What managed care contracts does your practice have? How is each contract similar and different?
- What are the reimbursement rates for CNMs/CMs in your practice?

Next, obtain a copy of your practice's encounter form. Familiarize yourself with its layout and learn in what areas you are responsible for completing the data. Ask to track an encounter form from provider through payment.

Table 11–7 For Your Professional Files

The ACNM has published three handbooks that the midwife can use with issues related to billing, coding, and getting Paid for services.
1. *Getting Paid: Billing, Coding and Payment for Midwifery Services* (2003)
2. *Nurse–Midwifery Today: A Handbook of State Laws and Regulations* (2002)
3. *Guidance for CNMs in Managed Care Contracting*

References

American Academy of Professional Coders. (2004). *Independent study program 2004*. Salt Lake City, UT: Author.

American College of Nurse–Midwives. (2002a). *Getting paid: Billing, coding and payment for midwifery services*. Washington, DC: Author.

American College of Nurse–Midwives. (2002b). *Nurse–midwifery today: A handbook of state laws and regulations*. Washington, DC: Author.

American Medical Association. (2003). *CPT 2004: Current procedural terminology*. Chicago: Author.

Buppert, C. (2003). *The primary care provider's guide to compensation and quality*. Sudbury, MA: Jones and Bartlett.

Department for Health and Human Services. (2003). *Medicaid at-a-glance 2003*. Washington, DC: Author. Retrieved July 20, 2006, from http://www.cms.hhs.gov/MedicaidEligibility/downloads/Medicaid%20At%20A%20Glance%202003.pdf.

Kongstvedt, P. (2001). *The managed health care handbook* (4th ed.). Gaithersburg, MD: Aspen.

Medicode. (2004). *ICD-9-CM Expert for Physicians, Volumes 1 & 2: International Classification of Diseases, 9th Revision: Clinical Modifications* (6th ed.). Salt Lake City, UT: Ingenix.

Nurse–Midwifery Service Director's Network. (1996). *An administrative manual for nurse–midwifery services* (2nd ed.). Dubuque, IA: Kendal/Hunt.

Ob-Gyn Practice Management. (1998). *The ob-gyn managed care maze—successful maneuvering tactics for ob-gyn practices and clinics in managed care*. Naples, FL: Author.

Slager, J. (2004). *Business concepts for healthcare providers: A quick reference for midwives, NPs, PAs, CNSs and other disruptive innovators*. Sudbury, MA: Jones & Bartlett.

CHAPTER 12

Quality Management

Lynette Ament, PhD, RN, CNM, FACNM

Jackie Tillett, ND, CNM

Learning Objectives

1. Define quality management, quality improvement, and utilization review.
2. Describe peer review and ACNM's guidelines for peer review.
3. Identify the ACNM position statement on quality management.
4. List benefits and impediments to quality management and peer review.
5. Discuss the ACNM benchmarking project.
6. Describe the purpose and function of JCAHO, NCQA, and HEDIS and how they interact with the profession.
7. Describe provider profiling and its uses.
8. Describe the Institute for Healthcare Improvement (IHI) and its quality initiatives that relate to midwifery and women's health.

This chapter is an introduction to the concepts of quality management, patient safety, and outcomes management. Under quality management, you will learn the basic principles of quality improvement and quality assurance and explore the use of such tools as provider profiling and Health Plan Employer Data and Information Set (HEDIS) measures to ensure quality. Patient safety, a very important aspect of quality management, has become a national focus. You will become familiar with the Institute of Medicine's reports on patient safety. Critical to all of these components is the use of evidence-based practice and outcomes management, reflected in the Agency for Healthcare Research and Quality's (AHRQ) clinical guidelines series. This chapter is designed to give you the necessary tools for safe clinical practice and the preliminary foundation to apply these tools.

Quality management is both an old and a new concept in health care. Florence Nightingale was one of the first in health care to have an organized program of quality improvement when she worked with British soldiers in the Crimean War. Avedis Donabedian

(1966) described and evaluated methods for assessing the quality of medical care. He suggested that when assessing medical care, outcome measures should not be the only criterion; one must also examine process and structure outcomes. Donabedian proposed sources and methods of obtaining information, sampling and selection of criteria, and indices of medical care. Modern quality management principles were developed in industry and manufacturing by William Deming. Deming (1986) studied quality improvement techniques in Japan and brought the principles he learned to the United States. Deming's work focused on employees—building quality into the product rather than inspecting for errors. He believed that managers must first promote quality efforts in order for staff to adopt its principles.

Quality as a concept is elusive and difficult to define. Because of rising concerns about patient safety in the late 20th century and early 21st century, the Institute of Medicine (IOM) launched an initiative focused on the assessment and improvement of the quality of care in the United States. The IOM defines quality as the degree to which health services for individuals and populations increase the likelihood of desired health outcomes and are consistent with current professional knowledge (Committee on Quality of Health Care in America, 2001). The IOM's Quality Initiative has three phases. The first phase is documentation of the problem of quality and patient safety. The second phase is the development of the IOM's vision for change. The third phase focuses on operationalizing the vision for change; in other words, measuring and improving the quality of health care in the United States. The IOM's vision for change is important for midwifery and for all health care disciplines, and focuses reform efforts on organizations and consumers of health care: the patients.

Definitions

Quality assurance describes activities that monitor and evaluate care according to specific indicators. *Total quality management* is a process that develops slowly and promotes a holistic approach to management, including the concept of *continuous quality improvement,* which takes the concept of planning from the initial design through implementation (Ament, 1996, p. 56). *Risk management,* on the other hand, involves making conscious decisions to decrease risk and financial losses (Ament, 1996).

Joint Commission on the Accreditation of Healthcare Organizations (JCAHO)

The mission of the Joint Commission on the Accreditation of Healthcare Organizations (JCAHO) focuses on quality: "to continuously improve the safety and quality of care provided to the public through the provision of health care accreditation and related services that support performance improvement in health care organizations" (Joint Commission on Accreditation of Healthcare Organizations [JCAHO], 2005). The Joint Commission on Accreditation of Hospitals (JCAH) was created in 1951 as a joint venture of the American College of Physicians (ACP), the American Hospital Association (AHA), the Canadian

Medical Association (CMA), and the American College of Surgeons (ACS) as an independent, not-for-profit organization whose primary purpose was to provide voluntary accreditation (JCAHO, 2006a). The ACS was formed in 1913, and in 1917 developed the Minimum Standards for Hospitals. In 1918, the ACS began on-site inspections of hospitals, and only 89 of the 692 hospitals inspected at that time met the minimum requirements. In 1987, JCAH changed its name to JCAHO to better reflect its expanded scope of activities. JCAHO now accredits organizations such as hospice care, long-term care facilities, and home health care agencies. Although accreditation remains voluntary, criteria for federal funding and other opportunities typically require accreditation. For example, in 1965 Congress recognized JCAH as the organization to set standards for hospitals receiving Medicare funds.

Consumers and health care professionals can locate and compare information about a health care organization's accreditation status. You can search for any accredited organization on the JCAHO web site. Data include the organization's accreditation status and comparisons of its patient safety and quality improvement efforts to national and statewide benchmarks (http://www.qualitycheck.org). Other issues addressed by JCAHO include public policy issues, such as emergency preparedness, pay-for-performance, health care professional education, tort resolution, and injury prevention.

In 1987, JCAHO integrated performance measurement data into the accreditation process through the implementation of the ORYX initiative to permit comparison of care across hospitals. One of the performance measures is the Pregnancy and Related Conditions Core Measure Set. This set contains three measures: vaginal birth after cesarean (VBAC), inpatient neonatal mortality, and third or fourth degree laceration (JCAHO, 2002). Other maternal care measures have been identified for potential future implementation: episiotomy rate, primary cesarean section rate, and maternal transfer to perinatal center.

National Committee for Quality Assurance

Another major player in the external assessment of quality is the National Committee for Quality Assurance (NCQA). The NCQA has a very different focus from JCAHO. The mission of NCQA is to improve the quality of health care, and it is a private, non-for-profit organization that accredits managed care organizations (MCOs). It began accrediting managed care organizations in 1991 in response to the need for standardized, objective information about the quality of these organizations (NCQA, 2005). NCQA evaluates MCOs in the areas of patient safety, confidentiality, consumer protection, access, service, and continuous improvement. There are 60 different standards, falling into five broad categories: access and service, qualified providers, staying healthy, getting better, and living with illness. Like JCAHO, NCQA accreditation is voluntary, but several states accept NCQA accreditation as meeting the needs of state review.

The NCQA has several programs. The Health Plan Employer Data and Information Set (HEDIS) tool measures performance on dimensions of care and service. There are more than 60 measures and they are designed to provide purchasers (typically employers) and consumers with information to compare the performance of MCOs (NCQA, 2005). Maternal and women's health indicators include breast and cervical cancer screening, access to prenatal and postpartum care, and frequency of ongoing prenatal care. HEDIS also includes the CAHPS 3.0H survey, which measures members' satisfaction with their care in areas such as claims processing, customer service, and getting needed care quickly. Quality Compass is a tool to assist consumers in selecting a health plan, conducting competitor analysis, evaluating quality improvement efforts, and examining benchmarking and health care research (NCQA, 2005). Quality Compass includes features such as trended data and customized reports.

Other Organizations Addressing Quality and Safety

Institute for Healthcare Improvement

The Institute for Healthcare Improvement (IHI) is a not-for-profit organization whose mission is to drive the improvement of health by advancing the quality and value of health care (Institute for Healthcare Improvement [IHI], 2005a). The IHI was founded in 1991 and is based in Cambridge, Massachusetts. The focus of IHI's work is on safety, effectiveness, patient-centeredness, timeliness, efficiency, and equity. Since 1995, its Breakthrough Series Collaboratives have helped health care organizations to make breakthrough improvements in quality while reducing costs. One current initiative is the Idealized Design of Perinatal Care, which is planning to redesign the perinatal care system to improve the reliability of the processes of care (induction, fetal monitoring, etc.) (IHI, 2005b). There are currently 16 health care teams examining two topics: elective induction and augmentation.

The Leapfrog Group

Composed of more than 170 public and private organizations that provide health care benefits, the Leapfrog Group works with medical experts from around the United States to identify problems and propose solutions that it believes will improve health care systems (Leapfrog Group, 2005). Its members work to reduce preventable medical mistakes, improve the quality and affordability of health care, encourage public reporting of health care quality and outcomes, reward doctors and hospitals for improving care, and help consumers of care make smart health care decisions. The Leapfrog Group was formed in 1998 and has focused on four hospital quality and safety practices: computer physician order entry, evidence-based hospital referral, ICU physician staffing, and the Leapfrog safe practices score. This score is based on 27 identified safe practices.

Consumers can search the Leapfrog Web site for hospitals to assess whether the hospital has implemented and/or made progress on Leapfrog's recommended quality and safety leaps. Each hospital included in the database has voluntarily submitted the information. As of July 1, 2005, 933 hospitals completed the Leapfrog Hospital Quality and Safety Survey, an increase of 23.5% over the 2004 response rate.

Patient Safety

The Committee on the Quality of Health Care in America was appointed in 1998 to identify strategies for improving the quality of health care in the United States. The committee's first report, *To Err is Human: Building a Safer Health System*, was released in 1999 and focused on patient safety. The committee's second report, *Crossing the Quality Chasm*, was released in 2001. This second report focused on how to redesign the health care system to improve care. The committee proposed six aims for improvement: health care should be safe, effective, patient-centered, timely, efficient, and equitable.

The Agency for Healthcare Research and Quality (AHRQ) has placed a high priority on health services research that improves patient safety and quality of care. AHRQ is a federal agency within the U.S. Department of Health and Human Services whose mission is to improve the quality, safety, efficiency, and effectiveness of health care for all Americans (Agency for Healthcare Research and Quality [AHRQ], 2005a). AHRQ provides resources for clinical information such as evidence-based practice, preventive services, and clinical practice guidelines. The guidelines contain evidence-based recommendations for breast, cervical, and ovarian cancer screening; screening for chlamydia infection; family and intimate partner violence; and behavioral interventions to promote breastfeeding.

AHRQ has several quality and patient safety initiatives. The Health Information Technology initiative includes $139 million in grants and contracts to 40 states to support investment in health information technology, particularly in rural and underserved areas (AHRQ, n.d.). The *National Healthcare Quality Report 2004* proposed final measure set examines the effectiveness of care in areas such as maternal and child health and mental health (AHRQ, 2005b). The maternal and child health category, maternity care, collects vital statistics data on the percentage of pregnant women who receive prenatal care in their first trimester, percentage of liveborn infants with low and very low birthweight, infant mortality, and maternal death rate. This report card was released in 2003 and annually thereafter, focusing on standardized quality measures.

Provider Profiling and Pay-for-Performance

One of the fastest growing tools for managed care organizations is that of provider profiling. Profiling will tell you, your employer, and your managed care credentialers about your prescription rates, referral rates, treatments, hospitalization rates, and rates of clients who receive standard screenings and primary care examinations. These data are used to determine how effective you are at using health care resources, both in terms of quality and of course, cost. To achieve more rapid changes in provider behavior to improve quality and patient safety, programs that offer structured incentives for practitioners to achieve benchmarks have been aggressively promoted. Pay-for-performance programs financially reward those providers who meet or exceed benchmarks, for example, number of patients receiving breast and cervical cancer screening. Managed care organizations also contribute to this incentive by giving providers tools to achieve benchmarks, such as information systems and patient education materials. Many providers who receive pay-for-performance incentives are using those monies to further improve their care. Data on the effectiveness of this incentive program continue to evolve.

Quality Management and Midwifery

Quality management activities are fundamental to midwifery practice. The Core Competencies for Basic Midwifery Practice include participation in self-evaluation, peer review, continuing education, and other activities that ensure and validate quality practice as a professional responsibility of Certified Nurse–Midwives and Certified Midwives (American College of Nurse–Midwives [ACNM], 2002). The Standards for the Practice of Midwifery state that midwifery care is evaluated according to an established program for quality management that includes a plan to identify and resolve problems (ACNM, 2003b). The mechanisms for this evaluation are delineated in **Table 12–1**. The ACNM Division of Standards and Practice includes a Quality Management section, which is charged with keeping abreast of trends in quality management, educating members on quality management practices, and integrating quality management principles into the other sections of the division, among other responsibilities.

The ACNM definition of quality is longer and more midwifery specific:

> Quality care advocates for, and provides easy access to, appropriate, satisfying and cost-effective midwifery care, which empowers women to make positive life choices. Care is accessible when women are able to obtain care where and when they need it. Appropriate care is the right care, delivered at the right time, in the right amount, and is culturally specific. Care is satisfying when the results of the care and the way in which it was delivered meet or exceed the woman's expectations. Cost-effective is the most effective use of resources needed to achieve the desired outcomes. (ACNM, 2003b)

Quality management in midwifery practice includes several processes to monitor and improve midwifery care. These processes include peer review, quality assurance, quality improvement, and benchmarking.

Several organizations have identified quality indicators for use in obstetrics, gynecology, and midwifery. The American College of Obstetrics and Gynecology has maternal in-

---

Table 12–1 Standards for the Practice of Midwifery: Quality Management

Standard VII (ACNM, 2003a)
Midwifery care is evaluated according to an established program for quality management that includes a plan to identify and resolve problems.
The midwife:
1. Participates in a program of quality management for the evaluation of practice within the setting in which it occurs.
2. Provides for a systematic collection of practice data as part of a program of quality management.
3. Seeks consultation to review problems, including peer review of care.
4. Acts to resolve problems identified.

dicators and neonatal indicators (see http://www.acog.org). JCAHO has developed a series of indicators for minimal performance by a health care organization. ACNM has a set of benchmarking indicators with practice information available to the members (see **Table 12–2**). Midwifery practices need to develop indicators for quality measurement and assurance within their own practice. The indicators developed by practices can be used as a starting point, but thresholds and achievement may vary between practices. Thresholds indicate the acceptable level of care, or predetermined standard of measurement, for certain indices of care, such as third-degree lacerations and epidural anesthesia.

Indicators can measure structure, process, and outcomes. Structural indicators measure the characteristics of the midwife and facility in which care is given and the capacity to provide care. They are usually monitored with a checklist. Structural standards require 100-percent compliance and are necessary to maintain a practice. Examples of structural indicators include licensure, staffing patterns, building codes, office space, equipment, and regulatory compliance.

Process indicators measure the way in which care is provided. They may often be measured by adherence to clinical guidelines and professional standards of care. Indeed, the written guidelines maintained by a midwifery practice are a good place to begin a program of quality management. Process indicators may include risk assessment tools, screening measures, and documentation. Examples of process indicators include patient flow, patient education procedures, referral process, and collaboration. If an outcome is difficult to measure, process indicators may serve as a proxy. Many processes of midwifery care can be monitored; the goal is to choose those processes that are critical to the health and well-being of midwifery clients. JCAHO requires monitoring of high-risk, high-volume, and problem-prone areas (Ament, 1999).

Table 12–2 ACNM Benchmark Categories

Total deliveries
Spontaneous vaginal deliveries
Total vaginal deliveries
Cesarean sections
Neonatal outcomes
   Apgar $1'' \leq 7$
   Apgar $5'' \leq 7$
Epidural anesthesia
Perineum outcomes
   Intact
   1st degree
   2nd degree
   3rd degree
   4th degree
   Episiotomy
Infant feeding
   Breast
   Bottle

Outcome indicators serve to monitor the direct results of care. Traditional outcome measures include the rates of normal spontaneous vaginal births, episiotomy, cesarean birth, and infant mortality. Outcome indicators are also used to examine sentinel events, such as eclamptic seizures or maternal deaths.

Indicators must be monitored by the midwifery practice on a regular basis. Rate-based indicators such as vaginal birth after cesarean or intact perineum provide a practice with valuable information. Monitoring of indicators can be as simple as a written log kept at each birth or can be assigned to one member of the practice.

Sentinel events should be reviewed to learn if changes in the care given might have led to an improved outcome. A sentinel event is defined as "any unexpected occurrence involving death or serious physical or psychological injury, or risk thereof" (JCAHO, 2006b). The JCAHO advocates for voluntary self-reporting of sentinel events. There is a defined subset of sentinel events that are subject to review by JCAHO. For maternal/child health, the unanticipated death of a full-term infant, discharge of an infant to the wrong family, or abduction of any individual are included in that subset (JCAHO, 2005).

Each outcome indicator needs a threshold. A threshold is a data point that can be a minimal performance standard or a target standard. Performance targets can be difficult to develop in midwifery practices. Every practice would like to have a 100-percent intact perineum rate, but a more reasonable target could depend on the population served, the skill and experience of the midwives, and the culture of the hospital, birth center, or area in which the midwives practice. Targets can be developed by looking at your current statistics and deciding within your practice if these rates are appropriate and/or acceptable or could be improved.

Thresholds and indicators need to be reviewed on a regular basis. Structural indicators may need only yearly review whereas process or outcome indicators may need review as often as every month. The review can determine whether care is above the preset standard, at the standard, or below the standard. Care determined to be below the standard will need to be analyzed and a quality improvement process developed.

Patient Satisfaction as a Quality Assurance Mechanism

Patient satisfaction is often used as a marker of quality in health care. Patient satisfaction is vital to maintain clientele and is positively related to better health care outcomes. Patients who are satisfied are likely to adhere to recommendations for treatment and more likely to return for follow-up. Measuring patient satisfaction is similar to other measures of quality. The practice must decide what to measure, how to measure it, when to measure it, and what to do with the information gathered. There are instruments available for use by midwives, including a simple tool in the *Quality Management Handbook* (ACNM, 2003a). Aspects of patient satisfaction that could be evaluated include whether staff introduce themselves, time from arrival at office to time seen by the midwife, comprehension of educational efforts, and compliance with follow-up instructions (Ament, 1999).

The ACNM Benchmarking Project

The health care environment today places great value on productivity and cost effectiveness. Midwifery practices have been pressured to meet productivity standards that were developed outside the profession of midwifery. Midwifery leaders saw the need for the development of standards for care and productivity that are identified by midwives themselves as important, pertinent, and achievable. The Service Directors Network provided seed money for the benchmarking project. In May 2002, ACNM released its benchmarking data from its pilot project. At this time, the benchmarking project tracks only obstetrical care, but work has begun on a gynecological benchmarking tool.

Using expert opinion, a tool was developed that is concise yet encompassing of the care midwives provide. Any practice can participate, and the information is collected yearly. Each midwifery practice should participate as part of its professional responsibility. The practice can provide valuable data and can receive valuable data. Each practice that participates receives a report comparing its data to data from the other participating midwifery practices. If a practice is designated as "best practice," other practices are invited to contact this practice for advice or consultation. Benchmarking practice data not only provides for an overall assessment of outcomes, but also provides the practice an opportunity to review its structure and process indicators in an effort to find better or different ways to deliver care.

Peer Review

Peer review in midwifery is an educational review in the absence of a suspected deficit in care. In other words, the care and outcomes of midwifery practice are reviewed on a periodic basis with predetermined criteria to assess for areas of strength and improvement. Peer review is done for the purposes of quality assurance and improvement, not for fault finding or punishment; it does not focus on negative events or outlier values. Peer review is the professional responsibility of all midwives.

Peer review differs from other quality management techniques in several ways. The reviews are conducted by other midwives only. They are confidential and not shared with others outside the reviewed practice. Discipline is not a goal of peer review, and the review should not be used punitively.

The concept of peer review in health care is often a topic of discussion and has even been mandated by the federal government. Health care providers are often reluctant to engage in peer review for several reasons. One reason for reluctance is discomfort with reviewing peers and possibly finding fault with one's peers. This reason is pervasive among midwives. There is also concern about the legal risks and possible legal consequences of performing peer review, especially with findings of a negative review.

Peer review has been found reliable in improving patient care, especially if the reviewers use specific and structured instruments. The use of two or more reviewers increases the reliability of the review. Reviewers who have been trained are more reliable than untrained reviewers. Midwives can receive training from peers who have already participated in peer review or from midwifery leaders, such as chapter chairs. Reviewers who can reach a consensus provide a more useful, reliable review than two or more independent reviews.

The reasons for participating in peer review are listed in **Table 12–3**. Although each midwifery chapter or practice can develop its own peer review instrument, the ACNM Quality Management section has developed reliable instruments for use by any midwifery practice or chapter. These instruments include forms for obstetrical and gynecological

Table 12–3 Reasons for Participation in Peer Review

1. To develop standards for midwifery practice in the state
2. To validate standards of quality midwifery care and function to update these standards
3. To act as a mechanism for identifying practice strengths and needs
4. To provide a forum in which problems can be constructively addressed in the process of review
5. To provide a venue for education, communication, and support
6. To provide consumers with quality care and be responsible to consumer protection needs
7. To assist midwives to develop and maintain adequate documentation of care
8. To demonstrate the ability of midwives to self-evaluate
9. To help to validate the competency of CNMs/CMs for licensure and prescriptive privileges

practices, office practices, and full scope practices. These forms can be found in the ACNM *Quality Management Handbook* (2003a).

When conducting peer review with another midwifery practice, the midwives conducting the peer review should request background data in anticipation of the visit. Examples of data collected prior to the review include a description of the scope of practice, practice guidelines, and practice statistics for the past year. Once at the practice site, the peer reviewers will review medical records for compliance with guidelines as established by JCAHO standards, state licensure standards, and ACNM standards. Random samples of records for the past 12 months may be reviewed by category of care, such as births, prenatal records, gynecological visits, and primary care visits. In addition, any cases with poor outcomes may also be reviewed. Examples of such cases might include low birth weight infants, premature births, fetal injury, fourth degree lacerations, or postpartum hemorrhage. Reviewers may also ask to verify midwifery licenses, collaborative practice agreements, position descriptions, and midwifery records of continuing competency participation.

Barriers to Quality Management Processes

Quality management processes reveal a wealth of information to a practice and are important for the maintenance and improvement of quality care to patients. But any process takes time and resources. Many midwifery practices are reluctant to invest the time, not realizing the tremendous benefit. Other barriers to quality management include a perception that quality management techniques are difficult, a reluctance to investigate less than optimal outcomes, a reluctance to share information with other competing practices, and a perception that care is already optimal and not in need of improvement.

Summary

Certified nurse–midwives have repeatedly demonstrated safety and quality in our delivery of care to women and families. Nurse midwifery care can also be said to be cost-efficient through lower rates of technological intervention, shorter lengths of stay in hospitals, and lower payroll costs for staff model HMOs. CNMs/CMs have worked hard to demonstrate the positive health care outcomes and cost savings of our work. It is relatively simple and self-evident to document this data in the short term. But if the profession of midwifery were to take into account the long-term effects of our care or examine the full range of resources we use, such as social services, labor sitting, and prevention education, the data may not be so self-evident. The next natural progression will be to demonstrate the cost-effectiveness of the interventions that are unique to the profession, be they models of care, providers of care, sites of care, or processes of care. Interventions can be linked with outcome measures to compare across multiple sites or to determine best practices. First and foremost, the development of a prototype that incorporates and recognizes midwifery quality and costs within the overall health care system must be accomplished.

Chapter Exercises

Case Example #1
Midwife Jones has been in solo full scope practice for a year. She keeps each birth in a birth log but does not know her rates of vaginal birth, vaginal birth after cesarean, or cesarean birth. The physician she collaborates with has a cesarean birth rate of 24% and assures Ms. Jones that her rates are "probably ok." Ms. Jones is unsure if she is "doing things right." How could she begin to quantify her practice and compare her statistics to other midwifery practices?

Case Example #2
The New Woman Midwifery Center staff are concerned about patient understanding and consent for a trial of labor after cesarean (TOLAC). The midwives are uneasy about the documentation in their patient charts. First, the midwives decide to survey the information. Each chart of a patient attempting a TOLAC during the last year is retrospectively reviewed for documentation of the elements of informed consent regarding vaginal birth after cesarean (VBAC). A tool is developed listing the elements of consent, the midwife seeing the patient, and the outcome of the birth. This tool measures process indicators and outcome indicators. They decide to set a threshold of 100 percent, given the importance and risk around the procedure. When the information is correlated, the midwives find that three of them are in compliance with accepted standards of documentation, one is not. How would you address the noncompliant midwife and promote a change in her practice? How and when would you evaluate whether progress/change has occurred?

Table 12–4 Quality Management Resources

HEDIS www.ncqa.org/programs/HEDIS
ORYX www.jcaho.org/accredited+organizations/hospitals/oryx

References

Agency for Healthcare Research and Quality. (2005a). *About AHRQ.* Retrieved April 7, 2006, from http://www.ahrq.gov/about

Agency for Healthcare Research and Quality. (2005b). *National healthcare quality report: 2004 proposed final measure set.* Retrieved April 7, 2006, from http://www.ahrq.gov/qual/nhqr04/premeasures.htm

Agency for Healthcare Research and Quality, National Resource Center for Health Information Technology. (n.d.). *Home page.* Retrieved May 25, 2006, from http://healthit.ahrq.gov

Ament, L. (1996). Risk management/continuous quality improvement. In S. Gardner & M. Hagedorn (Eds.), *Maternal child risk management* (Chapter 6). Menlo Park, CA: Addison-Wesley.

Ament, L. (1999). Quality management activities in the obstetric triage setting. *Journal of Nurse–Midwifery, 44*(6), 592–599.

American College of Nurse–Midwives. (2002). *Core competencies for basic midwifery practice.* Washington, DC: Author.

American College of Nurse–Midwives. (2003a). *Quality management handbook.* Washington, DC: Author.

American College of Nurse–Midwives. (2003b). *Standards for the practice of midwifery.* Washington, DC: Author.

Committee on Quality of Health Care in America, Institute of Medicine. (2001). *Crossing the quality chasm: A new health system for the twenty-first century.* Washington, DC: National Academies Press.

Deming, W. (1986). *Out of crisis.* Cambridge, MA: MIT Press.

Donabedian, A. (1966). Evaluating the quality of medical care. *Millbank Memorial Fund Quarterly, 44*(3), 166–206.

Institute for Healthcare Improvement. (2005a). *About us.* Retrieved April 7, 2006, from http://www.ihi.org/ihi/about

Institute for Healthcare Improvement. (2005b). *Perinatal care.* Retrieved April 7, 2006, from http://www.ihi.org/ihi/topics/perinatalcare/

Joint Commission on Accreditation of Healthcare Organizations. (2002). *A comprehensive review of development and testing for national implementation of hospital core measures.* Retrieved May 25, 2006, from http:www.jointcommission.org/NR/rdonlyres/48DFC95A-9C05-4A44-AB05-1769D5253014/0/AComprehensiveReviewofDevelopmentforCoreMeasures.pdf

Joint Commission on Accreditation of Healthcare Organizations. (2005). *JCAHO Web site.* http://www.jcaho.org

Joint Commission on Accreditation of Healthcare Organizations. (2006a). *A journey through the history of the Joint Commission.* Retrieved April 7, 2006, from http://www.jointcommission.org/AboutUs/joint_commission_history.htm

Joint Commission on Accreditation of Healthcare Organizations. (2006b). *Sentinel event.* Retrieved April 7, 2006, from http://www.jointcommission.org/SentinelEvents

Kohn, L. T., Corrigan, J., & Donaldson, M. S. (2000). *To err is human: Building a safer health system.* Washington, DC: National Academies Press.

Leapfrog Group. (2005). *Leapfrog Group Web site.* Retrieved April 7, 2006, from http://www. leapfroggroup.org

National Committee for Quality Assurance. (2005). NCQA's Quality Compass. Retrieved April 7, 2006, from http://www.ncqa.org/info/qualitycompass/index.htm

Press, I. (2004). The measure of quality. *Quality Management in Health Care, 13*(4), 202–209.

Stichler, J. F., & Weiss, M. E. (2001). Through the eye of the beholder: Multiple perspectives on quality in women's health care. *Journal of Nursing Care and Quality, 15*(3), 59–74.

Vincent, D., Hastings-Tolsma, M., & Park, J. H. (2004). Down the rabbit hole: Examining outcomes of nurse midwifery care. *Journal of Nursing Care and Quality*, 19(4), 361–367.

CHAPTER 13

Historical Perspectives on Research and the ACNM

Lisa L. Paine, CNM, DrPH, FACNM

"The contribution that midwifery throughout the world can make to scientific research is almost beyond our imagination. . . ."

—*Ernst, 1964*

Learning Outcomes

1. Describe the importance of research to midwifery and women's health.
2. Discuss the importance of research to clinical practice.
3. Identify factors that enhance or impede midwifery research, and discuss the importance of compiling data about midwifery and midwifery practice for all midwives.
4. Describe the origin and ongoing development on the nurse–midwifery minimum dataset, and discuss other datasets in which midwifery-related events are compiled.
5. Describe the evolution of research within ACNM, including the Division of Research, and discuss how the current Division of Research agenda relates to the ACNM strategic priorities.

Research is important to midwifery and women's health in infinite ways. It may come as a surprise to some that this is not a new phenomenon brought about by the recent focus on evidence-based research and practice, but rather by centuries of experience on the part of our foremothers, who recognized early-on that without "evidence" to support practice, women and their families would not be well served. Today's midwife must be knowledgeable about the growing body of "scientific evidence" about them, the women they serve, and the care they seek to provide, and they must be aware of the long-standing conditions that enhance or impede this effort. Midwives must also recognize, embrace, and be well voiced about their own role and inherent responsibility in advancing midwifery research (Albers & Sedler, 2004; Craigin, 2005; Kennedy, 2005; Paine, 1991; Raisler, 2000b).

Historical Perspective

More than three centuries ago, Parisian midwife Louyse Bourgeois (1563–1636) used theory to support clinical practice as evidenced in her writings, which contain guidelines for sound clinical practice as well as an ethical code for such practice (Dunn, 2004; Kalish, Scobey, & Kalish, 1981). Bourgeois's instructions about the interface among education, practice, research, and ethics provide a contemporary blueprint for midwives today who seek to advance midwifery research (Dunn, 2004; Paine, 1991). Writing about midwives' practice in colonial America was done by men in positions of power, and often with impudence in large part because of the religious and political environment. This is well documented in Governor John Winthrop's 17th-century accounts of births attended by colonial midwives, most specifically the highly skilled midwife and articulate, outspoken religious reformer, Anne Hutchinson (Dunn, Savage, & Yaendle, 1996; LaPlante, 2004; Paine, 2000).

A century later, Frisian midwife Vrouw Catherine Shrader (1693–1740) contributed to the written documentation about midwives' practice by counting her births, as well as writing extensive case notes about them (Shrader, 1700s/1987). Another half-century later, American midwife Martha Ballard meticulously documented her practice in both exquisite and ordinary notes in the form of a diary, emerging as one of the first American midwives to write about her practice (Kennedy, 2005). Martha Ballard's diary entries, and thus the record of her midwifery practice, would not have been known without the work of Pulitzer-prize-winning historian and author Laurel Thacher Ulrich, who published Martha Ballard's diary in 1990 (Ulrich, 1990). Another American midwife, immigrant Hannah Porn, whose birth records from the early 1900s were examined by Declercq and published in the *American Journal of Public Health,* demonstrated the safety of her practice (including a neonatal mortality rate less than half that of local physicians), yet it was not enough to prevent her case from leading to abolition of midwifery in Massachusetts (Declercq, 1994).

As Kennedy affirms in her 2005 editorial about the history of nurse–midwifery/midwifery research, there was minimal documentation about midwifery practices and outcomes in the United States before the 20th century (Kennedy, 2005). Groundbreaking work in the early 20th century, conducted and funded in large part by those outside of the profession, confirmed midwives' commitment to the care of vulnerable and marginalized populations, as well as the excellent outcomes that resulted from that care (Kennedy, 2005; Raisler & Kennedy, 2005; Rooks, 1997; Thompson, 1986; Levy, Wilkinson, & Marine, 1971). Attention was also drawn to the work of midwives in other ways, both scientific and artistic (Breckenridge, 1981; Life Magazine, 1951; Metropolitan Life Insurance Company, 1960; Paine, 2005; Paine, Greener, & Strobino, 1988).

Research on midwifery and midwives advanced during the latter part of the 20th century for a variety of reasons, including the early value placed on research by leaders of the new professional organization called ACNM, an increasing number of midwives and subsequent rise in their participation in clinical care, inclusion of midwifery and childbirth in the agendas of feminist and women's health activist groups, and the pursuit of research-oriented academic degrees on the part of midwives.

Research and the American College of Nurse–Midwives

"We are a generation bombarded with information."

—*Hemschemeyer, 1956, p. 6*

In evolving and iterative ways, the American College of Nurse–Midwives (ACNM) incorporated research into its agenda and activities from the very beginning, and that commitment remains ever-present in the ACNM's bylaws: "to promote research and develop literature in the field of nurse–midwifery, as practiced by CNMs and CMs" (American College of Nurse–Midwives [ACNM], 1997). One of the most illustrative examples of the early ACNM research lies within the ACNM Archives at the National Library of Medicine in Bethesda, Maryland, wherein one can find the original copy of the first American College of Nurse–Midwifery membership survey conducted in 1955 under the direct influence of ACNM's first president, Hattie Hemschemeyer. Brief results of the study were published in Volume 1, Number 2 of the *Bulletin of the American College of Nurse–Midwifery* in March 1956 in the form of a table entitled "Positions Held by Members of the College"; review of subsequent membership surveys—and there have been many—shows that the topic of positions held by members of the college, in addition to characteristics of their practice, has remained a topic of great interest (ACNM Research Committee, 1969; Adams, 1989; Rooks & Fischman, 1980; Runnerstrom, Cramer, Fischman, Matousek, & Nissen, 1971).

Hemschemeyer's vision about the need for data collection and dissemination to document professional practice outcomes is one that has been shared by the college's leaders over time (Fullerton, Schuiling, & Sipe, 2005). Kennedy (2005) recently reviewed every editorial published in our professional journals (first the *Bulletin of the American College of Nurse–Midwifery,* later the *Journal of Nurse–Midwifery,* and now the *Journal of Midwifery & Women's Health*); she found that research was either the focus or was referenced in more than 30 of them. An even closer examination of past issues of our professional publications reveals a treasure trove of evidence about the inextricable concept of research by and about midwives, as well as the populations they serve (Shah, 2005; Shah, Barger, & King, 2005). These publications confirm that research, as we know it today, was an integral part of the infrastructure of the college from the very beginning, with connections that reflected the issues faced by midwives, their colleagues, and their populations.

As ACNM's membership and activities have grown in size and scope, its research activities have grown as well; the coordination of research activities has also grown and evolved. In 1956, Ruth Doran was authorized to chair a committee, choosing her own membership to set up a form and coding system for gathering membership data for statistical purposes after reviewing 1955 questionnaires and getting statistical consultation (ACNM, 1957).

Subsequently, in 1956, the ACNM Special Committee on Statistics, chaired by Ruth Doran, was established. The committee's name changed to Special Committee on Research in 1963, and in 1964, it became the Special Committee on Research & Statistics. Eventually, it became a standing Committee on Research & Statistics. The college's research activities were organized for years within the structure of these various committees, yet the membership of ACNM was still relatively small and its members held a wide range of positions in universities and government settings in which funding was available to support various research activities. In addition, the midwives involved possessed the skills to conduct the research as well as acquire the funding, especially from funding sources interested in the long-standing public health contributions made by nurse–midwives, such as the Maternal and Child Health Bureau, the Robert Wood Johnson Foundation, and the ACNM Foundation, Inc. (Kennedy, 2005).

The ACNM Division of Research Is Born

"The major event of [my presidency] was the creation of the Division of Research."

—Elizabeth Bear (Fullerton et al., 2005)

By the mid-1980s, nearly 30 years after Hattie Hemschemeyer proclaimed in her address to the membership that: "We are a generation bombarded with information" (Hemschemeyer, 1956, p. 6), the ACNM Research & Statistics Committee presented the Board of Directors with the following problem statement in their proposal for a Division of Research: "Nurse–midwives are in the midst of an information explosion. The need for research related services, activities, and above all, information about and for CNMs, had surpassed the ability of the ACNM to supply such information" (Paine, 1987). The ACNM Research & Statistics Committee, led by Chair Claire Andrews, had for several years believed that if they were to function as a division rather than a committee "thereby broadening their role, responsibilities, and ability to attract outside funding," the ACNM could more effectively respond to such things as mounting criticism of nurse–midwifery; better respond to an increased national focus on birth outcomes and the effectiveness of certified nurse–midwives (CNMs); effectively document nurse–midwifery practices in order to positively influence health policy, legislation, and marketing strategies; and utilize rapidly growing computer technology and information gathering. So, in 1987, when the Research & Statistics Committee, now chaired by Lisa Paine, proposed to the Board of Directors that a Division of Research (DOR) was needed, the board approved the committee's proposal, with some clarification regarding plans to seek outside funding (Paine, 1987). Like her presidential predecessors, ACNM President Betty Bear, CNM, PhD, strongly supported the proposal to strengthen the college's research capacity; her argument in support of the proposal was compelling, unfailing, and firm. In May 1988, the ACNM membership heeded Betty Bear's call, and voted nearly unanimously to establish a Division of Research (DOR) within the ACNM.

The early structure of the DOR addressed the needs of the ACNM, especially in regards to collection and analysis of data about CNMs and their practices. By design, it also addressed the needs of the membership as determined in a needs assessment designed and conducted in 1987–88 for that very purpose (Greener, Paine, LeeDecker, & Gray, 1989; Paine & Greener, 1989). The survey provided information used to set the initial priorities for the division's work, which included the development and subsequent computerization of the Nurse–Midwifery Clinical Dataset, something that the membership had perceived as their greatest need and had been viewed as a priority by the ACNM Research & Statistics Committee since the early 1970s (Greener, 1990).

In addition to these priorities, the DOR also maintained responsibility for the coordination, analysis, and dissemination of such data as salaries for CNMs, demographic and practice characteristics, and populations served by CNMs (Lehrman & Paine, 1990). In the early years, the division also pursued the development and dissemination of resources for CNMs, including an annotated bibliography about midwifery research, which were particularly important because many early midwifery studies were not readily available because they were published in literature that was not recognized by Index Medicus (Kennedy, 2005); in fact, it was not until 1981 that the *Journal of Nurse–Midwifery* was officially accepted into Index Medicus (Shah, 2005).

Another major accomplishment of the DOR during that period included a 1991 Robert Wood Johnson Foundation grant for the population-based study entitled "Nurse–Midwifery Care for Vulnerable Populations in the United States," with seed money for its preparation from the ACNM Foundation, Inc. (Paine, Scupholme, DeJoseph, & Stobino, 1993). This landmark population-based study resulted in widely disseminated research results to a variety of audiences (Declercq, Paine, DeJoseph, & Simmes, 1998; Paine, 1994; Paine, Johnson, et al., 2000; Paine, Lang, et al., 1999; Scupholme, DeJoseph, Stobino, & Paine, 1992; Scupholme, Paine, Lang, Kumar, & DeJoseph, 1994; Scupholme & Walsh 1994).

By the mid-1990s, the DOR, chaired by Linda Walsh, presented the ACNM Board of Directors with annual research priorities, which exemplified the division's evolving role as a policy-oriented advisory group. Priorities were presented in the areas of clinical practice, education, and policy. In addition to its important responsibility in making recommendations for research priorities, the division continued to play an essential role in the review of requests for use of the ACNM mailing list for research purposes, a role the division continues today.

By 2000, during the presidency of midwife researcher and scholar Joyce Roberts, the DOR entered another evolutionary phase. A series of meetings were convened to review the purpose, structure, and future priorities of the division, during which the importance of the division was reaffirmed and a new structure was defined and approved by the ACNM Board of Directors. The DOR would now be governed by a board, and it would include three distinct sections: 1) Development and Conduct of Research, 2) Dissemination of Research, and 3) Midwifery Data, including the ACNM Data Set Series and midwifery surveys. Jeanne Raisler was appointed division chairperson in February 2000, after which she announced that the ACNM DOR was "reorganizing, expanding, and reaching out to involve more midwifery researchers (including students)" (Raisler, 2000a). It was also during this time that the DOR expanded its formal connection with the international midwifery community (Kennedy, 2005).

This reassessment of the Division of Research coincided with an ever-increasing demand for an evidence-based perspective in research and clinical care (Albers, 2001; Barger, 2001; Murphy, 1997; Rooks, 1997), an evolution of the need for and use of a nurse–midwifery clinical dataset (ACNM, 1996; ACNM, 1997), the proliferation of information technology resources, and mounting interest outside of the midwifery profession about the advancement of midwifery research (Raisler, 2000b). Most notably, the UCSF Center for Health Professions (and Pew Health Professions Commission) 1999 Taskforce on Midwifery made two distinct recommendation for midwifery research, as well as 12 additional recommendations in midwifery education, practice, regulation, and policy (Dower, Miller, O'Neil, & The Taskforce on Midwifery, 1999). The sole policy recommendation—the proposed overarching plan—called for an existing body (such as the Institute of Medicine) to address the key areas of midwifery workforce supply and demand, interstate differences in regulation, funding for midwifery education and research, and disparate federal policies and programs that affect midwives (Paine & Dower, 1999). To date, this plan has not been fulfilled, but little evidence suggests that it is no longer valid.

ACNM and Research in the 21st Century

> "We must be creative to conduct research that documents 'how' we practice and 'why' it is related to positive health outcomes."
>
> —*Kennedy, 2005*

In 2003, Holly Powell Kennedy was appointed chair of the ACNM Division of Research at a time when the ACNM had begun to broaden and reinvigorate its strategic agenda development and evidence-based care had become the gold standard in clinical practice (Starr & Chalmers, 2003; "Using Evidence," 2000), bringing with it both excitement and challenges for the midwifery community (Kearney, 2005; King, 2003; Murphy, 2005; Sakala, 2003). In addition, the focus of much of the history of midwifery research until this time had been on qualitative data, so the research leadership and qualitative research expertise brought by Dr. Kennedy has been timely (Kennedy, 2000; Kennedy & Lowe, 2001). The most recent DOR history is also characterized by greater coordination between and among various ACNM committees and divisions, as well as an emphasis at the ACNM national office on communication, including updated and expanded Web resources. (See **Table 13–1** for a list of the contents of the current DOR Web site.) Currently, the Division of Research is organized into five sections: Research Advisory, Research Development & Dissemination, Networking, International, and Data & Information. (See **Table 13–2** for a description of the activities of the various DOR sections.) Section chairs, along with the DOR chair, comprise the Governing Board; liaison members from the ACNM Board of Directors and ACNM national office staff further support the DOR's work.

Table 13–1 ACNM Division of Research Web Site Resources, 2005

The Mission and Overview of the DOR
- DOR Sections
- Organizational Chart of the DOR
- Quarterly Report

ACNM Research Agenda
- Explanation of Development of Research Agenda in Alignment with the ACNM Strategic Priorities

Who's Who in Midwifery Research?
- Profiles of Midwifery Researchers
  - List of Research by Topic
  - Alpha List of Researchers by Name

Resources for Evidence-Based Practice
- Definition of Evidence-Based Practice
- Critiquing the Evidence: How Do I Know if I Can Use the Evidence?
- Links to Evidence-Based Practice Information
  - Links to centers Supporting Evidence-Based Practice
  - Links to Information on appraising Evidence
  - Links to resources on Evidence-Based Practice
- International Sites for Midwifery Practice
- Links to Research Centers and Organizations Supporting Women's Health

Resources for Research
- Practice-Based Research Networks
- Minimal Data Sets
- The Optimality Index—U.S. Working Group

Source: American College of Nurse–Midwives. (2005). *Division of research.* Retrieved September 23, 2005, from http://www.midwife.org/abou.cfm?id=258.

The current mission of the ACNM Division of Research—unchanged since the reorganization of 1999—is that it "contributes to knowledge about the health of women, infants and families and advances the profession of midwifery by promoting the development, conduct and dissemination of research" (ACNM, 2005). The DOR's role is to "inspire, facilitate, disseminate, coordinate, and link research activities within the ACNM, as well as with other national and international midwifery research organizations." The DOR focuses on "research that investigates, elucidates, and advances midwifery practice and education" and aims "to develop a midwifery research agenda, and disseminate it widely" (ACNM, 2005). The DOR also "helps develop the research interests and abilities of ACNM members, and fosters communication among midwifery researchers, clinicians, the media, policy makers, health planners, and funders" and advises the ACNM about "research issues, including membership surveys, research priorities, and evaluation of research proposals that require ACNM endorsement or support" (ACNM, 2005). The DOR also "works closely with other entities within the ACNM, including the Program Committee, DSOP, DOE, Public Relations, the International Health Committee,

Table 13–2 ACNM Division of Research Section Descriptions (2005)

Research Advisory Section—Works with the ACNM on membership survey issues; advises ACNM national office on survey research issues.

Research Development & Dissemination Section—Facilitates the growth and development of a research culture within the ACNM; coordinates ACNM-recognized research activities at the Annual Meeting; develops specific activities to assist members in developing research skills such as research modules for the membership and *Quickening* articles.

Networking Section—Links midwifery research by developing a Midwifery Researchers' Directory; sponsors student research committee; promotes interdisciplinary networking (public health, CDC, etc.); manages DOR membership and maintains current membership lists.

International Section—Coordinates international research endeavors for the DOR; liaisons with Research Standing Committee of the ICM; networks with other international organizations; liaisons with the ACNM International Health Committee & Global Outreach; encourages international research presentations at the ACNM Annual Meeting; seeks to obtain funding for midwives from low income countries to attend.

Data & Information Section—Encourages the systematic collection of data for midwifery practice and education, including use of the ACNM minimum data sets; explores the use of technology in the collection of midwifery data; supports the development of practice-based research networks (PBRN).

Source: American College of Nurse–Midwives. (2005). *Divisions: Division of research.* Retrieved September 23, 2005, from http://www.midwife.org/about.cfm?id=56.

Global Outreach, and the ACNM Foundation" (ACNM, 2005) toward a goal—"to use research to inform clinical midwifery practice and care, for the benefit of women, infants, and the midwifery profession" (ACNM, 2005).

Recently, the ACNM Division of Research, at the direction of the ACNM Board of Directors, developed a research agenda in relation to the board's current strategic areas of focus, which include policy, evidence-based practice, education, collaboration, visibility/message, and organizational/leadership development. The DOR's long-standing focus on research priority setting and research policy development, combined with the DOR's careful process of seeking input from key ACNM leaders and the membership (Kennedy, Schuiling, & Murphy, 2005), resulted in a superbly integrated research agenda that is intended to guide the organization's research direction over the next 5 years (Kennedy et al., 2005). The current ACNM Research Agenda, also available online, can be seen in **Table 13–3**.

While the ACNM and DOR look to the future with these ambitious goals, they also celebrate the past, especially in preparation for the 50th Anniversary of the ACNM (Kennedy, 2005; Levy, Wilkinson & Marine, 1971; Raisler & Kennedy, 2005). With the support of the DOR, a unique service learning project was recently conducted for the purpose of identifying midwifery's research heritage (Farley, 2005); midwife scholars identified the top ten studies that are historically or currently important to midwifery practice, which can be seen in **Table 13–4**. While this list is limited by the fact that most midwifery research in

---

Table 13–3 ACNM Research Agenda, 2005

Research Priorities by ACNM Strategic Focus:

Policy: *Pursue legislative, political and legal strategies to promote the hallmarks of midwifery as the standard for women's health care.*
- Examine members' perceived barriers to practice.
- Critical analysis of state legislation restrictive and conducive to midwifery practice.
- Identify thriving and struggling midwifery services to examine their practice environment for common and discordant issues. This would include but not be limited to reimbursement avenues, malpractice, credentialing processes, level of autonomy, regulations, and internal policies.

Research/Evidence-Based Practice: *Promote excellence in clinical midwifery practice that is founded on the best available research evidence.*
- Develop a systematic approach to collecting clinical practice data across the membership.
- Promote research that describes and links midwifery processes of care to specific outcomes.
- Describe women's decision-making processes on choice of provider and procedures during pregnancy and birth.
- Development of research on VBACs and epidurals.

Education: *Provide a strong foundation for midwifery practice and women's health through basic midwifery education programs, continuing education and the education of consumers.*
- Describe the reasons for the declining pool of midwifery applicants.
- Examine schools with thriving and struggling applicant pools for common and discordant issues.

Collaboration: *Strengthen coalitions with individuals, organizations, and agencies that focus on or impact women's health (physicians, other midwives, nurses, other health professions, government agencies, NGO, etc.).*
- Explore practice environments where collaboration is especially strong among differently prepared and licensed midwives.
- Establish a common research goal with the MANA Board of Directors.

Visibility/Message: *Increase visibility and demand for midwifery services and a midwifery model of health care.*
- Describe what women believe, and how they learned, about midwives and midwifery practice.
- Describe what legislators and insurance (both health reimbursement and liability) executives believe, and how they learned, about midwives and midwifery practice.

Organizational/Leadership Development: *Enhance communication and optimal functioning among and between ACNM's members, volunteer leaders and staff.*
- Examine the reasons midwives (a) do not join, or (b) leave the ACNM.
- Identify each member's top priority to be addressed by the ACNM.

Source: American College of Nurse–Midwives. (2005). *Research agenda: Research priorities by strategic focus.* Retrieved September 23, 2005, from http://www.midwife.org/sitefiles/Publications/ACNMResearch Agenda2005.pdf.

---

the past 50 years has been retrospective and descriptive, its findings are important. As noted by Kennedy (2005) in the editorial that accompanied the article: "It provides a glimpse of the past to help guide the future." Hopefully, the same can be said about this chapter, which is focused on historical perspectives, research, and the ACNM.

Table 13–4 Top Ten Studies Historically or Currently Important to Midwifery Practice, 2005

---

1. a. Rooks, J. P., Weatherby, N. L., Ernst, E. K. M., Stapleton, S., Rosen, D., & Rosenfield, A. (1989). Outcomes of care in birth centers: The National Birth Center Study. *New England Journal of Medicine, 321,* 1804–1811.
    b. Rooks, J. P., Ernst, E. K., & Weatherby, N. L. (1992). The National Birth Center Study: Part 1 methodological and prenatal care and referrals. *Journal of Nurse Midwifery, 37,* 222–253.
    c. Rooks, J., Ernst, E. & Weatherby, N. (1992). The National Birth Center Study: Part II. Intrapartum and immediate postpartum and neonatal care. *Journal of Nurse–Midwifery, 37,* 361–397.
    d. Rooks, J., Ernst, E., & Weatherby, N. (1992). The National Birth Center Study: Part III. Intrapartum and immediate postpartum and neonatal complications and transfers, postpartum and neonatal care, outcomes and client satisfaction. *Journal of Nurse–Midwifery, 37,* 361–397.
2. Albers, L., Schiff, M., & Gorwoda, J. (1996). The length of active labor in normal pregnancies. *Obstetrics and Gynecology, 87,* 355–359.
3. Levy, B. S., Wilkinson, F. S., Marine, W. M. (1971). Reducing neonatal mortality rates with nurse–midwives. *American Journal of Obstetrics and Gynecology, 109,* 50–58.
4. Kennedy, H. P. (2000). A model of exemplary midwifery practice: Results of a Delphi study. *Journal of Midwifery & Women's Health, 45,* 4–19.
5. Metropolitan Life Insurance Company. (1958). Summary of the tenth thousand confinement records of the Frontier Nursing Service. *FNS Quarterly Bulletin, 33*(4), 44–55.
6. Greulich, B., Paine, L. L., McClain, C., Barger, M. K., Edwards, N., & Paul, R. (1994). Twelve years and more than 30,000 nurse–midwife attended births: The Los Angeles County and University of Southern California Women's Hospital Birth Center experience. *Journal of Nurse–Midwifery, 39,* 185–196.
7. a. Roberts, J. E., Goldstein, S. A., Gruener, J. S., Maggio, M., & Mendez-Bauer, C. (1987, January/February). A descriptive analysis of involuntary bearing-down efforts during the expulsive phase of labor. *Journal of Obstetrics, Gynecological, and Neonatal Nursing,* 48–55.
    b. Roberts, J. E., Mendez-Bauer, C., Blackwell, J., Carpenter, M. E., & Marchese, T. (1984). Effects of lateral recumbency and sitting on the first stage of labor. *Journal of Reproductive Medicine, 29,* 477–482.
    c. Aderhold, K. J. & Roberts, J. E. (1991). Phases of second stage labor. *Journal of Nurse–Midwifery, 36,* 267–275.
8. Murphy, P. A., & Fullerton, J. (1998). Outcomes of intended home births in nurse–midwifery practice: A prospective descriptive study. *Obstetrics and Gynecology, 92,* 461–470.
9. MacDorman, M. F., & Singh, G. K. (1998). Midwifery care, social and medical risk factors, and birth outcomes in the USA. *Journal of Epidemiology and Community Health, 52*(5), 310–317.
10. Scupholme, A., DeJoseph, J., Strobino, D. M., & Paine, L. L. (1992). Nurse–midwifery care to vulnerable populations. Phase 1: Demographic characteristics of the national CNM sample. *Journal of Nurse–Midwifery, 37,* 341–347.

Source: Farley, C. (2005). Midwifery's research heritage: A Delphi survey of midwife scholars. *Journal of Midwifery & Women's Health, 50*(2), 122–128.

References

Adams, C. J. (1989). Nurse–midwifery practice in the United States, 1982 and 1987. *American Journal of Public Health, 79,* 1038–1039.

Albers, L. L. (2001). "Evidence" and midwifery practice. *Journal of Midwifery & Women's Health, 46*(3), 130–136.

Albers, L. L., & Sedler, K. D. (2004). Clinician perspectives on participation in research. *Journal of Midwifery & Women's Health, 49*(1), 47–50.

American College of Nurse–Midwives. (1957). Summary of minutes of the Executive Board Meetings 1956. *Bulletin of the American College of Nurse–Midwifery, 2*(1), 13.

American College of Nurse–Midwives, Research Committee. (1969). Nurse–midwifery statistics. *Bulletin of the American College of Nurse–Midwives, 14*(3), 70–75.

American College of Nurse–Midwives. (1996). *ACNM data set—Intrapartum.* Retrieved September 23, 2005, from http://www.midwife.org/about/dor.cfm

American College of Nurse–Midwives. (1997). *Articles of incorporation.* Washington, DC: Author.

American College of Nurse–Midwives. (1999). *ACNM data set—Antepartum care.* Retrieved September 23, 2005, from http://www.midwife.org/about/dor.cfm

American College of Nurse–Midwives. (2005). *Division of research.* Retrieved September 23, 2005, from http://www.midwife.org/about.cfm?id=258

Barger, M. K. (2001). Evidence-based practice: New opportunities, new responsibilities [Editorial]. *Journal of Midwifery & Women's Health, 46*(6), 352–353.

Breckinridge, M. (1981). *Wide neighborhoods: A story of the Frontier Nursing Service.* Lexington: University Press of Kentucky.

Cesario, S., Morin, K., & Santa-Donato, A. (2002). Evaluating the level of evidence of qualitative research. *JOGNN, 31,* 708–714.

Craigin, L. (2005). Conference proceedings: Abstracts from research forums presented at the ACNM 50th Annual Meeting 2005. *Journal of Midwifery & Women's Health, 50*(5), 361–362.

Declercq, E. R. (1994). The trials of Hanna Porn: The campaign to abolish midwifery in Massachusetts. *American Journal of Public Health, 84*(6), 1022–1028.

Declercq, E. R., Paine, L. L., Simmes, D. R., & DeJoseph, J. F. (1998). State regulation, payment policies, and nurse–midwife services. *Health Affairs, 17*(2), 190–200.

Dower, C. M., Miller, J. E., O'Neil, E. H., & the Taskforce on Midwifery. (1999, April). *Charting a course for the 21st century: The future of midwifery.* San Francisco: Pew Health Professions Commission and the UCSF Center for the Health Professions.

Dunn, P. M. (2004). Louise Bourgeois (1563–1636): Royal midwife of France. *Archives of Disease in Childhood, Fetal and Neonatal Edition, 89,* F185–F187.

Dunn, R. S., Savage, J., Yaendle, L., (Eds.). (1996). *The journal of John Winthrop, 1630–1649—Unabridged.* Boston: Harvard University Press.

Ernst, E. K. M. (1964). How the midwife can contribute to scientific research. *Bulletin of the American College of Nurse–Midwifery, 9,* 1–7.

Farley, C. (2005). Midwifery's research heritage: A Delphi survey of midwife scholars. *Journal of Midwifery & Women's Health, 50*(2), 122–128.

Fullerton, J., Schuiling, K. D., & Sipe, T. A. (2005). Presidential priorities: 50 years of wisdom as the basis of an action agenda for the next half-century. *Journal of Midwifery & Women's Health, 50*(2), 91–101.

Greener, D. L. (1990). *Technical reports: The Nurse–Midwifery clinical dataset.* Washington, DC: American College of Nurse–Midwives.

Greener, D. L., Paine, L. L., LeeDecker, C. A., & Gray, C. A. (1989). Nurse–midwives speak out on the ACNM. Results of the 1987–88 needs assessment survey, Part 1. *Journal of Nurse–Midwifery, 34*(1), 21–30.

Hemschemeyer, H. (1956). Miss Hattie Hemschemeyer, first president of the college, sends message to members. *Bulletin of the American College of Nurse–Midwifery, 1*(2), 5–6.

Kalish, P. A., Scobey, M., & Kalish, B. J. (1981). Louyse Bourgeois and the emergence of modern mid-wifery. *Journal of Nurse–Midwifery, 26*(4), 3–17.

Kearney, M. H. (2005). Seeking the sound bite: Reading and writing clinically useful qualitative research [Editorial]. *JOGNN, 3,* 417.

Kennedy, H. P. (2000). A model of exemplary midwifery practice: Results of a Delphi study. *Journal of Midwifery & Women's Health, 45,* 4–19.

Kennedy, H. P. (2005). Reflections on the past and future of midwifery research. *Journal of Midwifery & Women's Health, 50*(2), 110–112.

Kennedy, H. P., & Lowe, N. K. (2001). Science and midwifery: Paradigms and paradoxes. *Journal of Midwifery & Women's Health, 46*(2), 91–97.

Kennedy, H. P., Schuiling, K., & Murphy, P. A. (2005). *Executive summary. Developing a research agenda for the American College of Nurse–Midwives.* Retrieved September 23, 2005, from http://www.mid-wife.org/sitesfiles/Publications/ACNMResearchAgenda2005.pdf

King, T. L. (2003). Clinical controversies: Applying evidence in practice. *Journal of Midwifery & Women's Health, 48*(4), 243.

LaPlante, E. (2004). *American Jezebel: The uncommon life of Anne Hutchinson, the woman who defied the Puritans.* San Francisco: HarperCollinsPublishers.

Lehrman, E. J., & Paine, L. L. (1990). Trends in nurse–midwifery. Results of the 1988 ACNM Division of Research Mini-Survey. *Journal of Nurse–Midwifery, 76*(1), 42–43.

Levy, B. S., Wilkenson, F. S., & Marine, W. M. (1971). Reducing neonatal mortality rate with nurse–midwives [Madera County Study]. *American Journal of Obstetrics and Gynecology, 109*(1), 50–58.

Life Magazine. (December 3, 1951). Nurse–midwife: Maude Callen eases the pain of birth, life, and death. *Life,* 23.

Metropolitan Life Insurance Company. (1960). Summary of the tenth thousand confinement records of the Frontier Nursing Service. *Bulletin of the American College of Nurse–Midwifery,* 5(1), 1–9.

Murphy, P. A. (1997). Evidence-based care a new paradigm for clinical practice. *Journal of Nurse–midwifery, 42* (1), 1–3.

Murphy, P. A. (2005). Grounding midwifery in evidence of all types. *Journal of Midwifery & Women's Health, 50*(5), 361–362.

Paine, L. L. (1987). *Proposal for the development of a Division of Research.* Washington, DC: ACNM.

Paine, L L. (1991). Midwifery education and research in the future. *Journal of Nurse–Midwifery, 36*(3), 199–203.

Paine, L. L. (2000, November). *Midwifery, childbirth, politics, and religion: Lessons from the case of Anne Hutchinson, colonial midwife.* Paper presented at the 128th Meeting of the American Public Health Association, Boston, MA.

Paine, L. L. (2005). The public health perspective in clinical midwifery research. In Diers, D. (Ed.), *Celebrating the contributions of academic midwifery* (pp. 60–67). New Haven: Yale University School of Nursing.

Paine, L. L., Dower, C. M., & O'Neil, E. H. (1999). Midwifery in the 21st century: Recommendations from the Pew Health Professions Commission/UCSF Center for Health Professions 1998 Taskforce on Midwifery. *Journal of Nurse–Midwifery, 44*(4), 341–348.

Paine, L .L., & Greener, D. L. (1989). Nurse–midwives speak out on research. Results of the 1987–88 Needs Assessment Survey, Part 2. *Journal of Nurse–Midwifery, 34*(2), 66–70.

Paine, L. L., Greener, D. L., & Strobino, D. M. (1988). Birth registration: Nurse–midwifery roles and responsibilities. *Journal of Nurse–Midwifery, 33*(3), 107–114.

Paine, L. L., Johnson, T. R. B., Lang, J. M., Gagnon, D., Declercq, E. R., DeJoseph, J. F., et al. (2000). A comparison of visits and practices of nurse–midwives and obstetrician–gynecologists in ambulatory care settings. *Journal of Midwifery & Women's Health, 45*(1), 37–44.

Paine, L. L., Lang, J. M., Strobino, D. M., Johnson, T. R. B., DeJoseph, J. F., Declercq, E. R., et al. (1999). Characteristics of nurse–midwife patients and visits, 1991. *American Journal of Public Health, 89*(6), 906–909.

Paine, L. L., Scupholme, A., DeJoseph, J. F., & Strobino, D. M. (1993). *Nurse–midwifery care for vulnerable populations in the United States: The final report.* Washington, D.C.: American College of Nurse–Midwives.

Paine, L. L., Scupholme, A., DeJoseph, J. F., & Strobino, D. M. (1994). *Nurse–midwives: Quality care for women and newborns.* Washington, D.C.: American College of Nurse–Midwives.

Raisler, J. (2000a, March/April). Division of Research enters active phase. *Quickening.* Washington, DC: ACNM.

Raisler, J. (2000b). Midwifery care research: What questions are being asked? What lessons have been learned? *Journal of Midwifery & Women's Health, 45*(1), 20–36.

Raisler, J., & Kennedy, H. P. (2005). Midwifery care of poor and vulnerable women, 1925–2003. *Journal of Midwifery & Women's Health, 50*(2), 113–121.

Rooks, J. P. (1997). *Midwifery and childbirth in America.* Philadelphia: Temple University Press.

Rooks, J. P. (1999). Evidenced-based practice and its application to childbirth care for low-risk women. *Journal of Nurse–Midwifery, 44*(4), 355–369.

Rooks, J. B., & Fischman, S. H. (1980). American nurse–midwifery practice in 1976–1977: Reflections of 50 years of growth and development. *American Journal of Public Health, 70*, 990–996.

Runnerstrom, L., Cramer, B., Fischman, S., Matousek, I., & Nissen, C. (1971). *Descriptive data: Nurse–midwives, USA.* New York: American College of Nurse–Midwives.

Sakala, C. (2003). New resources for evidence-based practice. *Journal of Midwifery & Women's Health, 48*(1), 69–71.

Scupholme, A., DeJoseph, J., Strobino, D. M., & Paine, L. L. (1992). Nurse–midwifery care to vulnerable populations in the United States. Phase 1. Demographic characteristics of the national CNM sample. *Journal of Nurse–Midwifery, 37*(5), 341–348.

Scupholme, A., Paine, L. L., Lang, J. M., Kumar, S., & DeJoseph, J. F. (1994). Time associated with components of clinical services rendered by nurse–midwives. Sample data from phase II of nurse–midwifery care to vulnerable populations in the United States. *Journal of Nurse–Midwifery, 39*(1), 5–12.

Scupholme, A., & Walsh, L. (1994). Home-based services by nurse–midwives. Sample data from phase II of nurse–midwifery care to vulnerable populations in the United States. *Journal of Nurse–Midwifery, 39*(6), 358–362.

Shah, M. A. (2005). The Journal of Midwifery & Women's Health 1955–2005: Its historic milestones and evolutionary changes. (2), 159–168.

Shah, M. A., Barger, M. K., & King, T. L. (2005). Editor's choice: The first 25 years of the journal. *Journal of Midwifery & Women's Health, 50*(2), 154–158.

Shrader, C. (1987). *Mother and child were saved* (H. Marland, Trans.). Amsterdam: Rodopi. (Original work published in early 1700s)

Starr, M., & Chalmer, I. (2003). *The evolution of the Cochrane Library, 1988–2003.* Retrieved October 6, 2004, from http://www.update-software.com/history/clibhist.htm

Thompson, J. E. (1986). Nurse–midwifery care: 1925 to 1984. *Annual Review of Nursing Research, 4,* 153–173.

Ulrich, L. T. (1990). *A midwife's tale: The life of Martha Ballard, based on her diary, 1785–1812.* New York: Knopf/Random House.

Using evidence on yourself. (2000). *British Medical Journal, 320*(7228), A.

Wegman, M. E. (1984). Annual summary of vital statistics—1983. *Pediatrics, 74*(6), 981.

CHAPTER 14

Professional Ethics

Joyce E. Thompson, RN, CNM, DrPH, FAAN, FACNM

"To be professional is to be ethical, and to practice ethically requires an understanding of ethics, values, and oneself."

—*J.E. Thompson & H.O. Thompson (1996)*

Learning Objectives

1. Define and distinguish between values, morals, ethics, ethical theories, moral development stages, moral reasoning, and the scientific method.
2. Discuss sources of personal and professional values and their influence on ethical decision making in midwifery care.
3. Describe the interface of law and ethics reflected in the concept of informed consent.
4. Analyze the components of moral reasoning and their application in ethical decision making.
5. Identify key ethical concerns facing women and midwives, reflecting a human rights framework for midwifery care.

Professional role acquisition in any health discipline begins and ends with the ethical concept of accountability, which is taking responsibility for making decisions with and for others, along with taking responsibility for the outcomes of those decisions made as a person and as a professional. Accountability is grounded in respect for self and others, maintaining competence in one's chosen profession, and a personal willingness/commitment to be a thoughtful, responsible human being at all times—especially in our interactions with others. Midwifery is a profession, though one might argue that not all midwives are professionals. As one is learning how to be a midwife, it is imperative that one understands what it means to be a professional, including how to be responsible for one's actions, behavior, and decisions. "To be professional is to be ethical, and to be ethical is to be professional" is a core belief of the author (Thompson & Thompson, 1996). To be ethical requires an understanding of ethics, values, moral reasoning, and ethical decision making.

An underlying assumption in learning new content is often that once presented or discussed or read about, the book or notes can be placed on a shelf and the "job" of learning is finished. This is *not* true with ethics education. It is, like midwifery content, an ongoing, ever-present engagement of the mind, heart, and soul of the learner. In other words, moral development and ethics education is a womb to the tomb endeavor; it is ever evolving as long as we are alive (Thompson & Thompson, 1993). As Sara Fry (1989) noted some years ago, the goal of teaching and learning ethics is to "produce a morally accountable practitioner who is skilled in ethical decision making" (p. 485).

Prior chapters have focused on elements of what it means to be a professional midwife, including educational and practice dimensions. This chapter focuses on what it means to be an ethical person (a moral agent, if you will) and to practice midwifery in an ethical manner. It will also explore some of the common ethical issues and dilemmas faced during midwifery practice at the beginning of the 21st century. The very nature of ethics requires one to focus on what it means to be human and how to interact with others in a respectful manner. It is important to note that this chapter is an introduction to ethics and moral reasoning. For the reader who is ready to delve into more detail, several texts (Bandman & Bandman, 2004; Beachamp & Childress, 2001; Tschudin, 2003) are suggested in the reference list along with key articles in professional journals that address a particular ethical concern relating to women and their health.

The chapter begins with definitions and key questions raised in ethics that set the stage for the content that follows. The very nature of human beings is moral (Thompson & Thompson, 1985), so it is important to understand our moral selves and how to develop the personal self into a professional/ethical midwife. The influences of personal and professional values and moral development on decision making are discussed, along with the interfaces of human rights and ethics and law and ethics. Specific attention is paid to the development of codes of ethics for midwives, one of the hallmarks of a profession that describe the moral ideals of professional behavior and provide guidelines for ethical practice. In addition, the concept of shared decision making is explored as an ethical standard for midwifery practice, based on the midwifery philosophy (American College of Nurse–Midwives [ACNM], 2004b; International Confederation of Midwives [ICM], 1990) and code of ethics (ACNM, 2004a; ICM, 1999a) and embodied within the ACNM *Standards for the Practice of Midwifery* (2003). A framework for the analysis of the ethical dimensions of midwifery practice and factors that can assist one in making ethical decisions is presented. The concluding portion of the chapter highlights some of the current ethical issues or concerns faced by midwives on a daily basis as they work with women and childbearing families. The emphasis in this chapter will be on everyday ethics rather than the newspaper headlines of ethics.

Definitions

The field of health care ethics is filled with many words or terms that are not commonly used in educational or practice settings. In addition, terms such as *values*, *morals*, and *ethics* have multiple definitions in the literature and can lead to confusion when a novice professional is studying this content for the first time. The following brief definitions of key terms are offered to frame the ethics discussion that follows.

Values

Though there are many different yet related definitions of values found in dictionaries and other sources, the author uses the following definition of *values* throughout this text: Values are beliefs and attitudes put into practice in our daily lives that help us define what is good or right behavior or action. This definition recognizes that we have far more beliefs than values. It is precisely those beliefs that we hold so dearly that influence or guide our actions and choices on a daily basis (Thompson & Thompson, 1990b).

Morals

Morals comes from the Latin word *moralis*, referring to customs or society-maintaining actions. For purposes of this chapter, the term morals refers to what a person *should or ought to do* in a given situation. Thus morals are the should and should nots of culture, education, family, God, humanity, nature, religion, society, or a variety of other sources. Morality consists of being and doing *good*.

Ethics

Ethics comes from the Greek word *ethos*, and also can refer to right action or behavior. In this chapter, however, ethics refers to the *reasons behind* the moral shoulds and oughts of behavior and action. Ethics is a philosophical approach to morality, answering the ever-present *why* of thought or action based in ethical theory (Thompson & Thompson, 1985).

Bioethics

Bioethics is the study of the ethics of all living things, including human beings, animals, plants, and the environment. In current usage, bioethics has been taken over by health professionals and refers to the ethics of working with or caring for human beings. Biomedical ethics is another common term for bioethics, though it relates more ethics applied to the practice of medicine.

Metaethics

Metaethics goes beyond ethics to ask such questions as, "Why be ethical? Why be professional? Why be good? Why study ethics?" Although these are important questions to think about and reflect upon, they will not be addressed in detail in this chapter. Suffice it to say, the primary reason for being ethical/professional is based on the mandate from society to any professional group licensed to practice their profession. The midwife's mandate from society, which is captured within the mission of the American College of

Nurse– Midwives (1992), is to provide the best quality of midwifery care to women and childbearing families.

Key Questions Related to the Study of Ethics

Why Study Ethics?

The study of ethics is important for understanding oneself, the nature of human interactions, and how best to relate to other individuals and groups (Thompson & Thompson, 1990a). In fact, the study of ethics is all about what it means to be a human being and how one should treat or interact with other human beings in a responsible manner. It is what we need to know and use every day as professionals. We study ethics to know ourselves and to know others. We study ethics to understand our values, our biases, and our patterns of thinking and doing in comparison with others and with prescribed norms of our society as well as global mandates for health (Tschudin, 2003; United Nations [UN], 2000). We study ethics to understand ethics.

Ethical behavior is neither automatic nor easily understood at times, given the great variation in human values, cultures, and definitions of *good* or *right* behavior that can pit one's personal and professional values against each other. As Tschudin (2003) noted in the Preface to the 3rd edition of her ethics text, "Ethics will always produce more questions than satisfactory answers. Ethics is therefore above all a venture in how to be human." An important addition to Tschudin's statement is that questions in ethics are getting harder, more complex, and sometimes elusive. Yet these questions do have answers if we are willing to take the time to reason through them, reflect, critically evaluate alternatives, and make a commitment to right action with right reasons, as noted below. We study ethics because we are professionals who make decisions with and for others, and we need to understand what constitutes a "good" or correct decision for everyone involved (Thompson, Kershbaumer, & Krisman-Scott, 2001; Thompson & Thompson, 1984).

What Is the Goal of Ethical Midwifery Practice?

Given the distinction between morals and ethics noted earlier, the goal of ethical midwifery practice is *to do the right thing* (the moral shoulds) *for the right reason* (ethical justification). It is obvious, then, that understanding ethics equates with understanding what it means to be a professional who is committed to right action and accountability and learning how to make ethical or good decisions as a midwife. How do we know what is the right or good thing to do? Some suggest they simply *know,* a form of intuitionism. Others consult a wise and trusted colleague to guide their decision making, an example of the conventional level of moral development (Kohlberg, 1981). And still others, through experience, have found the study of moral reasoning and ethical theory very helpful in dealing with the complex situations midwives face on a daily basis in their work with women (Frith, 1996; Thompson & Thompson, 1985). The goal of midwifery practice is to promote the health and well-being of women and childbearing families, wherever they reside, raising cultural, value, and ethical concerns that need to be respected and understood before making a final decision on a plan of care or action in the political arena.

Midwives study behavioral and physical sciences. They study the bio-psycho-social aspects of what it means to be a woman and to carry out one's reproductive roles. Midwives also study philosophy and ethics, political processes and leadership. At some point, these abstract theories must be put into practice. Knowing *how* to make good decisions as well as *why* these decisions were made constitutes ethical midwifery practice. If a person agrees to carry out others' decisions without understanding or questioning the basis for that decision or knows how to apply a piece of technology without understanding how that technology works, that person is merely a technician and not a professional. Professionals make their own decisions based on solid rationale and understand how technology works, including its limitations and risks, before using it on others (Thompson & Thompson, 1985).

What Are the Primary Ethical Theories?

When one attempts to understand the *why* of ethical action, it is helpful to look for answers in psychology, moral theology, and moral philosophy. In Western societies, ethical theories tend to be classified within philosophical thought as: 1) descriptive, 2) normative or prescriptive, 3) virtue-based, and 4) applied or practical ethics (Davis, Aroskar, Liaschenko, & Drought, 1997; Thompson & Thompson, 1985; Tschudin, 2003).

Simply stated, *descriptive ethics* describes what is—the values of individuals, institutions, professions, or societies and levels of moral development. In everyday use, the term *values* is often used interchangeably with *ethics*, though they are distinct concepts. Values are related to and can influence ethical reasoning, but they are not the same (Thompson & Thompson, 1990b). In other words, one's values may lead to a preferred choice of action, but that action may be wrong or inappropriate for others in the situation because there is a conflict of values (Thompson, 2003) or the attitude that says "my way is not your way so it is wrong." This highlights personal preferences driving choices rather than a reflective and critical evaluation of the ethical justification for choice or action. For example, the midwife may value autonomy or self-determination and expect the women she works with to hold that same value. Some women have been value programmed to let others decide for them and will not willingly participate in making decisions about their own health care. In some cultures, the mother's brother makes such decisions and in other cultures the mother-in-law or husband is the decision maker. This variation in views of self-determination across or within cultures is neither right nor wrong; it simply is.

Moral development is another aspect of descriptive ethics, coming primarily from psychology. Many years ago, psychologist Lawrence Kohlberg (1981) addressed a century-long debate about whether human beings are good by nature or whether we learn to be good. He began observing young children and followed them for years to explore how they developed their understanding of right and wrong, building upon the earlier work of Jean Piaget who concentrated on intellectual development. Both Piaget and Kohlberg have suggested that morality is both internal and external (Thompson & Thompson, 1985). In other words, the primary response to the nature–nurture debate is that humans are born with the capacity to be and to do good, influenced by the environment in which they live. This suggests that the teaching of values and ethics along with creating an environment that is safe for learning and sharing personal values and ethical discourse is vital to the ongoing development of professional midwives.

Stage theories of moral development (Gilligan, 1982; Kohlberg, 1981) can be used to further understand how humans determine what is right based on who or what they use as their source of moral authority (e.g., policemen, law, parent, ethical principles such as justice or fairness). Individuals functioning primarily at the preconventional level of moral development tend to make decisions based on what will get them a reward and avoid punishment, or ensure a return favor from another person (reciprocal). Midwives who are concerned about losing their job if they "rock the ethical boat" by disagreeing with a hospital policy (e.g., continuous electronic fetal monitoring or IV) that does not fit the needs of healthy childbearing women will not take the risk (punishment) of attempting to change such a policy. Their reward is continued employment, though the women in their care may not receive evidence-based, appropriate care, and may leave the encounter less than satisfied with their care and caregiver.

Individuals functioning primarily at the conventional level of moral development make choices based on what a wise and trusted colleague (personal authority) or the law suggests is right. Continuing the example above, the midwife in this situation may follow the hospital policy because she truly believes it is the right thing to do, not out of fear of losing her job (a different level of reasoning). Finally, those who function primarily at the post-conventional level of moral development use universal ethical principles (justice, fairness) to guide their decision making (Thompson & Thompson, 1985). A midwife functioning at the postconventional level of moral development and facing the same situation above will work to use scientific evidence and moral reasoning to push for needed change in hospital policies based on the ethical principles of doing good, avoiding harm (no ambulation with EFM can lead to increased incidence of dysfunctional labors or unnecessary discomfort for the laboring woman), and using scientific evidence. Another example of the postconventional level of moral development is the large group of midwives devoted to providing care for vulnerable populations based on the ethical principles of social justice or equity.

Understanding how individuals who function at different levels of moral development make moral choices helps explain, in part, how very caring, sensitive, intelligent persons can make decisions in a similar situation that are quite different. Respect for others requires that the midwife understand the values and moral development levels of herself and others when approaching choices and decision making (Thompson, 2003; Thompson & Thompson, 1985). It is important to understand, however, that respect does not imply that the midwife must agree with the proposed choices or even support these choices in every situation. An example is the woman/family who has chosen to birth at home with the midwife's decision that her health status is appropriate for home birth. However, when a potentially dangerous situation arises unexpectedly and the woman refuses to be transferred to a hospital setting, the midwife is caught in the ethical (and legal) dilemma of understanding the woman's choice but not agreeing with it. More on making good decisions in the face of disagreements can be found in the Thompson & Thompson (1988) article on how to accept ethical decisions with which one disagrees.

Normative ethics sets standards for ethical behavior or action that require individuals to go beyond what they may have normally done or chosen without thinking about whether that choice or action is in the best interests of others. For midwives, these others are women and families seeking midwifery care. Sometimes it is helpful to ask oneself, "What if I did this with/to all women?" in order to focus attention on broader ethical norms. This is often referred to as the principle of universalizability (Thompson & Thompson, 1985). In other words, normative ethics prescribe what one should do based on deontological, utilitarian, or natural law reasoning (Bandman & Bandman, 2004; Davis et al., 1997; Tschudin, 2003).

Deontology or rule ethics uses principles such as respect for human dignity, beneficence (do good), nonmaleficence (do no harm), quality of life, sanctity of life, justice, privacy, truth-telling, fidelity, and others as the basis or ethical justification for decisions. Although theoretically there is no limit to the number of ethical principles, some of the more common ones used during midwifery and women's health care are listed in **Table 14–1**. Beachamp and Childress (2001) defined four key or umbrella ethical principles under which they suggest all other principles fall. These umbrella principles are 1) autonomy, 2) beneficence, 3) nonmaleficence, and 4) justice. Immanuel Kant, a Prussian philosopher in the 19th century, thought that people had an imperative to do and be good at all times (categorical imperative; Kant, 1965). This deontological imperative was based on the ethical ideal that human beings are ends themselves and never should be used as a means to someone else's end. Simply put, midwives should not use the women they care for to meet their own needs for nurturing, parenting, maintaining control, or the like. Midwives must view women and their health needs as ends in themselves, worthy of respect and caring. This ethical ideal is vital to understand when working with women because it forms the justification for treating all women as human beings, rather than as objects to be used and abused by others (Thompson, 2002; Thompson, 2004).

Utilitarianism offers justification for good or right actions based on the choice(s) that will promote the greatest good or happiness for the greatest number of people. Health care institutions function primarily on a utilitarian ethic, a concern for structuring the environment to meet the needs of the great majority of patients and workers, not the individual's need. This type of ethical justification may help midwives understand why the institutional model of care for people with illnesses is very difficult to change to accommodate healthy childbearing women (the minority of individuals in hospitals). On the other hand, if one were to use utilitarian reasoning, it is difficult to justify using the model of care designed

---

Table 14–1 Common Ethical Principles

Respect for human dignity	Confidentiality
Autonomy/self-determination	Privacy
Do good (beneficence)	Quality of life
Do no harm (nonmaleficence)	Sanctity of life
Justice as fairness	Basic human rights
Social justice	Accountability/responsibility
Truthtelling/veracity	

for women experiencing a high risk pregnancy (about 5–8%) with the 92–95% of women who are healthy and expect a healthy outcome of childbearing.

Another aphorism used to describe utilitarianism is that the end or result of the decision justifies whatever was used (means) to reach that decision or outcome. This is a helpful system of ethical thought for midwives in that one can find oneself, for example, in a situation requiring major surgery (cesarean section) to save the life of the newborn or mother, yet are aware that performing surgery is harmful to the woman's body. This immediate harm of surgery (the means) is justified on the basis of saving a life (a good outcome or end).

Some authors suggest that deontology is primarily concerned with *how* good decisions are made (the process or means) supported by principles, whereas utilitarianism is more concerned with a good *outcome* (end) than with how one arrived at this outcome. Most individuals use a mix of deontological and utilitarian reasoning in arriving at the good or right decision. Others may use Natural Law reasoning, which suggests what is good or right is what occurs in nature—an argument often used against the development and use of artificial methods of contraception (Thompson & Thompson, 1985). Still others suggest that none of these philosophical theories of ethics are a good fit with women's health care, and one should focus on feminist ethics, often referred to as an ethic of care (Noddings, 1984; Thompson, 2003; Tong,1998; Tschudin, 2003). This author has defined the ethic of care with three essential components: competence, compassion, and covenant fidelity. If you truly care about another person, you will always remain competent in midwifery practice. If you truly care about another person, you will be compassionate in your interactions. And if you truly care about another person (women) you will always be faithful in the relationship going beyond the legal aspects of contract to the ethical aspects of covenant fidelity.

Virtue-based theories of ethics describe what kind of person one should be; for example, what virtues a *good* or *moral* midwife should have, such as integrity, compassion, trustworthiness, and kindness (Bandman & Bandman, 2004; Davis et al., 1997; Thompson, 2003; Tschudin, 2003). Feminist ethics and the ethics of caring reflect many aspects of virtue-based ethics. *Applied or practical ethics* refers to the use of normative and virtue-based theories in the practice of one's profession (e.g. midwifery ethics).

How Do Values Affect the Practice of Midwifery?

Values are directional signals, if you will, for what we believe we should or ought to do or choose as a *good* person because our values are based on our most deeply held beliefs about life and its meaning. Individuals come to the profession of midwifery with deeply held personal values. It is important to understand that we acquire values from a variety of sources. Children observe the world and begin to take on values espoused by parents, religion, peers, educational settings, media, and their geographic location. Massey (1981) called these early values "gut-level," with over 90% acquired by the age of 10. Recent generational theory suggests differences in the way health professionals approach their work ethic depending on when they were born and how they were value programmed (Duchscher, 2004). Such different values attached to work can create conflict between older and younger midwifery clinicians as well as between faculty and students. Adult values are added as we are exposed to others in our peer groups, as well as through professional socialization. Professional values are often embodied in a statement of moral behavior, which is a code of ethics as described later in this chapter.

It is helpful to understand that values can be changed. The process of changing one's values or adding new ones begins with an understanding of the values we currently hold dear. Next one needs to be exposed to different values, beginning to prefer the new ones, and then deliberately choosing to adopt and integrate the new value into our daily lives. In addition, depending on the situation, some values will become more dominant at a given time (value hierarchy) and less so at another time (Thompson & Thompson, 1985). For example, midwives holding key values of honesty, integrity, family, and service to others may have to put the needs of others (their clients) ahead of personal family needs at times. This does not imply that the midwife replaces or loses her value of family, but that the immediate patient need (e.g., labor) that caused her to miss her son's soccer game this week will be shared with her son as she explains what happened and why. It is this ability to shift value emphasis that allows midwives (and all people) to balance life's competing demands and understand how to make choices in keeping with our dominant values. Ignoring these values leads to personal and professional discomfort, and if ignored too long can result in apathy and loss of joy in living.

Personal and professional values are an integral part of who we are as individuals. These values are often congruent, with personal values often leading to the choice of one's career. For example, individuals who grow up valuing family, self-determination/autonomy, caring, and service to others often choose a health career such as midwifery. One must be aware that these values are not always shared by others, and can lead to conflict in relationships or communication. The midwifery philosophy, model of care, and code of ethics stress respect for women, active participation in decisions about their health care, and responsibility for the outcomes of these decisions (ACNM, 2003; ICM, 1999a). This is referred to as a shared decision-making model. Some midwives may not be comfortable with this decision model as they prefer to be "in control," and some women really want the midwife to make decisions for them when they are very capable of making their own decisions. This is one of those moments when the midwife needs to stop, reflect on choices available, and use ethical theory to validate how she should proceed in collaboration with the women seeking midwifery care. Critical thinking, negotiation, compromise, and standards of practice are the tools that every midwife needs to develop to a high level in order to address everyday ethics.

Every person has a unique value lens through which the world is viewed. It is our obligation as professionals to know our dominant values, to understand how these might influence what we say and do with others, and how these values could bias us against other individuals with different values (worldviews) that lead to different choices than we would make. One cannot provide nondiscriminatory midwifery care, an ethical obligation, if she is ignorant of her own values and value biases. It is also considered unethical to impose one's values on others unconsciously, without thinking (hence the need to know one's self).

Why Is It Important to Understand Human Rights and Health?

Anyone working with women to promote their health and well-being must be mindful of the important roles that gender, economics, status, and human rights play in women's lives and the effects on their health. In several World Health Organization (WHO) publications since the 1994 International Conference on Population and Development (ICPD) and the 4th World Conference on Women in 1995, the world health community has focused directly on the important role that women play in the health and development of nations. In fact, the Millennium Development Goals (MDGs) adopted by member states of the United Nations in 2000 address women's health and women's rights, especially Goal 3, the empowerment of women. (See http://www.un.org/millenniumgoals for full discussion of goals and targets.) These WHO-commissioned and UN reports focus on the persistent denial of basic human rights for many of the world's women and what this has done to their health and well being (Cook, 1994; UN, 1979, 1996). In all of these publications, the direct link between health and human rights emerges (Cook & Dickens, 2002; World Health Organization [WHO], 2002) and therefore must be acknowledged as an integral part of professional ethics (Commonwealth Medical Association [CMA], 1997).

Basic human rights that impact directly on one's health include such things as the right to security of person (no violence); respect for one's humanness (personhood) and dignity (self-determination); food and nutrition; shelter; privacy; freedom from any form of discrimination; the right to health and equitable access, when needed, to health and illness services of high quality; and the benefits of scientific progress (Thompson, 2004). One of the main reasons that women are often denied these basic human rights can be attributed to the dominant patriarchal view of women as objects or chattel, rather than as persons (Thompson, 2004). When women are objectified, they and their wishes can easily be discounted. Even female health care providers have participated in this form of objectification of women when they refuse to listen to the woman's health concerns, use technology when it is not indicated (abuse), fail to obtain informed consent before treatment (coercion), or determine that they "know what is best" for the patient rather than allowing the woman to determine what is best for herself. Cook and Dickens (2002) have pushed the international agenda to place safe or healthy motherhood as a basic human right, noting that the persistent denial of basic human rights has resulted in continuing high level of unnecessary maternal deaths and disability, especially in developing countries.

Thompson (2004) described the link between human rights and ethics and its implications for midwifery practice. The human rights framework for midwifery practice embodies the values, culture, and human rights of both women and midwives within the larger context of ethics. The ICM *International Code of Ethics for Midwives* (1999) incorporated the human rights mandate, as did the 2004 revision of the ACNM *Philosophy and Code of Ethics* (see **Table 14–2**). You might be wondering why linking human rights and ethics is so important for midwives. The bottom line is that if women are not respected as persons with full human rights, then their care and caregivers will be compromised. This is an unethical situation at best, and a devastating health outcome at worst.

Summary

Understanding values, moral development, human rights, and the ethical foundations or principles for good decision making in all aspects of our lives require time, reflection, study, and practice along with guidance from one's professional organization and mentors.

Table 14–2 ACNM Code of Ethics

Code of Ethics of the American College of Nurse-Midwives
Accepted by the ACNM Board of Directors
December 12, 2004

The *Code of Ethics* sets forth values, ethical principles, and standards to which professionals aspire and by which their actions can be judged. The purpose of this code is to identify the moral obligations of all certified nurse-midwives and certified midwives inherent in their professional roles. Specifically, midwives are obligated to support and maintain the integrity of the profession of midwifery in order to promote the health and well-being of women and newborns within their families and communities.

Midwives in all aspects of professional relationships will:
1. Respect basic human rights and the dignity of all persons.
2. Respect their own self worth, dignity, and professional integrity.

Midwives in all aspects of their professional practice will:
3. Develop a partnership with the woman in which each shares relevant information that leads to informed decision making, consent to an evolving plan of care, and acceptance of responsibility for the outcomes of their choices.
4. Act without discrimination based on factors such as age, gender, race, ethnicity, religion, lifestyle, sexual orientation, socioeconomic status, disability, or nature of the health problem.
5. Provide an environment where privacy is protected and in which all pertinent information is shared without bias, coercion, or deception.
6. Maintain confidentiality except where disclosure is mandated by law.
7. Maintain the necessary knowledge, skills, and behaviors needed for competence.
8. Protect women, their families, and colleagues from harmful, unethical, or incompetent practices by taking appropriate action that may include reporting as mandated by law.

Midwives as members of a profession will:
9. Promote, advocate for, and strive to protect the rights, health, and well-being of women, families, and communities.
10. Promote just distribution of resources and equity in access to quality health services.
11. Promote and support the education of midwifery students and peers, standards of practice, research, and policies that enhance the health of women, families, and communities.

The rest of this chapter will focus on key details of how to make good/ethical decisions in today's world with both ongoing and new challenges to our understanding of ethics and midwifery practice with women and childbearing families.

Ethical Duties and Obligations of Midwives: Codes of Ethics

Codes of ethics (moral behavior) are grounded in normative ethical theory. Codes define what a midwife should do, how she should interact with others, and what the profession of midwifery should promote for the good of society. The importance of defining the moral ideals of midwives and midwifery practice rest with the societal mandate to promote the health and well-being of women and newborns within their families and communities (ACNM, 1992).

As one hallmark of a profession, groups set forth the moral ideals of behavior and action that members of society can expect from the practitioners of that profession. Midwives have responded to this need by issuing a variety of codes of ethics in countries throughout the world. Usually these codes consist of moral obligations or duties to self, to those seeking midwifery care, to other members of the profession and team members, and to society at large. The *International Code of Ethics for Midwives* was first adopted by the International Confederation of Midwives (ICM) Council in 1993 and was most recently updated in 1999. (See http://www.internationalmidwives.org for the complete text.) The ACNM *Code of Ethics for nurse–midwives* was first adopted in 1990, and was revised in 2004 (see **Table 14–2**). The similarities are many, as one would expect, including the mandates to respect and promote human rights, to respect the dignity of all persons, to support self-determination and a partnership model of care, to maintain confidentiality, to act without discrimination, and to promote and develop the profession through education, research, and policy making for the good of women and society.

When one reads a code of ethics, it becomes clearer that the statements of the code relate to the moral shoulds and oughts of relationships and behaviors. Each of these statements must be supported by ethical justification or reasons, often embodied in explanatory notes such as the ACNM code or in the *Interpretive Statements* of the *ANA Code of Ethics for Nurses* (American Nurses Association [ANA], 2001). This allows the practitioner and the public to understand the ethical why or reason for the moral obligation. As an example of the reflection and thought processes that went into the most recent revision of the ACNM code, the deliberations on the wording of the 11 statements took nearly a year, and were coordinated with the working group refining the ACNM philosophy as well as multiple consultations with key stakeholders. The explanatory notes took somewhat less time because the working group continually assessed the ethical justification for each code statement as these were developed. Further analysis of the ethical justification for statements 1 and 2 resulted in viewing them as the foundation for the nine other statements that follow. This happened because the ethical rationale for "respect basic human rights and the dignity of all persons" and "respect for self" are grounded in the ethical principles of respect, human dignity, personhood, self-determination, doing good, social justice, non-discrimination, and self-worth. The rest of the code statements are grounded in these overarching principles and the utilitarian concept of doing the most good for the most people. Confidentiality, competence, protection, advocacy, caring, and continuation of the profession all relate to what it means to respect and be respected, and to be treated fairly as a human being.

Reviewing the codes of ethics of the midwifery profession reveals more clearly how midwives view women and their health, childbearing families, and the midwife's and profession's obligation to promote just distribution of resources and equity in access to quality health services in any society. Entering this woman- and family-centered profession requires a commitment to these values and moral behavior, including reciprocal, trust-based relationships as well as the virtues of being a good person.

There are important caveats to understanding professional codes of ethics and how they can be used. First and foremost, codes of ethics describe the *ideal* of behavior and action that all strive to meet on a daily basis. However, as human beings with inherent flaws and the capacity to make mistakes, we do not always reach the ideals of ethical behavior or action. In these instances, the code reminds us of the goal for what one should do the next time. Another important caveat in using the code of ethics is to understand that following the moral mandates prescribed in the code will not guarantee an ethical answer to a given dilemma one is facing. The code offers guidance in knowing what to do or how to act, but a caring person will always have to use their own critical thinking processes to analyze the specifics of the situation along with their commitment to ethical action by applying the tenets of moral behavior.

Moral Reasoning and Ethical Decision Making

Moral reasoning and ethical decision making are also grounded in the normative or prescriptive theories of ethics, notably deontology, utilitarianism, and natural law. These theories provide the ethical *why or rationale* for choices or action. As noted earlier, the goal of ethical practice is to do the right thing for the right reasons. We are now into a discussion of the process (how to) of making good or ethical decisions in midwifery practice.

As bioethics and biomedical ethics became popular in the 1960s, philosophers and theologians were often consulted by health professionals in situations where the individuals involved (professionals, patients, family members) could not agree on a course of action. Hospital ethics committees were formed and gradually health professionals took on the role of ethical arbitrators along with clergy, lawyers, and philosophers/ethicists. Decision theories from business and mathematics were used to help predict the potential outcome of treatment decisions as well as the chances of survival with a given illness. These decision theories, however, could not replace the need for consideration of values, ethics, and critical thinking to approach the inevitable moral questions, "What *should* we do in this situation? How *should* we decide? Who owns the problem? Who *should* decide the course of action?

These questions require understanding of how individuals reason morally as distinct from scientific reasoning. The concept of moral reasoning addresses the process for making ethical decisions, including analyzing, weighing, justifying, choosing, and evaluating each available choice prior to taking action (Thompson & Thompson, 1985). One will note the similarity of the moral reasoning process with the scientific and midwifery care processes in that several steps in sequence need to be followed, referring back to a previous step as more information is obtained or the situation changes. The scientific process, however, primarily uses evidence from research and clinical practice for justifying choices, whereas the moral reasoning process is focused on what it means to be human (values) and how to relate to others, and uses ethical principles or theory to justify the right or good action to be taken. Moral reasoning helps us choose the most appropriate response from among the reasoned alternatives.

Thompson and Thompson Bioethical Decision-Making Model 2004

The development of a bioethical decision-making model over the past two decades has resulted in the framework for decision making presented in **Table 14–3**. This model is grounded in the understanding of how values and levels of moral development can influ-

---

Table 14–3 Thompson & Thompson Bioethical Decision-Making Model

Adapted from Thompson & Thompson, 1985.
Updated January 2004.

Step 1: **Review the situation** to determine:
1. Health problems—physical, spiritual, mental, psychosocial.
2. Decision/actions needed immediately and in near future.
3. Ethical components of situation and decision/action.
4. Key individuals potentially affected by the decision/action and outcomes.
5. Any potential human rights violations in situation.

Step 2: **Gather additional information** to clarify and understand:
1. Legal constraints, if any.
2. Limited time to thoroughly explore.
3. Decision capacity of individual(s).
4. Institutional policies that affect choices in situation.
5. Values inherent in choice of information.

Step 3: **Identify the ethical issues or concerns** in the situation:
1. Name the ethical concern.
2. Explore historical roots of each.
3. Identify current philosophical/religious positions on each issue.
4. Discuss societal/cultural views on each issue.

Step 4: **Define personal and professional moral positions** on ethical concerns:
1. Review personal biases/constraints on issues raised.
2. Understand personal values affected by situation/ethical issues raised.
3. Review professional codes of ethics (moral behavior) for guidance.
4. Identify any conflicting loyalties and/or obligations of professionals and family in the situation.
5. Think about your level of moral development operant in this situation.
6. Identify the virtues needed for professional action.

Step 5: **Identify moral positions of key individuals** in the situation:
1. Think about levels of moral development operant in each participant.
2. Identify any communication gaps or misunderstandings.
3. Provide guidance in clarifying varying levels of moral development.

Step 6: **Identify value conflicts,** if any:
1. Provide guidance in identifying potential conflicts, interests, or competing values.
2. Work toward possible resolution of conflict based on respect for differences.
3. Seek consultation if needed to resolve key conflicts.

Step 7:   Determine who should make needed decision:
1. Clarify your role in the situation.
2. Who "owns" the problem/decision?
3. Who stands to lose or gain the most from the decision/action?
4. Is the decision to be made by a single individual or a group?

Step 8:   Identify the range of actions with anticipated outcomes of each:
1. Determine the moral justification for each potential action.
2. Identify the ethical theory that supports each action.
3. Apply concepts of beneficence and fairness to each potential action.
4. Attach outcomes to each potential action and determine best outcome.
5. Are additional actions/decisions required as a result of each action?

Step 9:   Decide on a course of action and carry it out:
1. Understand why a given action was chosen.
2. Help all involved understand these reasons.
3. Establish a time frame for review of the decision/action and expected outcomes.
4. Determine who can best carry out the chosen action/decision.

Step 10:   Evaluate/review outcomes of decisions/actions:
1. Determine whether expected outcomes occurred.
2. Is a new decision or action needed?
3. Was the decision process fair and complete?
4. What was the response to the action by each key individual?
5. What did you learn from this situation?

ence decision making. It requires critical thinking, reflection, time, caring, integrity, and use of moral reasoning to sort out the key aspects of the situation, alternatives for action, and moral mandates from professional codes that can provide direction to the decision making. This decision model also requires that participants consider the ethical rationale for each potential choice before proceeding to action, weighing and justifying each one much the same as the midwifery care process requires a rationale for proposed action before a final decision is made. An important caveat to the use of this or any other decision model is that following the steps will not automatically guarantee a good outcome—critical thinking, reflection, and commitment to doing the right thing are required, similar to the requirements for the effective use of the midwifery care process (Thompson & Thompson, 1990a). It is also helpful to use the decision model within groups for practice in sharing values, morality, and use of ethical theories to justify moral action. Respect and mutual trust are required when analyzing the ethical dimensions of a clinical situation as individuals risk sharing their most deeply held values and innermost thoughts. Success in making ethical decisions in midwifery practice requires time, experience, compassion, understanding, a commitment to reason and reflection, knowledge of self and others, and competence in midwifery. The case study at the end of the chapter illustrates the use of the decision model in midwifery care. Narrigan (2004) also used this model in her examination of a cross-cultural clinical encounter.

Ethical Issues in Midwifery

The practice of midwifery focuses on working primarily with women during their repro-ductive years. As such, midwives are faced with the majority of contemporary ethical issues or concerns. These ethical concerns begin prior to pregnancy with questions of when, with whom, how, and whether a woman should conceive. Ethical issues surrounding contracep-tion, abortion, and adolescent sexuality are added to those relating directly to conception. Lack of basic human rights to health, education, economics, and safety affect young girls and women more often than they affect young boys and men, creating the need to promote these basic human rights for all persons rather than accepting the continued disparities (Braverman, Egerter, Cubbin, & Marchi, 2004; Thompson & Thompson, 1997, 2001). Adult issues surrounding genetics made more complex by the mapping of the human genome and our developing knowledge of genetic markers for such conditions as breast cancer have made decisions and choices more complex, especially with healthy women (Van Riper & McKinnon, 2004). On the other hand, end-of-life decisions and the allocation of scare resources are rare occurrences in the practice of midwifery, with the exception of sick newborns (Penticuff, 1998), as midwives concentrate most of their practice in health promotion activities and with normal life-cycle events during a woman's lifetime. This chapter provides a brief overview of ethical issues raised during the practice of midwifery and is organized around three major themes that permeate most of the specific ethical con-cerns raised previously. These themes in women's health and midwifery are 1) technology, 2) informed consent, and 3) health as a basic right for all.

Technology

Health care ethics in the Western world gained renewed public attention in the 1960s, stim-ulated in part by the technological revolution in illness detection and treatment (Patel & Rushefsky, 2002). Newer questions raised by the specter of new technologies resulted in such ethical concerns as whether we should use the technology on everyone just because we could, rather than only when indicated (Thompson & Thompson, 1985). The Techno-logical Imperative was born and then quickly challenged, "Just because we can do some-thing, should we?" Women's health care, especially related to reproductive health, focused this ethical discussion on the use and abuse of reproductive technologies, and raised the risk–benefit questions of who was obtaining the benefits of such technologies and who was shouldering most of the risk (Thompson & Thompson, 2001).

Midwives face the ethical concern of whether and when to use technology on a daily basis in their practice. They understand that much of reproductive technology, including the development of female contraceptive methods or the multiple methods of assisted re-production, were designed and tested with less than acceptable research methodologies (Stanworth, 1987). The diethyl-stillbesterol (DES) off-label use for maintaining pregnan-cies resulted in untoward side effects in daughters and sons of women taking DES. Several intrauterine contraceptive devices had to be pulled from use based on harm done to the users that were not tested for in advance. The overuse of electronic fetal monitoring (EFM) leading to unnecessary cesarean sections is well known to all. What will be the next harmful technology for women? Will it be the overuse of ultrasonography during pregnancy or the continuation of unnecessary hysterectomies or mastectomies when other forms of treatment are available and proven reliable? Will it be the continued push to have all babies born in hospitals based on the unwarranted and unsubstantiated concern for safety? Will it be the discrimination practices that can result from new genetic knowledge? These questions are a reminder that science and ethics must be viewed together if ethical midwifery care is to result. In fact, technology was and is developed as an adjunct to clinical decision making, not as a replacement for judgment and critical thinking (Thompson & Thompson, 2001).

Midwives, like other health professionals, need to avoid the temptation of using technology when it is not indicated. In fact, there are several ethical questions that must be addressed in order to determine whether to use technology in the care of women. These include:

- Can the practitioner obtain the needed information in some other way (e.g., use of hands for fetal size rather than ultrasound or ears rather than EFM for fetal heart)?
- Do the benefits from use of the technology far outweigh the risks (known and potential) of using the technology?
- Does the woman understand the risks and limitations of the technology proposed?
- Is the technology really indicated? (Thompson & Thompson, 2001)

The thrill or glitz of technology is eye-catching and seductive. Overuse of technology when working with women can be viewed as another attempt to treat women as objects, rather than persons who are intelligent, educated, autonomous human beings and who deserve our best science and morality during their health care encounters. The ethical use of technology, whether drugs, devices, or surgical procedures, is based on the deontological principles of respect for human dignity, doing good while avoiding harm, honesty and integrity (admit the limits of knowledge about the proposed technology), and scientific evidence.

Informed Consent: An Interface of Law and Ethics

As patients began to be valued for the expertise they brought to the professional encounter, concepts such as active participation in decisions about health and illness care leading to informed consent came to the fore. The changing relationship between health care professional and patient/client from a patriarchal system of decision making (the professional knows best) to a shared process in which all participants are of equal worth and their perspectives respected is one example of the interface between law and ethics. For example, many years ago the courts determined that an adult of sound mind had the right to determine what would be done or not done to them in the course of medical treatment. Building on the Nazi war criminal trials, the legal concept of informed consent was championed, particularly in research, and gradually took its rightful place in everyday decisions in health and illness care. It is important to note, however, that the model of shared decision making in midwifery care predated by centuries the modern concept of informed participation in health and illness care decisions and consent. Midwives, working "with women" as the name implies, have and continue to use shared decision making as the norm.

In daily practice, the midwife is often called upon to make decisions with and for others. Davis et al. (1997) noted that the decisions we make in clinical practice can be both ethical and legal, or can be legal but not ethical, or ethical and illegal. This awareness of how ethics and the law intersect in clinical practice is important for professionals. It is also important to understand that individuals who function primarily within the conventional level of moral development are more likely to make choices directed by legal policies of the practice setting, even if that choice is not in the best interests of an individual woman. Midwives who work primarily with vulnerable populations often push for social justice or equity in health policies and access to needed services, reflecting a postconventional level of moral development. This ethical stance may require the midwife to go beyond what is legally mandated for care and services.

The concept of informed consent is an important example of the interface of law and ethics (Mann, 2004). This interface results in both a moral and a legal obligation for the midwife to provide information about proposed treatment; alternatives, if any; and risks and benefits of each in an understandable manner, and then obtain needed consent from the woman before proceeding to touch her or prescribe any treatment. Why is consent needed, and what does it mean to be "informed" before giving consent (Lowe, 2004)? Briefly, the concept of informed consent is grounded in the deontological principle of autonomy or self-determination and requires respect for others' views, choices, and preferences. Autonomy does not mean that individuals can do anything they want, and respecting another's preferences does not mean one has to agree with them. Autonomy implies a reasoned choice based on principles and reflection, not simply whim, along with a willingness to accept the consequences of those choices. Generally speaking, autonomy related to health care decisions means having the ability to receive and understand health care information, reflect on its meaning, and retaining the right to agree or refuse suggested treatment or care. The key elements of informed consent are noted in **Table 14–4**.

Health as a Basic Right for All

In 1948, the Charter of the United Nations included the Universal Declaration of Human Rights, which stated that "Everyone has a right to a standard of living adequate for the health and well-being of himself and his family . . . including medical care . . ." (UN Charter, 1948). Since this time there has been much discussion of what it would mean if everyone had a *right* to health, including access to health and illness care. As noted throughout this chapter, women have often lacked basic human rights because they were viewed as less than human,

---

Table 14–4 Key Elements of Informed Consent

1. Proposed treatment
2. Full and unbiased information
3. Use of language that is understood
4. Risks and benefits of each proposed action
5. Verification that information given was understood
6. Obtain consent to deny or proceed with proposed action

less than persons, by many societies. Maternal death and disability is a tragic example of the persistent denial of women's rights and of women's personhood (Cook, 1994). Violence against women during times of war and civil unrest perpetuate the myth that women are to be viewed as property or the spoils of war, and not as fully human (see ICM *Position Statement on Women, Children, and Midwives in Situations of War and Civil Unrest*, 1999b). Domestic violence (Garcia-Moreno, 2002; United Nations Population Fund, 2001) and the rising incidence of HIV/AIDS in women is another example of what happens to women when they have no right to safety in their own homes or within partner relationships.

In order for women to be healthy and valued for themselves, not as a producer of children, a sexual playmate, or a spoil of war, they must be given the same status as men in society (ICM, 1990). Women also must demand equal treatment and equal rights to health and well-being. Midwives, predominantly women themselves, have a pivotal role to play in advancing the status of women and their basic human rights. When the midwife speaks to other women with respect, when she touches others only after obtaining consent, when she acknowledges the woman's values and preferences during health encounters, and when she actively encourages and supports women as partners in decision making, the midwife is advancing the cause of health for women as a right and women as deserving of this basic human right. This is the ethical ideal of midwifery care. This is ethics in action.

Summary

This chapter has attempted to cover a range of ethical concerns and topics, beginning with key definitions. The main topics covered were:

- Philosophical systems of ethics
- Sources and influence of personal and professional values
- Moral mandates for the profession of midwifery embodied in codes of ethics
- Human rights framework for midwifery practice
- Ethical and legal concept of informed consent
- Ethical use of technology in women's health care
- Bioethical decision-making model for the analysis of the ethical dimensions of midwifery practice

It is hoped that the reader has been stimulated to read other sources, to take seriously the moral mandates of the profession of midwifery, and to strive for ethical decision making daily. Better health and health care for women is the result, and it is gratifying to know that one has played an important role in achieving this goal though ethical midwifery practice.

Chapter Exercises
Using the Thompson and Thompson Decision-Making Model

T.M. is the midwife on-call in a community hospital labor and delivery unit. As she begins her night rounds, she is called to the admissions area to evaluate a 32-year-old G4P3003 who just arrived in active labor at term. The woman, in obvious discomfort, requests an immediate epidural to "get rid of the pain." T.M. completes her initial evaluation quickly. She quietly reassures the woman that all is progressing well, and that she will give birth shortly. The woman again asks for an epidural, and begins to yell at T.M. that she wants a real "doctor" right away. T.M. explains that her request for an epidural cannot be granted as the baby's head is crowning and delivery is imminent. She urges the woman to gently push and a healthy, 8-pound baby girl is born. Both mother and infant are in good condition, but the woman is still very upset at not receiving an epidural and wants to speak to the "doctor in charge."

Using the Thompson and Thompson Decision Model, identify the ethical issues in this situation and proceed to determine what T.M. should do.

1. The notable health concern is the woman's apparent mental distress at not having her wish for an epidural granted. T.M. needs to decide how to proceed with the woman's demand to speak to the doctor in charge at 3 a.m. The key individuals in the situation are the woman, her newborn, the midwife, the physician, and other potential staff of the hospital. The woman may think that having an epidural is her "right" even though the timing was not optimal and the anesthesiologist had to be called in from home.

2. As time is limited for reflecting on this situation, the midwife may wish to determine if there is someone who brought the woman to the hospital whom she would like to be with. The midwife may also wish to know about the woman's past labors and births and try to understand why having an epidural was important to this woman.

3. The major ethical concerns in this situation revolve around the self-determination or autonomy of the laboring woman, her decision capacity in active labor, and the midwife's professional responsibility to attend to the impending birth to assure safe passage of the newborn, understanding that she was going against the choice of the woman for an epidural. Professional accountability and patient choice are in conflict in this situation.

4. In this step, the reader is asked to assess his or her own personal and professional values about use of epidural in late labor and the value placed on client self-determination even when a choice may appear to be unsafe or inappropriate. The reader is encouraged to look at the ACNM *Code of Ethics for Nurse–Midwives 2005* for guidance, including a review of the Explanatory Notes.

5. Step 5 is difficult to complete without talking with the key individuals.

6. Both the woman and midwife could value self-determination or choices, but in this situation, the midwife's concern for the safety of the birth overrides the client's request for an epidural (self-determination). This is not a violation of the woman's right of choice—it is placing safety of the baby at a higher level of importance than the mother's choice for

pain relief. The mother may or may not share this view. The hierarchy of values changes depending on the situation, and this case illustrates the importance of good communication and understanding of each other's perspectives.

7. Due to the potential emergent situation of impending birth, the midwife was the most appropriate person in this situation to decide whether an epidural was to be used. She has a duty to explain her decision making to the woman once the birth was completed along with her reasons for the decision.

8. The decision at hand is how to handle the woman's anger and whether to awake the physician on-call to come and talk with the woman. There are many possible courses of action that could be justified with ethical reasoning, including what would promote the greatest "good" in the situation and the least "harm." The midwife could begin with her explanation for her decision, using both scientific evidence (timing of epidural) and the concern for the safety of the newborn. The midwife could agree to call the physician, though she may question if it is worth waking her (conflicting loyalties). Respect for the woman and her anger requires understanding and listening to why the epidural was so important at the time of birth. Reciprocal respect for the midwife and her choice also requires that the woman listen to the midwife, though she does not need to agree. Mutual concern for the welfare of the infant might suggest that both pay attention to the newborn and agree to talk about the epidural in the morning. Shared decision making on how to proceed with the request to talk with the physician would support many ethical principles.

9. The reader is encouraged to reflect on what she or he would do in this situation and why (the ethical justification).

10. Evaluation is always important for the midwife who is concerned about doing what is best for the patient (in this case, two patients). One can learn from this situation what may be helpful to do in a similar situation in the future.

Table 14–5 For Your Professional Files: Web Sites for Professional Documents

---

American College of Nurse–Midwives: www.midwife.org
   Mission Statement, December 2003
   Philosophy of the American College of Nurse–Midwives, September 2004
   Code of Ethics of the American College of Nurse–Midwives, December 2004
   Standards for the Practice of Midwifery, March 8, 2003

International Confederation of Midwives: www.internationalmidwives.org
   Vision for Women and Their Health, 1990
   International Code of Ethics for Midwives, 1999
   Midwives, Women and Human Rights: ICM Position Statement, 2002
   Women, Children, and Midwives in Situations of War and Civil Unrest, 1999

References

American College of Nurse–Midwives. (1992). *Mission*. Washington, DC: Author.

American College of Nurse–Midwives. (2003). *Standards for the practice of midwifery*. Silver Spring, MD: Author.

American College of Nurse–Midwives. (2004a). *Code of ethics of the American College of Nurse-Midwives*. Silver Spring, MD: Author.

American College of Nurse–Midwives. (2004b). *Philosophy of the American College of Nurse-Midwives*. Silver Spring, MD: Author.

American Nurses Association. (2001). *Code of ethics for nurses with interpretive statements*. Washington, DC: Author.

Bandman, E. L., & Bandman, B. (2004). *Nursing ethics through the life span* (4th ed.). Stamford, CT: Appleton & Lange.

Beachamp, T. L., & Childress, J. (2001). *Principles of biomedical ethics* (5th ed.). New York: Oxford University Press.

Braverman, P. A., Egerter, S. A., Cubbin, C., & Marchi, K. S. (2004). An approach to studying social disparities in health and health care. *American Journal of Public Health, 94*(12), 2139–2148.

Commonwealth Medical Association. (1997). *Declaration on ethics and a woman's right to health*. London: Author.

Cook, R. J. (1994). *Women's health and human rights*. Geneva: World Health Organization.

Cook, R. J., & Dickens, B. M. (2002). Human rights to safe motherhood. *International Journal of Gynaecology and Obstetrics, 76*, 225–231.

Davis, A. J., Aroskar, M. A., Liaschenko, J., & Drought, T. S. (1997). *Ethical dilemmas and nursing practice* (4th ed.). Stamford, CT: Appleton & Lange.

Duchscher, J. E. B. (2004). Multigenerational nurses in the workplace. *Journal of Nursing Administration, 34*(11), 493–501.

Frith, L. (Ed.). (1996). *Ethics and midwifery*. Oxford, England: Butterworth Heinemann.

Fry, S. T. (1989). Teaching ethics in nursing curricula. *Nursing Clinics of North America, 24*(2), 485–497.

Garcia-Moreno, C. (2002). Dilemmas and opportunities for an appropriate health service response to violence against women. *Lancet, 359*, 1509–1514.

Gilligan, C. (1982). *In a different voice: Psychological theory and women's development.* Cambridge, MA: Harvard University Press.

International Confederation of Midwives. (1990). *Vision for women and their health.* The Hague, The Netherlands: Author.

International Confederation of Midwives. (1999a). *International code of ethics for midwives.* The Hague, The Netherlands: Author.

International Confederation of Midwives. (1999b). *Position statement on women, children and midwives in situations of war and civil unrest.* Retrieved April 7, 2006, from http://www.internationalmidwives.org/Statements/War%20and%20Civil%Unrest.htm?OSTNUKESID=32a40d469fbOa7388f6612cb2de51bf7

Kant, I. (1965). The metaphysical elements of justice. *The metaphysics of morals. Part 1.* Indianapolis, IN: Bobbs-Merrill.

Kohlberg, L. (1981). *Essays on moral development. Vol. 1. The philosophy of moral development.* San Francisco: Harper & Row.

Lowe, N. K. (2004). Context and process of informed consent for pharmacologic strategies in labor pain care. *Journal of Midwifery & Women's Health, 49*(3), 251–259.

Mann, R. J. (2004). The interface between legal and ethical issues in reproductive health. *Journal of Midwifery & Women's Health, 49*(3), 182–187.

Massey, M. (Director) (1981). *What you are is . . .* [Series of 3 videotapes on values]. Farmington Hills, MI: Magnetic Video.

Narrigan, D. (2004). Examining an ethical dilemma: A case study in clinical practice. *Journal of Midwifery & Women's Health, 49*(3), 243–249.

Noddings, N. (1984). *Caring: A feminine approach to ethics and moral education.* Berkeley: University of California Press.

Patel, K., & Rushefsky, M. E. (2002). *Health care policy in an age of new technologies.* Armonk, NY: M. E. Sharpe.

Penticuff, J. H. (1998). Defining futility in neonatal intensive care. *Nursing Clinics of North America, 33*(2), 339–352.

Smith, S. J., & Davis, A. J. (1980). Ethical dilemmas: Conflicts among rights, duties, and obligations. *American Journal of Nursing, 80*(8), 1463–1466.

Stanworth, M. (Ed.). (1987). *Reproductive technologies: Gender, motherhood, and medicine.* Minneapolis: University of Minnesota Press.

Thompson, F. E. (2003). The practice setting: site of ethical conflict for some mothers and midwives. *Nursing Ethics, 10*(6), 588–601.

Thompson, J. B. (2004). A human rights framework for midwifery care. *Journal of Midwifery & Women's Health, 49*(3), 175–181.

Thompson, J. E. (2002). Midwives and human rights: Dream or reality? *Midwifery, 18*, 188–192.

Thompson, J. E., Kershbaumer, R. M., & Krisman-Scott, M. A. (2001). *Educating advanced practice nurses and midwives.* Chapter 3: Ethics, values and moral development in teaching. New York: Springer.

Thompson, J. E., & Thompson, H. O. (1984). Why should nurses study ethics? *Scholar and Educator, 8*(1), 51–61.

Thompson, J. E., & Thompson, H. O. (1985). *Bioethical decision making for nurses*. Norwalk, CT: Appleton-Century-Crofts. (Reprinted in 1992 in Lanham, MD: University Press of America).

Thompson, J. E., & Thompson, H. O. (1988). Living with ethical decisions with which you disagree. *MCN, 13*, 245–250.

Thompson, J. E., & Thompson, H. O. (Eds.). (1990a). *Professional ethics in nursing*. Malabar, FL: Kreiger Publishing Company.

Thompson, J. E., & Thompson, H. O. (1990b). Values: Directional signals for life choices. *Neonatal Network, 8*(4), 83–84.

Thompson, J. E., & Thompson, H. O. (1993). *Moral development and education*. Delhi: ISPCK.

Thompson, J. E., & Thompson, H. O. (1996). *Handbook of ethics for midwives*. Philadelphia: University of Pennsylvania School of Nursing.

Thompson, J. E., & Thompson, H. O. (1997). Ethics and midwifery. *World Health, 2*, 14–15.

Thompson, J. E., & Thompson, H. O. (2001). Ethical aspects of care. In L. Walsh (Ed.), *Midwifery: Community based care during the childbearing year* (Chapter 29). Philadelphia: Saunders.

Tong, R. (1998). The ethics of care: A feminist virtue ethics of care for health practitioners. *Journal of Medical Philosophy, 23*, 131–152.

Tschudin, V. (2003) *Ethics in nursing* (3rd ed.). Edinburgh: Butterworth Heinemann.

United Nations. (1979). *Convention on the elimination of all forms of discrimination against women*. New York: Author.

United Nations. (1996). *Beijing declaration and platform for action*. New York: Author.

United Nations. (2000). *Millennium development goals*. Retrieved (May 2, 2006) from http://www.un.org/millenniumgoals

United Nations Charter. (1948). *Universal declaration of human rights*. New York: Author.

United Nations Population Fund. (2001). *A practical approach to gender-based violence*. New York: Author.

Van Riper, M., & McKinnon, W. C. (2004). Genetic testing for breast and ovarian cancer susceptibility: A family experience. *Journal of Midwifery & Women's Health, 49*(3), 210–219.

World Health Organization. (2002). *25 questions and answers on health and human rights*. Geneva: Author.

CHAPTER 15

Women's Health and Midwifery

Debbie Jessup, CNM, FACNM

Learning Objectives

1. Describe how feminist health activism helped shape political reform in the twentieth century.
2. Explain the changes in Congress that brought about a women's health legislative agenda.
3. Discuss the history and current status of women's health in the agencies of the Department of Health and Human Services.
4. List women's health advocacy groups that have played a role in advancing gender equity in health research and services.
5. Discuss the documents and activities of the American College of Nurse–Midwives that address women's health policy and leadership.

A life cycle approach to the health of women is a precariously new tradition in the historical development of health care. Descriptive terminology, like *gynecology, reproductive health,* and *women's health,* are often interchanged by contemporary practitioners without a clear understanding of the fundamental philosophical and social changes these words represent. In fact, women's health in 21st century America represents the evolution of a paradigm that has been significantly impacted by the confluence of three forces: health professional development, social feminism, and political reform.

Midwifery practice falls within this paradigm of women's health. But more importantly, the philosophy of the American College of Nurse–Midwives asserts "a commitment to individual and collective leadership . . . to improve the health of women and their families worldwide" (American College of Nurse–Midwives [ACNM], 2004b). In order for midwives to be effective leaders in women's health, it is important that we understand the social, political, and professional forces that have shaped and continue to impact women's health. The purpose of this chapter is to give midwives a more thorough understanding of the historical evolution of women's health, and the processes and organizations that define it today.

Women's Health in the Twenty-First Century: The Evolution of a Paradigm

Health Professional Development and Women's Health

MEDICAL SPECIALIZATION

Medical interest in gynecological matters can be traced back to ancient Egypt. The earliest known references to the care of women outside of childbirth is found in translations of papyrus that describe treatment for prolapse of the uterus and remedies to prevent shrinkage of the breast (O'Dowd & Phillips, 1994).

During the mid-nineteenth century increasing consideration was given to the treatment of diseases and disorders that were specific to women. This practice became known as "gynecology," and in the United States its development is usually attributed to a physician named J. Marion Sims. Sims gained recognition by developing a surgical treatment for vesico-vaginal fistula in his southern slave patients. In 1855 Sims moved his practice north, and supported by a group of women reformers, established the first Women's Hospital of the state of New York. It was here that surgical techniques for female disorders were perfected, and the foundations for the specialty were laid down. In 1876 Sims, as president of the American Medical Association, co-founded the American Gynecological Society (McGregor, 1998).

The marriage of obstetrics and gynecology did not take place until 1930 when the American Board of Obstetrics and Gynecology incorporated the two practices into a single specialty. Centering primarily on surgical intervention and the management of potential obstetric complications, the specialty grew rapidly over the next 25 years. In 1951 the American College of Obstetricians and Gynecologists was established as the first national professional organization open to all qualified applicants (American College of Obstetricians and Gynecologists [ACOG], 2006).

During the last twenty years, an interesting contrast has taken place in the profession of obstetrics and gynecology (Ob/Gyn). In response to a change in health management and payment systems requiring a primary care gatekeeper to many specialty services, ACOG has argued for the recognition of obstetrician-gynecologists as primary care providers. At the same time, the medical specialty continues to develop more narrow areas of focus in reproductive health. Today, many Ob/Gyn physicians choose subspecialty concentrations in maternal-fetal medicine, reproductive endocrinology/infertility, gynecologic oncology, and female pelvic medicine/reconstructive surgery.

MIDWIFERY

Nurse–midwifery in the United States has its roots in public health nursing, and as such has a long history of providing primary care to women and families. In 1925, Mary Breckenridge established the first successful nurse–midwifery service in rural Kentucky.

The midwives of the Frontier Nursing Service functioned as primary public health nurse providers to over 1200 families in a 700 square mile radius of the Appalachian Mountains. In addition to attending births, their time was spent conducting school health examinations, providing health education on environmental sanitation, triaging health concerns, and providing primary care for minor illnesses (Breckinridge, 1981; Stone, 2000). The first five schools of nurse–midwifery also had public health origins. From 1931 to 1950, these programs took public health nurses and trained them to meet the primary care and obstetrical needs of special populations. Although practice opportunities in cities were extremely limited in availability and scope, the graduates of these programs brought high-quality, family-centered primary care to medically underserved communities (Rooks, 1997).

During these early years of nurse–midwifery, a dramatic change was taking place in the practice of American obstetrical health care. By 1950, childbirth was firmly entrenched within the hospital, and the fledgling profession of nurse–midwifery was struggling to define its role in this medicine-dominated system. Midwives, seeking entrance into these physician-controlled environments, found that their scope of practice was being defined by the setting and supervisory nature of their relationships with physicians. In 1961, the first practice definition adopted by the membership of the American College of Nurse–Midwives delineated nurse–midwifery management as the care of normal mothers and babies within the maternity cycle (Stone, 2000).

In 1970, Congress passed Title X of the Public Health Service Act, which provided authority and funding for family planning services to indigent populations. Midwives, with a long history of providing services to underserved populations, began to incorporate family planning services into their scope of practice. In 1977, the ACNM redefined nurse–midwifery practice to include the care of normal newborns and women, antepartally, intrapartally, postpartally, and gynecologically (Burst, 1998; Miller & Tsui, 1997). In the 1980 first edition of *Nurse–Midwifery,* Varney described this expanded scope of practice, known as the interconceptional period, as "the primary health care of women who are between menarche and menopause as it relates to the female reproductive system" (Varney, 1980).

During the 1980s, increasing numbers of nurse–midwives expanded their practices to include care of the perimenopausal and menopausal woman. In the last decade of the millennium, federal health reform efforts brought the concept of the primary care provider into the mainstream of the health marketplace. At this point, the profession of nurse–midwifery came full circle in reclaiming its primary care roots (Burst, 1998; Sullivan, 2000). A 1992 ACNM Position Statement asserted the role of the CNM as a "provider of primary health care for women and newborns" (ACNM, 1992). In 1997, the Core Competencies were revised to reflect the expanded primary care scope of practice (Stone, 2000).

Feminist Social Activism and Women's Health

The women's health movement is frequently equated with the women's rights movement and, most frequently, with the feminist social protests of the 1970s. In fact, women in this country have a much longer history of health reform. Each of the social reform movements of the last two centuries have had components of women's health activism that have helped reshape health care institutions and medical practice, influence health policy, and ultimately improve the status of women in our society (Weisman, 1998a).

Two periods of health activism in the 19th century are of notable interest. The popular health movement in the 1830s and 1840s brought an increased focus on health education and disease prevention. It also included a reaction against a male-dominated medical system and an endorsement of the gentler healing styles of female lay practitioners and midwives. In the post-Civil War period, there was a significant increase in the number of women attending medical schools. Since these female physicians were largely excluded from mainstream hospitals, they began to develop women's hospitals that focused on obstetrical and gynecological care for women by women (Weisman, 1998b).

The Progressive era of the 1920s and 1930s was the time of the women's suffrage movement. Three significant changes occurred in women's health during this time. The first involved women's quality of life and the development of disposable menstrual products. The other two represented fundamentally different views on women's societal roles. The birth control movement, led by Margaret Sanger and other birth control advocates, fought to remove legal restrictions on birth control information and supplies, thereby giving women some control of their reproductive health. The last change, rather than seeking to limit pregnancies, promoted healthy childbearing by improving access to and quality of prenatal care and child health services. This was highlighted by the establishment of the Children's Health Bureau in 1912 and the passage of the first governmental support of maternal and infant health in the Shepard Towner Act in 1921 (Department of Health and Human Services, 2002; Weisman, 1998b).

The feminist movement of the 1960s and 1970s challenged a multitude of societal standards, including female fashion stereotypes and male physician authority in the delivery of women's health care. Legal action against gender discrimination opened the doors for increased female admissions to medical schools. Feminist health advocates questioned long held beliefs about childbirth procedures and overuse of surgical measures such as mastectomy, hysterectomy, and cesarean section. Women's reproductive rights were extended in the areas of legalized abortion, product safety protection, and the expansion of self-help materials (Department of Health and Human Services, 2002; Weisman, 1998b).

Political Reform and Women's Health

The last decade of the 20th century saw unprecedented resources directed toward national women's health policy. With increasing numbers of women filling key leadership positions in government, academia, research, and health services administration, and with the support of a highly organized feminist health advocacy community, significant changes in gender health equity began to emerge. The passage of The Women's Health Equity Act in 1989 called for increased focus on women's health services, research, and prevention activities. Women's health offices were established throughout the government, and a Coordinating Committee on Women's Health was directed to synchronize activities for the best possible outcomes (Department of Health and Human Services, 2002; Weisman, 1998b).

A FEDERAL AGENDA FOR WOMEN'S HEALTH

Congress and Women's Health

During the 1990s, Congress gave unparalleled attention given to the subject of women's health. In 1989, the Women's Health Equity Act set the stage for an augmented focus on women's health services, prevention, and research. In the 17 years since then numerous bills addressing women's health issues have been introduced into the House and Senate during each congressional session. Several important pieces of legislation have been enacted during this time. In 1990, the Breast and Cervical Cancer Mortality Prevention Act authorized mammograms and pap smears for underserved women. In 1992, the Mammography Quality Standards Act established national standards and quality control systems for mammography clinics, and the Infertility Prevention Act authorized funding for screening, treatment, and follow-up of STDs that can lead to infertility. In 1994, the Violence Against Women Act defined violence against women as a federal crime and increased penalties for the offender. In 2000, the Breast and Cervical Cancer Prevention and Treatment Act increased services to women eligible for Medicaid (Department of Health and Human Services, 2000).

Some of this increased interest in women's health can be attributed to feminist social reform efforts, and some to health professional activism. But one internal change in Congress played a large role in bringing women's health issues to the forefront of Congressional attention.

The Congressional Caucus on Women's Issues

On April 19, 1977, when the number of women in the House of Representatives totaled 18, 15 of that number met in the Congresswomen's Reading Room to discuss spousal abuse. In the months that followed, the women formed a bi-partisan group to promote women's legislative issues. Led by Representative Elizabeth Holtzman (D-NY) and Representative Margaret Heckler (R-MA) the group became known as the Congresswomen's Caucus, and was influential in extending the ratification deadline of the Equal Rights Amendment (Hall, 2003).

The caucus continued to meet over the next several years, discussing such issues as retirement income reform, the importance of child care, moving women off welfare, and discrimination against women in the military. In 1981, the group decided to invite their male colleagues to join them, and changed the name of the caucus to the Congressional Caucus for Women's Issues (CCWI). In 1993, when the number of women on Capitol Hill nearly doubled, the CCWI membership included 43 of the 48 women House members and 117 male House members. In 1995, however, the House voted to abolish all 28 legislative service or caucus organizations, and to eliminate their budget and staff. Thirty-eight congresswomen reorganized themselves into an informal members organization with the same name. As a result, there are no longer male members of the caucus (Hall, 2003).

In 1989, the Congressional Caucus for Women's Issues introduced The Women's Health Equity Act and in 1990 initiated an investigation by the National Institutes of Health (NIH) into the exclusion of women from clinical trials. Since that time, the caucus has been responsible for the appropriation of several billion dollars for research and prevention activities in women's health. Today the CCWI continues to be a driving force in the passage of a number of significant women's health legislations. The caucus helps inform their male colleagues in Congress of important women's health and policy issues through its series of legislative briefings and hearings that have included topics such as women and heart disease, breastfeeding in the workplace, Tamoxifen use, and contraceptive technology (Hall, 2003; Lockwood-Shabat, 2003).

Staying abreast of the numerous pieces of health legislation affecting women that are introduced during each congressional session is a formidable task. Two nonprofit organizations offer resources that can help midwives to track and evaluate the issues and current legislations.

The Kaiser Family Foundation

The Kaiser Family Foundation (KFF) is a nonpartisan, nonprofit foundation that collects and analyzes health information for policymakers, the health care community, and consumers. The foundation conducts policy research, produces health communications programs, and offers an extensive list of publications. In addition, Kaisernetwork.org serves as an online resource for in-depth, timely health policy news and debates. The multimedia service offers a number of features, including three daily online reports, calendars of health policy events, public opinion polls on health issues, links to hundreds of reports and publications, and HealthCast recordings of both live and archived key meetings and congressional hearings (Kaiser Family Foundation, 2006).

One focus of the Kaiser Family Foundation is its Women's Health Policy Program. This division of the foundation offers information and analysis about health financing and delivery policies that affect women at both the federal and state levels. In addition, the Women's Health Policy Program identifies emerging women's health priority areas, organizes legislative briefings for policymakers and staff on current women's policy debates, and offers consumers side-by-side comparisons of candidates' platform areas that affect women's health policy. An excellent resource for midwives is *Women's Access to Care: A State-Level Analysis of Key Health Policies,* a 2003 comprehensive report that can be accessed from the KFF Web site (Kaiser Family Foundation, 2004).

Women's Policy, Inc.

Women's Policy, Inc. (WPI) is a nonpartisan and nonprofit organization that was founded in 1995 to track congressional action on women's issues and to promote informed political decision making at the federal, state, and local levels. WPI monitors women's policy issues and conducts legislative research, disseminating its findings through issue summaries, a weekly publication, and legislative briefings. WPI works in conjunction with the Women's Caucus to sponsor a congressional briefing series that has included such topics as Women and HIV/AIDS, Women and Medicare, Social Security, Violence against Women in Conflict Settings, and Diversity in the Workplace (Women's Policy, Inc., 2004).

WPI's weekly publication, *The Source on Women's Issues in Congress*, provides a detailed description of political action on a wide range of women's issues including health, education, child care, business, and international concerns. It is available as an online subscription, or can be accessed through the WPI Web site. In addition to *The Source,* WPI has another publication that is of particular interest to midwives. *Women's Health Legislation in the 107th Congress* is the second in an ongoing series of publications that detail women's health legislation that was introduced in a 2-year congressional session. The publication addresses women's health in three critical areas for legislation: research, preventative health services, and access to health care coverage (Lockwood-Shabat, 2003; Women's Policy, Inc., 2004).

Federal Programming and Women's Health

In order to understand the impact of the federal government on women's health in this country, it is helpful to briefly examine the roots of federal intervention in health care. Since the appointment of a chemist to serve in the Department of Agriculture by President Lincoln in 1862, there has been a constant presence in the government to address the health of the public. The cabinet-level Department of Health, Education and Welfare (HEW) was authorized in 1953 under President Eisenhower. In 1980, when the Department of Education was created, HEW became the Department of Health and Human Services (DHHS). Today, DHHS encompasses 10 agencies and includes more than 300 programs. It is responsible for more federal expenditures than all other federal agencies combined, and accounts for almost one quarter of the total federal budget (Department of Health and Human Services [DHHS], 2004b).

Since the passage of The Women's Health Equity Act in 1989, a number of changes across the agencies of the Department of Health and Human Services have altered the federal priorities and programming in regards to women's health. There is currently an office on women's health or a designated liaison on women's health issues in each of the department's 10 agencies. Each of these participates in a monthly meeting of a Coordinating Committee on Women's Health in order to synchronize efforts and priorities. Midwives may want to familiarize themselves with several of the larger agency efforts in women's health.

NIH Office of Research on Women's Health (ORWH)

Three months after the release of the Government Accounting Office (GAO) findings that there was slow and ineffective implementation of the policy requiring inclusion of women in clinical trials, the NIH established the Office of Research on Women's Health. The office had a threefold mandate: 1) to establish a research agenda for NIH by determining gaps in the current scientific knowledge about gender disparities in disease and specific disorders and health conditions that affect women, 2) to ensure the appropriate inclusion of women in clinical trials, and 3) to increase the numbers of women in all levels of biomedical careers including executive leadership. Since the establishment of the office in 1991, Dr. Vivian Pinn has been the full-time director of the ORWH (Pinn & Chunko, 1999).

In 1999, the ORWH published a report entitled *Agenda for Research on Women's Health for the 21st Century*. This report serves as the guideline for establishing yearly research priorities in women's health, and can be accessed through the ORWH Web site. The ORWH partners with other NIH institutes and centers to develop research initiatives that further these priorities. In addition, the office coordinates data collection and reporting methodologies to track inclusion of women in clinical trials. By 2003, approximately 60.7% of all subjects enrolled in extramural clinical research were women (Office of Research on Women's Health, 2004; Pinn & Chunko, 1999).

The ORWH sponsors a number of programs designed to increase opportunities for women in biomedical careers. The office also developed and implements an interdisciplinary research advancement program called Building Interdisciplinary Research Careers in Women's Health (BIRCWH) that pairs junior researchers with senior investigators. To date there are 24 BIRCWH centers that have included at least two nurse–midwifery researchers. Additionally, the ORWH offers free to the public a women's health seminar series that features nationally prominent speakers on timely topics in women's health (Office of Research on Women's Health, 2004; Pinn & Chunko, 1999).

Public Health Service Office on Women's Health (OWH)

The Office on Women's Health was established in 1991 to coordinate a comprehensive women's health agenda across the agencies of the department of Health and Human Services. It does not fall within one of the agencies of the department; rather it is one of 10 offices that report to the Assistant Secretary of Health within the Office of Public Health and Science. In this location it serves as the champion for women's health issues within the government and strives to abolish disparities in education, research, and health care services. The OWH is directed by the Deputy Assistant Secretary for Health (Women's Health), Dr. Wanda Jones, who has served in that capacity since 1998 (ACNM, 2004b; Pinn & Chunko, 1999).

The OWH is the second oldest DHHS office dedicated to women's health issues. During its first decade the office focused its efforts on establishing women's health as a focal point for government attention and action. The OWH expanded its outreach in women's health by establishing regional women's health coordinators (RWHCs) in each of the 10 public health service regions. The RWHCs identify regional needs, direct initiatives and programs, and coordinate women's health activities at the regional, state, and local levels. The OWH promotes innovations in women's health care through its partnership with academic health centers in the National Centers of Excellence in Women's Health (COEs) program. These are interdisciplinary and fully integrated comprehensive care centers for women that promote research, public health education, and community outreach. Since 2000, the OWH has also established National Community Centers of Excellence (CCOEs) that promote the same model of care at local clinics and community hospitals. One of the CCOEs has a midwifery base, with the Yale Women's Health and Midwifery Practice serving as the Clinical Care Center for the Griffin Hospital CCOE (ACNM, 2004b; Jones, 1999; Office on Women's Health, 2004).

A primary function of the OWH is health promotion and outreach. In the fall of 1998, the office launched the National Women's Health Information Center (NWHIC), a comprehensive online women's health education site and toll-free call center that receives more than 5 million consumer visits and calls per year. NWHIC serves as a national clearinghouse of federal and private sector health education resources including over 4000 publications, 2000 organizations, and 800 health topics. The office sponsors National Women's Health Week every May to focus attention on the positive impact of establishing preventive and positive health behaviors in everyday life. Since 2001, the Pick Your Path to Health campaign has promoted healthy behaviors among women of color. Additionally, the OWH sponsors numerous issue-specific health campaigns to reduce disparities in women's health. These include the Cardiovascular Education Campaign Initiative, the National Bone Health Campaign, Girl Power! (a national public health education campaign for girls ages 9–14), and the National Breastfeeding Campaign (ACNM, 2004b; Jones, 1999).

CDC Office of Women's Health (CDC OWH)

The Centers for Disease Control and Prevention established its Office of Women's Health in 1994. Located in the Office of the Director of the CDC, the mission of the CDC OWH is to ensure coordination of women's health efforts across the CDC and to expand its women's health activities. The associate director for women's health is in charge of leading and coordinating the CDC OWH efforts, and currently that position is filled by a certified nurse–midwife, Yvonne Green (Pinn & Chunko, 1999).

The CDC OWH has been responsible for a number of national projects and campaigns to improve women's health. In 1999, the office established The National Sexual Violence Resource Center, a clearinghouse for statistics, education, and resources related to sexual violence. The CDC OWH launched and directed A National Agenda for Action: The National Public Health Initiative on Diabetes and Women's Health in 2000 in order to unite partners for diabetes prevention and control, and to develop strategies, policies, and research to reduce the disease burden of a rapidly growing women's public health problem. The Healthy Women: State Trends in Health and Mortality project collates and publishes yearly state health data of women by race/ethnicity and age (Centers for Disease Control and Prevention [CDC], 2004).

THE ROLE OF MIDWIFERY IN THE FEDERAL AGENDA

In this country, women receive health care from a number of different provider types in both the private and public domain. Access, payment, and regulation for this health care are directly influenced by the legislative and executive branches of our government. As midwives we are challenged by our philosophy and code of ethics to play a leadership role in improving women's health. A primary venue for exercising both individual and collective leadership to impact women's health is through our political system at both the state and national levels.

When we think about impacting health care in this country, what comes to mind for most people is the policy legislation process. Our political system is one that allows personal advocacy in the form of direct communication with legislators. In this way, regardless of one's political interest or leanings, every midwife can exercise individual leadership in women's health. Midwives should make an effort to stay informed on policy questions that impact women's health. Regular communication through phone calls, emails, and letters to an elected official is one way to have a midwifery voice heard on these issues. Working to elect or re-elect politicians who champion women's health causes is another way to have an impact.

A very significant, but much less recognized avenue for impacting women's health is through the executive branch of our government. The agencies of the Department of Health and Human Services play an enormous role in regulating the health care of the public. In the early years of midwifery practice and education there was a strong bond between nurse–midwifery and the public health community. When practice opportunities were limited, midwives frequently took positions of leadership within public health. Over the years, however, as midwifery practice opportunities expanded and clinical competencies became more complex, midwifery became more defined by a set of skills and functions than by its knowledge and philosophy. Midwives who moved away from clinical practice into government leadership positions seemed to lose their identity and connection to midwifery.

Today this culture is beginning to change. The ACNM recognizes the importance of strengthening its ties with the federal public health community. Nurse–midwives in government leadership positions are reconnecting with the college and helping to mentor younger midwives into public health positions. ACNM is working to establish connections with the Office on Women's Health within DHHS so that a midwifery voice can be heard on issues of women's health research and programming.

CONSUMER ADVOCACY IN WOMEN'S HEALTH

The First Amendment of the U.S. Constitution grants and protects the rights of individuals to peaceably assemble and petition the government to address their grievances and concerns. As our democracy has matured, this right has evolved into the existence of formalized interest groups, which, loosely defined, are collections of individuals organized around some common interest or purpose who seek to influence policy. In the political system today, organized interest groups are the most effective demanders of public policy (Lindblom & Woodhouse, 1993; Longest 2002).

In health advocacy, two types of organizations have developed at the national level. The first type focuses on health issues that affect an entire population group, such as women, Hispanics, or lesbians. The second type of advocacy group directs its efforts to a single health issue. Both play an important role in promoting health policy for women.

WOMEN'S HEALTH ADVOCACY ORGANIZATIONS

A Web search will reveal a vast array of health advocacy groups that appear to speak for women. The midwife wishing to make a scholarly assessment of these organizations should first attempt to determine their mission, philosophy, and basis of support; the extent of their advocacy agenda; and the length of time they have been in existence. There are a few advocacy organizations that have set themselves apart because of their longevity and the reliability of the information they produce. Four organizations are delineated here.

Our Bodies, Ourselves (OBOS)

In 1969, a group of laywomen came together in the Boston area to discuss their lives, their bodies, their experiences with doctors, and women's health. The result of their discussions was the underground publication of a radical women's health booklet called *Women and Their Bodies*. In 1972, the group adopted the name the Boston Women's Health Book Collective (BWHBC) and commercially marketed that booklet as the landmark publication *Our Bodies, Ourselves* (Norsigian et al., 1999).

What began as a collective involving 12 women with a common philosophy and passion has evolved into a nonprofit public interest organization with a unionized staff and designated leadership positions. In 1980, the group brought together its publications and correspondences into one office and formed a Women's Health Information Center (WHIC). The influence of the organization expanded to include advocacy projects and political activism in local, national, and international arenas (Norsigian et al., 1999).

Today, the BWHBC is also known as Our Bodies, Ourselves (OBOS). For over 30 years, it has inspired the women's health movement through its efforts in health education, consulting, and advocacy. The original publication is now in its eighth edition with more than 4 million copies having been sold to date. The organization also boasts a Spanish adaptation of the book called Nuestros Cuerpos, Nuestras Vidas, and has collaborated on the production of nearly 20 foreign language editions of Our Bodies, Ourselves. The most recent project is a book on menopause that is expected to be published in late 2006. In addition, OBOS offers consulting services and speakers on a number of women's health issues and sponsors a project called The Latina Health Initiative that supports health prevention awareness and network building in Spanish-speaking communities (Norsigian et al., 1999; Our Bodies, Ourselves, 2004).

The National Women's Health Network (NWHN)

In 1975 a group of five feminists—an author, a PhD therapist, a political activist, a pediatrician, and a community organizer—envisioned a communication and political activism network to champion the cause of the women's health movement. The National Women's Health Network was born out of a desire to unite the rapidly growing number of women's health groups that were developing across the country and to give the women's health movement a political voice in Washington. Incorporated as a nonprofit educational organization, in its early years it represented over 100 health groups in the United States, and championed such issues as safe contraception, DES hazards, sterilization abuses, and legal abortion services (Norinsky et al., 1979).

Thirty years later, and with a membership of over 8000 individuals and organizations, the NWHN continues to advance the cause of optimal women's health through consumer education and political activism. It monitors the actions of federal agencies, health professions, and industry groups, and produces a bimonthly publication called *The Women's Health Activist,* designed to present the feminist viewpoint on current women's health issues. In addition, the NWHN publishes position papers, health information packets, and fact sheets that are available to consumers through its Web site (National Women's Health Network, 2004).

The Black Women's Health Imperative

Several national women's health advocacy organizations focus their efforts on specific racial or cultural groups to reduce disparities in health care for these women. The oldest and most active is the Black Women's Health Imperative, formerly known as the National Black Women's Health Project (NBWHP), which was founded in 1981 to improve the health status of African American women across the lifespan. The primary focus of the group is to encourage self-advocacy through the dissemination of health education and the promotion of self-care prevention programs.

In addition to conducting national and international conferences, the NBWHP has produced several self-help instructional videos and published the book *Our Bodies, Our*

Voices, Our Choices: A Black Women's Primer on Reproductive Health and Rights. Since 1990, the group has been involved in policy advocacy, collaborating with groups such as the Congressional Black Caucus Health Braintrust and the U.S. Senate Black Legislative Staff Caucus (Kaiser Family Foundation, 2004). Their most recent project is an interactive online health resource, established in 2002 (Black Women's Health Imperative, 2004).

Society for the Advancement of Women's Health Research (SWHR)

The Society for the Advancement of Women's Health Research was founded in 1990 to focus national attention on the historical exclusion of women from clinical trials and the problem of gender disparities in disease prevalence and expression. It is a nonprofit and nonpartisan organization that promotes a women's health research agenda in its attempts to shape public policy and impact professional education. The society sponsors a Women's Health Research Coalition that brings together leaders from medical academia, health organizations, and scientific institutions. Its official publication is the *Journal of Women's Health* (Greenberger, 1999).

The society hosts meetings for various audiences that encourage discussions of sex differences in topics such as clinical trials, nutrition, and stroke. It also sponsors an annual conference entitled Sex and Gene Expression. The SWHR reaches consumers through a Web page that informs women about federal legislation impacting women's health. Among its priority issues is the authorization of permanent women's health offices at the CDC, FDA, and DHHS (Society for Women's Health Research, 2004).

Single Issue Advocacy Groups

In addition to the national groups that focus on general woman's health, there are numerous issue-specific groups that concentrate their education and advocacy in one specialized area. Some of these are disease- but not gender-specific, but may have projects or special efforts that address women. Since 1940, the American Diabetes Association (ADA) has worked for prevention and cure of diabetes while concurrently improving the lives of those affected by the disease through education, research, and advocacy. The ADA is one of the cosponsors of the National Public Health Initiative on Diabetes and Women's Health, a comprehensive national effort to reduce the incidence of diabetes and decrease complications from the disease among women (American Diabetes Association, n.d.).

The American Heart Association was founded in 1924 to promote research in cardiovascular disease. Today its primary activities have expanded to include education and advocacy as it strives to reduce disability and death from cardiovascular diseases and stroke. The American Heart Association sponsors the Go Red for Women Campaign to encourage women to take charge of their heart health through education, awareness, and lifestyle change (American Heart Association, 2006).

Other advocacy groups are both issue- and gender-specific. The National Breast Cancer Coalition (NBCC) is the nation's largest breast cancer advocacy organization. Founded in 1991, the organization has been instrumental in increasing federal funding for breast cancer research six-fold and in developing the National Action Plan on Breast Cancer (National Breast Cancer Coalition, 2006). The Ovarian Cancer National Alliance was formed in 1997 when seven ovarian cancer groups joined forces to increase their influence and scope. The goal of this relatively young organization is to coordinate an advocacy effort towards policy makers and women's health care leaders that would move ovarian cancer education, treatment, and research more prominently onto the national agenda (Ovarian Cancer National Alliance, 2006). Other issue-specific advocacy groups in women's health address a range of topics from HIV/AIDS and endometriosis to hysterectomy and exercise.

MIDWIFERY AND ALLIANCES IN WOMEN'S HEALTH AND POLICY

When members of special interest groups share concordant interests in a particular policy issue, they form networks or coalitions to increase their political influence in that domain (Lindblom & Woodhouse, 1993; Longest, 2002). In its 50-year history, the ACNM has joined forces with a number of midwifery, nursing, and medical professional associations to support legislation that is beneficial to women's health. The college has been less proactive in forming coalitions with women's health advocacy organizations. In order to understand the rationale for determining interorganizational affiliations, it is important for the nurse–midwife to understand the process that an organization follows in becoming involved in networking and policy activities.

Interorganizational networking has significant outlays associated with it in terms of monetary costs and staff resources. When the ACNM considers involvement with another organization there are a number of considerations that must first be addressed. Are the goals of the organization consistent with those of the ACNM? What is the expected duration of the affiliation? What resource commitment will the liaison require in terms of meeting attendance and availability of staff or volunteers? What are the desired outcomes of the relationship (ACNM, 1989a)?

Throughout its history, the ACNM has had both formal and informal alliance relationships with organizations that address women's health. Informal alliances usually occur when a member or group of members belong simultaneously to another organization that promotes women's health. These members provide visibility for the ACNM by their participation and leadership in the meetings and activities of the other organization. They are not given financial compensation for their activities, nor do they speak officially for the ACNM at those meetings. Official liaisons, on the other hand, are appointed by the Board of Directors (BOD) of ACNM and are selected on the basis of qualifications, experience, and proximity to the proposed activity. They are delegated to speak in an official capacity for the college. There may be some financial reimbursement for the cost of participation in the meetings, and they are expected to provide an official report to the BOD on their activities (ACNM, 1990).

Determination of networking relationships is an ongoing challenge for the ACNM. As the number of professional and lay organizations that address women's health issues in policy arenas increases, it becomes crucial for the college to continually assess the benefits and costs of affiliating with individual organizations.

The Role of Midwifery in Women's Health

WOMEN'S HEALTH ISSUES

The ACNM, as a membership organization, is a special interest group that exists to advance the needs of its members. When considering potential political activity and affiliations, Feldstein (2001) argues that a special interest group must weigh the costs of political organization and activity against the expected value of the legislative outcome. This is evidenced in the evolution of the ACNM's political activity. Throughout its 50-year history, the college has been very involved in initiating and supporting legislation that would protect and expand the practice of nurse–midwifery. Issues involving women's health have been addressed as they intersect with midwifery scope of practice. However, as issues of licensing, regulation, and prescriptive authority have been successfully addressed in most states, the ACNM has been able to expand its attention to larger issues of women's health at the federal level.

The American College of Nurse–Midwives has a long history of joining forces with other provider organizations to support increased access to care for the uninsured and a patient's bill of rights. But when considering support of single-issue efforts in women's health, the processes and considerations are much the same as those discussed for potential interorganizational networking. First the proposed policy must be deemed congruent with the ACNM's mission and philosophy, code of ethics, strategic priorities, and any relevant position statements. Then it must be prioritized in terms of financial costs to the organization, staff commitments, and availability of volunteer representatives (ACNM, 2002b). Smaller organizations must choose their issues and causes wisely so as not to overcommit either their budget or womanpower.

There are several areas of women's health that have commanded particular attention by the ACNM over the years. To some degree, they coincide with the professional development of the practice of midwifery. A brief look at these women's health issues and the responses and activities they have generated within the college is important to the midwife's understanding of professionalism and leadership in women's health.

Contraception

The provision of family planning services has been a basic component of nurse–midwifery practice since the early 1970s, when the first midwifery modular curriculum developed at the Mississippi program included a module on family planning (Burst, 1998). ACNM core competencies require all midwives to have essential knowledge and management skills in "barrier, hormonal, mechanical, chemical, physiologic, and surgical conception control methods" (ACNM, 2002a).

Throughout its 30-year history of providing family planning services, the ACNM has consistently held the belief that all women should have equal access to contraceptive information and services. The college asserts the following three positions: "that every woman has the right to make reproductive choices; that every woman has the right to access to factual, unbiased information about reproductive choices, in order to make an informed decision; and that women with limited means should have access to financial resources for their reproductive choices" (ACNM, 1997a). In 1997, the Political and Economic Affairs Committee (PEAC) began the process of proactively defining policy positions for the college. One of the health policy position papers developed during that time was on family planning services, and made the following recommendations: that the ACNM support full funding for Title X and expansion of family planning services for Medicaid recipients; that the college support state and federal legislation mandating inclusion of contraceptive services, devices, and prescriptions to privately insured women; and that the ACNM oppose any limitations to the ability of clinicians to address the full scope of family planning services.

The ACNM continues to monitor the political climate regarding family planning services. After the FDA approved emergency contraceptive pills (ECPs) as safe and effective in preventing pregnancy, the ACNM took the position that barriers to the immediate availability of ECPs should be removed. The college supports "increased education for consumers and professionals, advance prescription of emergency contraceptive pills, direct pharmacy access, FDA approval of over-the-counter distribution, and insurance coverage for all prescriptive methods of contraception" (ACNM, 2001b).

Abortion

Abortion policy has been one of the most divisive issues that the ACNM has had to deal with in its 50-year history. When abortion became legalized in 1971, the college was asked to address the role of nurse–midwives in the provision and support of abortion services. At that time the Board of Directors approved a statement prohibiting nurse–midwives from performing abortions by supporting an ACOG statement describing abortion as an operative procedure only to be performed by a physician with hospital privileges (ACNM, 1971). In a response to a 1989 Supreme Court decision that upheld the constitutionality of Missouri's more restrictive abortion statutes, ACNM took the following position: "Recognizing the cultural and religious diversity of certified nurse–midwives, the American College of Nurse–Midwives does not have a position on Webster vs. Reproductive Health Services" (ACNM, 1989b).

In 1990, the ACNM reaffirmed its abortion position statement, changing only the wording that referred to physician control of the procedure. However, a floor resolution at the 1991 Annual Meeting recommended rescinding the statement that prohibited midwives from performing abortions. This was followed by a mail ballot that confirmed the desire of a majority of members to change the prohibitive statement. Although the statement was rescinded in 1992, allowing midwives to incorporate abortion into their practices by utilizing the proceedures outlined in the document "Guidelines for the Incorporation of New Procedures into Nurse–Midwifery Practice" (currently found in the Core Competencies), the college has never issued another position statement or policy brief that directly addresses abortion (ACNM, 2003b; Summers, 1992). The ACNM maintains a relatively neutral position on the issue of abortion, referring instead to the blanket terminology of "reproductive choice" and to the policy positions outlined in the similarly named position statement (ACNM, 1997a).

Primary Care

The ACNM's involvement in primary health care policy has taken a somewhat different approach. Since 1991, the college has nominated a midwife to the U.S. Public Health Service Primary Care Policy Fellowship each year, and every year except one that nominee has been chosen to be a part of the fellowship class. During a 6-month program this growing number of midwife fellows have had a chance to interact with an interdisciplinary group of scholars and leaders, study the policy-making process, and present a primary care policy issue to the Secretary of Heath and Human Services.

The Primary Care Policy Fellowship (PCPF) was created in 1991 to develop a politically competent and unified cadre of professionals who would be impassioned to speak for primary health care services, training, and research. Approximately 30 fellows are selected each year from over 70 professional organizations and associations. The fellows learn the fundamentals of the policy-making and health care financing processes, are introduced to the programs and initiatives of the DHHS agencies, and work within multidisciplinary groups to develop interdisciplinary approaches to primary health care problems (DHHS, 2004a; Hassmiller, 1995).

The Society of Primary Care Policy Fellows (SPCPF) was created to carry the mission of the PCPF beyond the 6-month duration of the fellowship. Its mission is to affect primary care policy, education, research, and service at the local, state, national, and international levels (Hassmiller, 1995). The 2003/2004 president of the SPCPF was a nurse–midwife, Heather Reynolds, and midwives continue to remain an active part of this alumni organization.

Special Projects and Global Outreach

As a professional organization, most of the work of the American College of Nurse–Midwives has been directed towards meeting the educational, licensing, accreditation, and practice needs of its membership. But in keeping with its mission to improve the health status of women within families and communities, the ACNM undertook a project to develop training programs for traditional birth attendants in 1982. This led to the establishment of a Special Projects Section whose mission was to improve the lives of women and children internationally by enhancing health outcomes in maternal and child health, family planning, and reproductive health. Since its creation, this department of the ACNM has provided technical assistance in over 20 developing countries, with projects that have included a Life Saving Skills Training Program, professional education of government and private sector midwives, strengthening of midwifery associations, and research on maternal mortality (ACNM, 2003a; Gordis, 2004).

Over the years, most of the work of the Special Projects Section was international in its focus. Partnership opportunities with the Department of Health and Human Services led ACNM to refocus its efforts domestically as well as internationally. In 1999 the name of the Special Projects Section was changed to the Department of Global Outreach to better reflect the mission and work of the department in both the domestic and international arenas ("Department gains new director and new name," 1999; Paluzzi & Houde-Quimby, 1996).

Violence Against Women

Two U.S.-based women's health projects of the Department of Global Outreach have been very noteworthy. The first was the domestic violence (DV) educational initiative. In October 1994, the ACNM received a grant from DHHS to promote DV awareness among student and practicing midwives by increasing the knowledge and skills necessary for universal screening. There were three educational components to the initiative: educator training programs, comprehensive CE workshops held both regionally and at the annual meeting, and a home study program published in the journal in 1996 (Paluzzi & Houde-Quimby, 1996).

During the 3-year initiative, Pat Paluzzi, CNM, served as the project director of the Domestic Violence Education Project. A library of written and audio-visual materials was created within the Special Projects Section, and the project director was available for phone and on-site consultation services. Other materials developed during this initiative included a domestic violence manual, packets of provider and patient information, and an information poster for use in clinical settings (Paluzzi, 1995). In 1997, the ACNM partnered with outside funding agencies to produce a two-volume training video and manual entitled *No Woman Deserves to Hurt* that was directed towards educating women's health care providers in the dynamics of DV (Saldinger, 1997).

As a part of the initiative, an ad hoc Committee on Violence Against Women was formed within the ACNM. This committee developed a membership position statement on violence against women that advocates a policy of zero tolerance for domestic violence and that promotes universal screening for violence. The committee made recommendations for the inclusion of DV content in the ACNM core competencies that were incorporated into the 1997 update (ACNM, 1997b; Paluzzi & Houde-Quimby, 1996). The ad hoc committee continues its work today within the Division of Women's Health Policy and Leadership, looking at expanded issues of family violence and practices of female genital cutting. Violence remains an important issue in the college, as evidenced by the fact that "Domestic Violence Awareness" was chosen as the theme for Nurse–Midwifery Week 2003.

Adolescent Health

A second major domestic initiative of the Department of Global Outreach was the THRIVE Project. In 2000, the ACNM received a second grant for a Providers Partnership Cooperative Agreement (PPCA) from the Maternal and Child Health Bureau of the Department of Health and Human Services. Providers Partnership I (1997–2000) had focused on establishing liaisons between private providers and public officials. Providers Partnership II was designed to build upon these cooperative agreements by developing innovative approaches to improving health in specific "at risk" populations. ACNM's grant described the development of an intergenerational health education program for young adolescent girls and their mothers and grandmothers: Teen Health Requires Interactions, Values and Education (THRIVE) (Swift-Scanlan, 2001b).

Kate Swift-Scanlan, CNM, served as the project manager of the THRIVE initiative, which had both an educational component and a networking/policy focus. As a part of the educational component, the ACNM developed and piloted educational packets for teens and their parent figures. A CD-ROM was produced that included listings of free and low cost adolescent health resources and references. An ongoing Web page serves as a link to other adolescent health sites. Three adolescent health sessions were held at annual meetings, and a home study program was published in the *Journal of Midwifery & Women's Health* in 2003 (Swift-Scanlan, 2001a, 2004).

The networking and policy focus of this initiative included the awarding of mini-grants to CNM–adolescent health coordinator partnerships in six states. These grants assisted in the planning and implementation of statewide meetings that focused on creative approaches to adolescent health. After the 3-year period of the PPCA II award, the ACNM continued its cooperative involvement as one of 16 partners in the Partners in Program Planning for Adolescent Health (PIPPAH) II initiative. PIPPAH II emphasizes making changes in the local, state, and national arena that support positive youth development as a basis for health intervention (Swift-Scanlan, 2003, 2004). The ACNM updated and revised a position statement on adolescent health care in 2001 that reflected its commitment to the provision of confidential services to adolescents, but with the promotion of intergenerational models of care, and to the support of legislation that increases health education programs in schools and communities and provides funding for improved access to care (ACNM, 2001a).

DIVISION OF WOMEN'S HEALTH POLICY AND LEADERSHIP

In 1999, the ACNM formed a task force to look at the potential for a new division within the college that would serve as a home for women's health and policy issues. The college was looking to increase individual and institutional capabilities and opportunities for leadership in these areas. The result was the development of a Division of Women's Health Policy and Leadership, commonly known as the DOW, whose mission is to "improve women's health at the community, national, and international levels through coordination of the development of public health and women's health policy initiatives" (ACNM, 2004a). The new division met for the first time at the 2000 annual meeting in Anchorage, Alaska.

There are five sections in the DOW. The Policy Development and Evaluation (PDE) section addresses women's health and policy issues and helps to develop a women's health policy agenda for the college. It serves as a home for the ACNM Primary Care Policy Fellows. The Women's Health Issues and Projects (WHIP) section identifies emergent issues in women's health and looks for partnership opportunities with local, state, national, and international groups to improve women's health. It serves as a base of coordination for public health issue project groups in women's health such as Violence against Women, Environmental Health, Breastfeeding, and Adolescent Health. The Leadership Development section (LDS) evaluates needs and develops activities to enhance leadership capabilities within the membership. It also works to facilitate interaction among CNM/CM leaders in maternal/child health and women's health, both nationally and globally. The Public Information section assesses needs and develops guidelines for consumer health education materials. The members of this section have interest and skills in writing public information materials and work with the Public Relations Committee and the National Office to create public information campaigns. The Networking section looks for opportunities to strengthen existing relationships and create new relationships between the ACNM and other women's and women's health organizations. It develops materials to prepare new organizational representatives and facilitates communication among current liaisons (ACNM, 2004a).

Summary

Women's health in twenty-first-century America represents the evolution of a paradigm, which has been significantly impacted by the confluence of three forces: health professional development, social feminism, and political reform. Although gynecology reflects a process of increased specialization, midwifery in America has grown throughout its 50-year history to return to its primary care public health roots. These changes in professionalism have been taking place against a backdrop of women's health activism that has helped reshape health care institutions and medical practice, influence health policy, and ultimately, improve the status of women in our society.

In 1989, the Women's Health Equity Act set the stage for an augmented focus on women's health services, disease prevention, and research. In the 17 years since then numerous bills addressing women's health issues have been introduced into the House and Senate during each congressional session. The Congressional Caucus for Women's Issues has played a pivotal role in bringing these women's health issues to the forefront of congressional attention. Staying abreast of the numerous pieces of health legislation affecting women that are introduced during each congressional session is a formidable task. Both the Kaiser Family Foundation and Women's Policy, Inc. offer resources that can help midwives track and evaluate the issues and current legislations.

Since the passage of the *Women's Health Equity Act* in 1989 a number of changes across the agencies of the Department of Health and Human Services have altered the federal priorities and programming in regards to women's health. There is currently an office on women's health or a designated liaison on women's health issues in each of DHHS's 10 agencies. The Office on Women's Health, established in 1991 within the Office of Public Health and Science to coordinate a comprehensive women's health agenda across the agencies of the Department of Health and Human Services, serves as the champion for women's health issues within the government, and strives to abolish disparities in education, research, and health care services.

In the political system today, organized interest groups are the most effective demanders of public policy. There are vast arrays of health advocacy groups that appear to speak for women, but a few advocacy organizations have set themselves apart because of their longevity and the reliability of the information they produce. For over 30 years the Boston Women's Health Book Collective (BWHBC) and the National Women's Health Network (NWHN) have inspired the women's health movement through their efforts in health education, consulting, and advocacy. Other national groups are the Black Women's Health Imperative and the Society for the Advancement of Women's Health Research (SWHR). In addition, there are numerous issue-specific groups that concentrate their education and advocacy on one specialized area.

As midwives we are challenged by our philosophy and code of ethics to play a leadership role in improving women's health. A primary venue for exercising both individual and collective leadership to impact women's health is through our political system at both the state and national levels. Midwives should make an effort to stay informed on policy questions that impact women's health. The ACNM needs to continue to strengthen its ties with the federal public health community so that a midwifery voice can be heard on issues of women's health research and programming.

When members of special interest groups share concordant interests in a particular policy issue, they form networks or coalitions to increase their political influence in that domain. ACNM has a history of both formal and informal alliance relationships with organizations that address women's health. However, interorganizational networking has significant outlays associated with it in terms of monetary costs and staff resources; determination of networking relationships is an ongoing challenge for ACNM.

Throughout its 50-year history, the ACNM, as a membership organization, has been very involved in initiating and supporting legislation that would protect and expand the practice of its members. As the organization has matured, it has been able to expand its attention to larger issues of women's health at the federal level. The Department of Global Outreach (formerly the Special Projects Section) has directed two U.S.-based women's health projects that have been very noteworthy: the domestic violence (DV) educational initiative and the THRIVE Adolescent Health Education Project. The Division of Women's Health Policy and Leadership was established in 2000 to help increase the college's individual and institutional capabilities and opportunities for leadership in women's health. Its five sections address women's health policy issues, leadership development strategies, priority and emergent issues in women's health, networking relationships, and public information initiatives.

Chapter Exercises

1. **Feminist Activism and Women's Health**

   Midwifery, nursing, and medical students of the twenty-first century may take for granted the significant advances in women's health education, practice, and research that have come about in a relatively short time. This could lead to complacency and the potential endangerment of these newly incorporated institutions, efforts, and rights. For this reason, it is important to reflect upon the past when considering the path for the future.

   • What impact did the women's suffrage movement have on changes in women's health in the 1920s and 1930s?

   • What societal standards and women's rights were altered by the feminist movement of the 1960s and 1970s?

   • Is there a need for feminist activism in health care today; if so, what do you consider the major areas of gender inequity in health care?

2. **Health Policy and Women's Health**

   In some countries, health care is a right for all citizens and the provision of health services is entirely a government responsibility. In the United States, government has played some role in health care since Lincoln's presidency, yet we remain a country that is fiercely dedicated to individual freedom and competitive enterprise. Regardless of where one stands on the issue of public responsibility or privatization of health care, a basic knowledge of the past, current, and potential future role of the government in the health of women should be a fundamental part of any midwifery education.

- What developments within the legislative branch of the government led to the proliferation of women's health legislation in the 1990s?
- How do the agencies within the Department of Health and Human Services support women's health today?
- How does the ACNM Code of Ethics challenge midwives to political advocacy, and what can an individual midwife do to impact women's health policy at the legislative and executive levels of government?

3. **Midwifery Leadership in Women's Health**

   In 2005, the American College of Nurse–Midwives celebrated its 50th anniversary. With their roots in public health, our founding foremothers were the original primary care specialists for women and children. But the 20th century was a time of proliferating medical specialization and increasing institutionalization of health care, and thus most of our 50-year history has been spent carving out the most basic of practice protections. With those protections now in place for most midwives, and our numbers having reached a critical mass, it is time once again for midwifery to be heard as the expert in, and champion of, women's health care.

   - What areas of women's health leadership are most compatible with midwifery training and expertise, and what visible products of leadership should the ACNM be engaged in to support these efforts?
   - What is the value of interorganizational networking, and what women's health professional and advocacy groups should the ACNM be forming liaisons with?
   - What role does the ACNM play in the international women's health arena, and where should this organization be in the next 10 or 25 years?

References

American College of Nurse–Midwives. (1971). *Abortion statement.* Washington, DC: Author.

American College of Nurse–Midwives. (1989a). *Guidelines for coalition participation.* Washington, DC: Author.

American College of Nurse–Midwives. (1989b). *Webster vs. Reproductive Health Services statement.* Washington, DC: Author.

American College of Nurse–Midwives. (1990). *Guidelines for the appointment of ACNM representatives to a special committee, task force or organization.* Washington, DC: Author.

American College of Nurse–Midwives. (1992). *Certified nurse–midwives as primary care providers position statement.* Washington, DC: Author.

American College of Nurse–Midwives. (1997a). *Reproductive choices position statement.* Washington, DC: Author.

American College of Nurse–Midwives. (1997b). *Violence against women position statement.* Washington, DC: Author.

American College of Nurse–Midwives. (2001a). *Adolescent health care position statement.* Washington, DC: Author.

American College of Nurse–Midwives. (2001b). *Emergency contraception: Expanding education and access position statement.* Washington, DC: Author.

American College of Nurse–Midwives. (2002a). *Core competencies for basic midwifery practice.* Washington, DC: Author.

American College of Nurse–Midwives. (2002b). *Guidelines for ACNM action on political issues, issuance of policy statements, and policy sponsorship* [Internal document]. Washington, DC: Author.

American College of Nurse–Midwives. (2003a). *Department of Global Outreach.* Retrieved October 10, 2004, from http://www.midwife.org/dgo

American College of Nurse–Midwives. (2003b). *Midwives and abortion services* [R&B Series]. Washington, DC: Author.

American College of Nurse–Midwives. (2004a). *Division of Women's Health Policy and Leadership SROPs.* Washington, DC: Author.

American College of Nurse–Midwives. (2004b). *Philosophy of the American College of Nurse–Midwives.* Washington, DC: Author.

American College of Obstetricians and Gynecologists. (2006). *ACOG.* Retrieved April 7, 2006, from http://www.acog.org/from_home/acoghistory.cfm

American Diabetes Association. (n.d.). *The American Diabetes Association.* Retrieved April 7, 2006, from http://www.diabetes.org/aboutus.jsp?WTLProo=HEADER_aboutus&vms=152585175006

American Heart Association. (2006). *About us.* Retrieved April 7, 2006, from http://www.americanheart.org/presenter.jhtml?identifier=1200029

Black Women's Health Imperative. (2004). *Home.* Retrieved October 20, 2004, from http://www.blackwomenshealth.org

Breckinridge, M. (1981). *Wide neighborhoods—A story of the Frontier Nursing Service.* Lexington: University Press of Kentucky.

Burst, H. V. (1998). The history of nurse–midwifery in reproductive health care. *Journal of Nurse–Midwifery, 43*(6), 526–529.

Centers for Disease Control and Prevention. (2004). *CDC/ATSDR Office of Women's Health.* Retrieved April 7, 2006, from http://www.cdc.gov/od/spotlight/nwhw/about.htm

Department gains new director and new name. (1999). *Quickening, 30*(6), 14.

Department of Health and Human Services. (2002). *A century of women's health 1900–2000.* Washington, DC: DHHS Office on Women's Health.

Department of Health and Human Services. (2004a). *DHHS Primary Health Care Policy Fellowship Program.* Retrieved November 20, 2004, from http://bhpr.hrsa.gov/interdisciplinary

Department of Health and Human Services. (2004b, April 16). *HHS: What we do.* Retrieved September 10, 2004, from http://www.hhs.gov/about/whatwedo.html

Feldstein, P. J. (2001). *The politics of health legislation* (2nd ed.). Chicago: Health Administration Press.

Gordis, D. (2004). DGO history and capabilities. In D. Jessup (Ed.) (pp. personal communication).

Greenberger, P. (1999). The women's health research coalition: A new advocacy network. *Journal of Women's Health and Gender Based Medicine, 8*(4), 441–442.

Hall, C. A. (2003). The Congressional Caucus for Women's Issues at 25; challenges and opportunities. In C. B. Costello, V. R. Wight, and A. J. Stone (Eds.), *The American Woman 2003–2004 Daughters of a Revolution—Young Women Today* (pp. 339–348). New York: Palgrave MacMillan.

Hassmiller, S. (1995). The Primary Care Policy Fellowship: An innovative model for interdisciplinary collaboration. *Journal of Health Administration Education, 13*(2), 277–286.

Jones, W. K. (1999). US Department of Health and Human Services. *Journal of the American Medical Women's Association, 54*(1), 41–42.

Kaiser Family Foundation. (2004). *Women's Health Policy.* Retrieved October 29, 2004, from http://www.kff.org/womenshealth/index.cfm

Kaiser Family Foundation. (2006). *About the Kaiser Family Foundation.* Retrieved April 7, 2006, from http://www.kff.org/about/index.cfm

Lindblom, C. E., & Woodhouse, C.E. (1993). Interest groups in policy making. In *The Policy-Making Process* (3rd ed., pp. 73–88). Englewood Cliffs, NJ: Prentice Hall.

Lockwood-Shabat, J. (2003). *Women's Health Legislation in the 107th Congress.* Washington, DC: Women's Policy Inc.

Longest, B. B. (2002). *Health policymaking in the United States* (3rd ed.). Chicago: Health Administration Press.

McGregor, D. K. (1998). *From midwives to medicine the birth of American gynecology.* New Brunswick, NJ: Rutgers University Press.

Miller, C. A., & Tsui, A. O. (1997). Family planning. In J. B. Kotch (Ed.), *Maternal and child health: Programs, problems and policy in public health* (pp. 69–84). Gaithersburg, MD: Aspen Publishers.

National Breast Cancer Coalition. (2006). *About NBCC and NBCCF.* Retrieved April 7, 2006, from http://www.natlbcc.org/bin/index.asp?strid=1&depid=1&btnid=0

National Women's Health Network. (2004). Retrieved November 1, 2004, from http://www.nwhn.org

Norinsky, M. (1979). A national voice for women's health concerns. *Health PAC Bulletin, 11*(2), 21–22.

Norsigian, J., Diskin, V., Doress-Worters, P., Pincus, J., Sanford, W., & Swenson, N. (1999). The Boston Women's Health Book Collective and *Our Bodies, Ourselves:* A brief history and reflection. *Journal of the American Medical Women's Association, 54*(1), 35–39.

O'Dowd, M. J., & Phillip, E. E. (1994). *The history of obstetrics and gynaecology.* New York: Parthenon.

Office of Research on Women's Health. (2004). *About the Office of Research on Women's health.* Retrieved November 3, 2004, from http://orwh.od.nig.gov/about.html

Office on Women's Health. (2004). *National Community Centers of Excellence in Women's Health.* Retrieved April 28, 2005, from http://www.4woman.gov/owh/CCOE/current.htm

Our Bodies, Ourselves. (2004). *Home page.* Retrieved November 4, 2004, from http://www.ourbodiesourselves.org

Ovarian Cancer National Alliance. (2006). *About Ovarian Cancer National Alliance.* Retrieved April 7, 2006, from http://www.ovariancancer.org/index.cfm?fuseaction=Page.viewPage&PageID=476&CFID=226419&CFTOKEN=59685053

Paluzzi, P. (1995). Domestic violence resources available. *Quickening, 26*(5), 13.

Paluzzi, P. A., & Houde-Quimby, C. (1996). Domestic violence: Implications for the American College of Nurse–Midwives and its members. *Journal of Nurse–Midwifery, 41*(6), 430–435.

Pinn, V. W., & Chunko, M. T. (1999). The NIH Office of Research on Women's Health and its DHHS partners: Meeting challenges in women's health. *Journal of the American Medical Women's Association, 54*(1), 15–19.

Rooks, J. P. (1997). *Midwifery and childbirth in America.* Philadelphia: Temple University Press.

Saldinger, M. (1997). Domestic violence video released with support from Pharmacia & Upjohn Foundation. *Quickening, 28*(1), 1, 21.

Society for Women's Health Research. (2004). Retrieved October 21, 2004, from http://www.womenshealthresearch.org

Stone, S. (2000). The evolving scope of nurse–midwifery practice in the United States. *Journal of Midwifery & Women's Health, 45*(6), 522–531.

Sullivan, N. H. (2000). CNMs/CMs as primary care providers: Scope of practice issues. *Journal of Midwifery & Women's Health, 45*(6), 450–456.

Summers, L. (1992). The genesis of the ACNM 1971 Statement on Abortion. *Journal of Nurse–Midwifery, 37*(3), 168–174.

Swift-Scanlan, K. (2001a). Educational materials and minigrants. *Quickening, 32*(6), 27.

Swift-Scanlan, K. (2001b). Providers partnership update. *Quickening, 32*(2), 11, 14.

Swift-Scanlan, K. (2003). ACNM partners with the American Nurses Association to improve adolescent health. *Quickening, 34*(6), 24.

Swift-Scanlan, K. (2004). A final report from THRIVE. *Quickening, 35*(1), 15.

Varney, H. (1980). *Nurse-midwifery.* Boston: Blackwell Scientific.

Weisman, C. (1998a, June 11). *Two centuries of women's health activism.* Paper presented at the History and Future of Women's Health Seminar, Washington, DC.

Weisman, C. (1998b, June 11). *Two centuries of women's health activism.* Retrieved May 1, 2004, from http://www.4women.gov.owh/pub/history/2century.htm

Women's Policy, Inc. (2004). About WPI. Retrieved November 1, 2004, from http://www.womenspolicy.org/about/

Table 15–1: For Your Professional Files   325

Table 15–1 For Your Professional Files

These documents from the American College of Nurse–Midwives are used in this chapter or are related to women's health issues addressed in this chapter. All can be found at www.acnm.org.

Descriptive Statements
- *Core Competencies for Basic Midwifery Practice* (2002)
- *Guidelines for the Incorporation of New Procedures into Midwifery Practice* (2003)

Position Statements
- *Adolescent Health Care* (2001)
- *Certified Nurse–Midwives and Certified Midwives as Primary Care Providers/ Case Managers* (1997)
- *Depression in Women* (2003)
- *Emergency Contraception: Expanding Education and Access* (2001)
- *Health Care for All Women and Families* (2004)
- *Human Immunodeficiency Virus (HIV) and Acquired Immunodeficiency Syndrome* (AIDS) (2003)
- *Immunization Status of Women and Their Families* (2004)
- *Reproductive Choices* (1997)
- *Violence Against Women* (1997)

Resources & Bibliography Series
- *CNMs as Primary Care Providers* (2003)
- *Colposcopy* (2003)
- *Immunization Resources* (2003)
- *Midwives and Abortion Services* (2003)
- *Oral Health* (2003)
- *Osteoporosis* (2003)
- *Women and Smoking* (2003)

Table 15–2 Advocacy Web Resources

Midwives may want to familiarize themselves with some of the major women's policy and women's health advocacy organizations. This is a partial listing with Web addresses:

Women's Policy Advocacy
- Women's Policy Inc.: http://www.womenspolicy.org
- Women's Research and Education Institute (WREI): http://www.wrei.org
- National Council of Women's Organizations (NCWO): http://www.womensorganizations.org
- National Women's Law Center: http://www.nwlc.org
- Legal Momentum: http://www.legalmomentum.org
- American Association of University Women: http://www.aauw.org
- YWCA: http://www.ywca.org

Women's Health Advocacy
- National Women's Health Information Center: http://www.4women.gov
- National Women's Health Network: http://www.womenshealthnetwork.org
- Our Bodies, Ourselves: http://www.ourbodiesourselves.org
- National Research Center for Women and Families: http://www.center4research.org
- Society for the Advancement of Women's Health Research: http://www.womenshealthresearch.org
- Black Women's Health Imperative: http://www.blackwomenshealth.org
- Kaiser Family Foundation: http://www.kff.org/womenshealth/index.cfm
- Jacob's Institute of Women's Health: http://www.jiwh.org

Single Issue Women's Health Advocacy
- American Diabetes Association: http://www.diabetes.org/home.jsp
- American Heart Association: http://www.americanheart.org
- National Breast Cancer Coalition: http://www.natlbcc.org
- Ovarian Cancer National Alliance: http://www.ovariancancer.org
- National Association of People with AIDS: http://www.napwa.org
- The Alan Guttmacher Institute (reproductive health issues): http://www.agi-usa.org

CHAPTER 16

Leadership in Midwifery

Barbara Hughes, CNM, MS, MBA, FACNM

Learning Objectives

1. Discuss organizational management issues.
2. Discuss effective group leadership skills and membership roles.
3. Discuss how to develop as a leader and the essential qualities of leadership.
4. Discuss the role of change in leadership.
5. Discuss the role of emotional intelligence in leadership.
6. Discuss competencies for effective leadership.
7. Discuss the influences of positive and negative uses of power.

As is typical in many professions, a highly competent midwife is often promoted into a leadership role because of outstanding technical knowledge or skill. Generally, the new midwifery leader does not have a basic understanding of leadership or organizational theory and accepts a leadership role with good intentions but no clear direction or knowledge about how to be an effective leader.

It is an important fact that leadership abilities are not innate, they are developed. "Leadership develops daily, not in a day" is a quote from John C. Maxwell's handbook entitled *Leadership 101: What Every Leader Needs to Know* (Maxwell, 2002). This simple statement sets the stage for this chapter about midwifery leadership. We will provide foundational information about leadership and will offer strategies to develop and grow as a leader.

Examples of Excellent Midwifery Leaders

The rich history of the ACNM highlights many powerful midwifery leaders. Hattie Hemschemeyer, Sister Angela Murdaugh, Kitty Ernst, Joyce Thompson, Joyce Roberts, and many others in both formal and informal roles have inspired those within and outside of the midwifery profession. When midwives are asked about specific qualities exhibited by leaders or mentors that have significantly impacted them in their careers, some of the common responses are: "She listened to me." "She provided me with support, even if I had made a mistake." "She trusted me." "She believed in me." "She did not judge me." "She cared about me." "She gave me feedback in a kind and constructive manner."

When asked about the behaviors exhibited by an important leader or mentor in their life, rarely do people cite examples of concrete technical tasks. The ability of a midwifery leader to deliver a baby over an intact perineum, to develop a sound clinical schedule for staff, or to produce a comprehensive business plan is not generally cited as the quality that made them a good leader. Indeed, many midwifery leaders are remembered for the significant contributions they have made to the profession in the areas of clinical excellence, educational strategies, business savvy, and policy development. However, it is a different set of leadership skills that significantly impact individuals and organizations that we will be examining in this chapter.

The Difference Between a Manager and a Leader

In today's complex health care environment, there are many terms used to describe an individual in a leadership role. Some examples include "lead midwife," "chief midwife," "head midwife," "midwifery manager," "service director," or "practice director." Leadership involves much more than the day-to-day management of a midwifery practice. Leadership is more than the "hard" skills, or management skills that have been addressed in prior chapters. Here are a few examples of the difference between a manager and a leader:

Managers minimize the fear of change whereas leaders maximize the excitement and challenge of change. Managers accept the status quo whereas leaders challenge it. Managers rely on systems and structure to reach goals whereas leaders focus on energizing people to overcome barriers, take risks, and experiment. Managers use a set of skills to work toward achieving a vision whereas leaders create the vision and a strategy to reach the vision. **Table 16–1** summarizes the differences between leadership and management and is adapted from Steven Covey's book, *The 8th Habit* (Covey, 2004).

As mentioned at the beginning of this chapter, a midwifery leader is often promoted into a leadership role because of technical competence. Indeed, one can also be asked to assume a leadership role because of demonstrated competence in various managerial skills. But, in order to be a good leader, one must move beyond the management role to a role that inspires others to make a commitment and take action towards a common vision.

I recommend that anyone considering or working in a midwifery leadership role spend some time understanding their leadership style and defining their personal leadership philosophy. There are numerous leadership assessment tools available in today's market that are based on sound research that can lead to an increased personal understanding of one's current leadership ability and style. Some of these tools are referenced in **Table 16–2**. Taking this knowledge to the next step involves the life-long process of seeking new knowledge and integrating new concepts that help the novice leader evolve over time into a highly effective, adaptable leader. The ability of a leader to grow and adapt will contribute to the success of the individual leader, their organization and the profession of midwifery as a whole.

Informal versus Formal Leaders

It is often assumed that an individual with a formal role or title is the true leader of the organization. Indeed, someone with a formal leadership role has the responsibility of per-

Table 16–1 Differences Between Leadership and Management

Leadership	*Management*
People	Things
Spontaneity	Structure
Empowerment	Control
Effectiveness	Efficiency
Programmer	Program
Investment	Expense
Principles	Techniques
Transformation	Transaction
Principle-centered power	Utility
Discernment	Measurement
Doing the right things	Doing things right
Direction	Speed
Top line	Bottom line
Purposes	Methods
Principles	Practices
On the systems	In the systems
"Is the ladder against the right wall?"	Climbing the ladder fast

forming various tasks and is often the one held accountable for performance of staff, clinical outcomes, or financial success. Often, individuals without a formal leadership role or title are the drivers behind the success of a midwifery practice. These informal leaders tend to be the relationship builders within and outside of the practice. They inspire the team to work together toward common goals and influence external partners to work with the team. As Cooper and Sawaf (1996) stated in *Executive EQ*: "The most important leadership trait for winning in business is not having the best technology, products, or services. It's having the best relationships." These relationships can be developed by every member of the team. In fact, if every member of a midwifery practice is developed and empowered to embrace their role as a "leader," imagine the potential for success!

Characteristics of a Good Midwifery Leader

What skills or attributes are needed to be a good midwifery leader? A sound understanding of the current health care environment, foundational knowledge of midwifery practice,

Table 16–2 Individual and Leadership Style Assessment Tools

Assessment Tool	*Resource Information*
DISC Style Assessment	www.discinsights.com
Myers-Briggs Type Indicator (MBTI)	www.cpp.com
The Thomas Concept	www.inpsyte.com
True Colors	www.truecolors.org
Winslow Personal Dynamic Profile	www.winslow-consulting.com

and basic communication skills are a good place to start. There is a core set of competencies that are needed for any individual in a leadership position. These competencies can be divided into "hard" and "soft" skills. Many of the hard skills have been addressed in detail in earlier chapters and include knowledge about:

- High-quality, cost-effective, evidence-based patient care
- Practice operations including patient flow and tracking
- Credentialing, both for hospital privileges and payers
- Quality management
- Marketing and practice promotion
- Billing, coding, and collections
- Budget development and management
- Human resource management
- Ethics

Soft skills are the foundational leadership skills that are critical for any leader. They include things such as:

- Communication
- Conflict management
- Developing and sustaining high-performance teams
- Inspiring others to grow and develop
- Recruitment and retention of staff

The soft skills are often the ones that are lacking in a new leader. Learning about and developing these skills is key to the success of any individual in a leadership role. In examining these skills further, they seem to be based upon human relationship skills. In fact, many of these skills are grounded in the behavioral science concept that is referred to as emotional intelligence or EI. The next section explores emotional intelligence and the relationship between EI qualities and successful leadership.

Emotional Intelligence and Leadership

The concept of IQ is common knowledge throughout our society, and is often thought of as the key to one's success. Most of us took standardized tests throughout our educational journey, and many continue to think that the individual with the highest test scores will be the most successful in their endeavors. In the last two decades Goleman (1994, 1998b, 2000, 2002), Bar-On and Parker (2000), Cooper (1997a, 2001, 2002), Cooper and Sawaf (1996), Essi Systems (1997), and many others have published numerous articles, books, and assessment tools addressing the issue of emotional intelligence. According to Cooper, "Emotional Intelligence is the ability to sense, understand, and effectively apply the power and acumen of emotions as a source of human energy, information, connection, and influence." One of the hallmarks of midwifery is the foundation of a trusting relationship with women and their families. The ability to listen to women and support them throughout pregnancy and birth through this trusting relationship relies on many characteristics of emotional intelligence explored in Cooper and Sawaf's book, *Executive EQ,* including emotional self awareness, emotional awareness of others, emotional expression, intentionality, creativity, resilience, interpersonal connections, constructive discontent, outlook, compassion, intuition, trust, personal power, and integrated self. The ability of a midwife to utilize these EI skills to influence healthy pregnancy and birth outcomes and patient satisfaction speaks clearly to the value of these soft skills.

Successful midwifery leaders skillfully use emotional intelligence qualities to influence relationships within and outside of their practice. They are able to recruit and retain highly satisfied staff as well as build strong, collaborative relationships with physician colleagues, hospital administrators, and community partners. Such leaders develop a practice philosophy, culture, and environment that attract patients and leave them so satisfied that they refer others for the same wonderful care. We have all heard of practices led by a technically skilled or business-savvy leader that were not able to survive challenging times. As is well documented in many other areas of business, I would suggest that the midwifery leader who has highly developed EI is more likely be successful, even in challenging times.

In *Primal Leadership: Realizing the Power of Emotional Intelligence,* Daniel Goleman (2002) describes leadership styles based on the underlying emotional intelligence capabilities that each style utilizes and links the style to outcomes. These styles are:

- Visionary
- Coaching
- Affiliative
- Democratic
- Pacesetting
- Commanding

It is critical for a midwifery leader to understand the leadership style that he or she uses most comfortably and the importance of transitioning to another style depending upon the situation. For example, an affiliative midwifery leader is one who believes that staff are valuable individuals and builds morale, loyalty, and a sense of team. In a time of crisis, facing funding cuts for example, this leader may need to transition to the pacesetting style, focusing on productivity and new opportunities. Without the ability to adapt one's leadership style to the situation, the affiliative midwifery leader may lead his or her team to its demise.

Organizational Structure and Culture

As discussed in Chapter 9, there are many models of midwifery practice. Some practices are independent and small with low volume whereas others are housed within a large and very complex organization and see tremendous volume. It is critical for a leader to take the organizational structure into account when determining the style of leadership that is the best fit for the success of the organization. The organizational chart is a graphical description of positions and chain of command in an organization. Horizontal and vertical relationships within an organization are even more clearly defined by job descriptions, and evaluation of the performance of individuals in these roles is addressed in a performance appraisal tool. A leader must understand how he or she fits within the organization and from there can determine the most appropriate leadership style and course of action to take.

The mission, vision, and values of an organization further help a leader assess the organizational landscape and the direction in which the organization is moving. One of the qualities of a leader that influences employee satisfaction is "leading through vision and values" (Developmental Dimensions International [DDI], 1996). This section addresses the concepts of mission, vision, and values and provides some suggestions for implementing the strategic planning process in your organization. One of the most important roles of every leader is to guide the team in defining their own vision, mission, and values statements and to use these statements as a charter upon which to design the day-to-day activities of the team.

One of the first and most important steps in an organization's strategic plan is defining the *vision*. Identifying the long-term overall vision, the "dream" or idealized scenario of what the future is for the organization, is a critical step in helping the whole team move forward in the same direction. Without a clear vision, it is a challenge for a leader to plan for steps to achieve the vision.

The *mission* of an organization is the organization's purpose and place in the world. It is the action-oriented statement that defines what we do and who we are. A leader must have a clear mission in order to keep on task and maintain focus on what actions need to be taken. Evaluation of an organization's success should focus on measurable goals that are based on the mission.

Finally, an organization must have a set of agreed upon *values*, principles that define the beliefs and behaviors that are expected by every member of the team. Without foundational values there are no guiding principles for the members of the team. Values such as excellence, integrity, respect, and teamwork are commonly found in organizational charters but are not consistently lived in daily practice. It is the responsibility of the leader to model the core values and to hold each member of the team accountable to exhibit behaviors that are in alignment with the values.

Table 16–3 lists common values statements. It is a useful tool to use with a team to help members define their own personal values and then expand to define team values. Ask members to select three to five core values that will be the foundation of all behaviors exhibited with team members and customers.

The culture of an organization is based upon the foundational values and is manifested by the "feel" of an organization. You may have been a customer in a business where you "felt" the enthusiasm, respect, and commitment of the employees. The needs of the customer are often placed at the center of these organizations and the employee behaviors and business processes are driven by the culture. You may also have experienced a business that left you with a "feeling" of having something missing. Negative employee attitudes, poor teamwork, and inadequate quality of work are often seen in organizations that do not have a healthy culture. Success is not likely when there is a conflict between the formal values statement and the behaviors exhibited by employees. This conflict impacts customer or client satisfaction and employee satisfaction, thereby causing employee turnover and finally impacting the quality of work or service provided.

A healthy midwifery practice has a vision and mission statement focused on excellent patient care and outcomes. There is also a core set of values that is consistently exhibited by every member of the team. It is the leader's role to help the practice develop a culture based

Table 16–3 Common Value Statements

Truth	Persistence	Resources
Efficiency	Sincerity	Dependability
Initiative	Fun	Trust
Environmentalism	Relationships	Excellence
Power	Wisdom	Teamwork
Control	Flexibility	Service
Courage	Perspective	Profitability
Competition	Commitment	Freedom
Excitement	Recognition	Friendship
Creativity	Learning	Influence
Happiness	Honesty	Justice
Honor	Originality	Quality
Innovation	Candor	Hard work
Obedience	Prosperity	Responsiveness
Financial growth	Respect	Fulfillment
Community	Fairness	Purposefulness
Integrity	Order	Strength
Peace	Spirituality	Self-control
Loyalty	Adventure	Cleverness
Clarity	Cooperation	Success
Security	Humor	Stewardship
Love	Collaboration	Support

on the mission, vision and values statements. This foundation will guide the rest of the strategy development, which will lead the practice through a journey of successful growth.

Building a Practice Team: The Role of the Leader

Some leaders are entrepreneurs, starting with an idea they develop a business and grow it into a large organization. Other leaders step into a well-established organization and are charged with the task of moving the organization to the next level. Some leaders inherit an organization rich with success and tradition whereas others step into a complex, dysfunctional group and are faced with conflict and poor performance. Regardless of the package we receive when we step into a leadership role, it is the responsibility of the leader to build a team of highly functional individuals who are the foundation of success for the organization.

Steven Covey, an internationally respected business consultant and author, published a classic business book titled *The 7 Habits of Highly Effective People* in 1989. An inspirational classic, Covey walks readers through his 7 Habits and how to improve personal, interpersonal, organizational, and managerial effectiveness. The 7 Habits as defined by Covey are:

- Habit 1:   Be Proactive
- Habit 2:   Begin with the End in Mind
- Habit 3:   Put First Things First

- Habit 4:   Think Win/Win
- Habit 5:   Seek First to Understand/Then to Be Understood
- Habit 6:   Synergize
- Habit 7:   Sharpen the Saw

Recently, Covey introduced the 8th Habit, "To Find Your Voice and Inspire Others to Find Theirs" (Covey, 2004). This concept moves beyond the organizational umbrella of vision, mission, and values to focus on the individual member of the team. Indeed, when investigating why employees leave an organization, the number one reason is a poor relationship with their direct supervisor. Therefore, in order for a leader to build a highly effective team, he or she must first seek to develop a relationship with each member of the team and learn what that individual needs to feel valued and heard. Very eloquently, Covey states, ". . . leadership is communicating to people their worth and potential so clearly that they come to see it in themselves." This critical step of relationship building with each member of the team must be accomplished in order to move the whole team to a higher level.

In a successful team there is respect for individual strengths and opportunities for collaboration. Every team member is acknowledged for the talents he or she brings to the team, and diverse strengths are valued. If every member of the team came from the same background, and had identical skills and similar weaknesses, the team would be greatly successful in some areas and woefully lacking in others. Often, individual members of a team do not understand their own personal strengths and vulnerabilities, never mind those of their teammates. Knowledge about one's self and one's teammates only serves to strengthen the team as a whole. When team members understand that they may need to adapt their communication style to better communicate with another member of the team, the quality of the relationship is improved. It is this ability of a team to better understand each other that leads to enhanced team performance and success.

Whether building a team from scratch or working with an existing team, once the leader has invested in getting to know each member of the team, the next step is to help the members of the team learn more about each other. There are numerous assessment tools and surveys that explore personality traits or styles. Common examples are the Myers-Briggs Type Indicator, the DISC Personality System, the Thomas System, and True Colors. Based on well-established behavioral science research, each of these tools provides a framework for identifying an individual's predominant personality style. In the context of a team, learning about the styles of teammates and how to best communicate with team members with differing styles enhances team relationships.

Consider the stereotypical midwife: caring and compassionate, a good listener and supporter, flexible, and respectful of the natural process of birth using technology only when indicated. Now, think about the skills that every midwife must have in order to be successful, such as clinical knowledge, competent technical skills, conflict management skills, and critical thinking ability. The midwife must balance her most comfortable skill set of listening and caring with technical ability in order to be a successful clinician. In any given team individuals come with strengths in certain areas, and the best team provides a balance of technical or hard skills with the people or soft skills. Some members of a midwifery practice bring very different skills than others. Acknowledgment of those whose strengths lie in developing forms and revising clinical practice guidelines is just as important as supporting those who like to teach students or represent the practice well in meetings with community agencies.

In Kenneth Blanchard's classic, *The One-Minute Manager Builds High Performing Teams* (Blanchard, Carew, & Parisi-Carew, 1990), the authors identify the following characteristics of high performing teams:

- Purpose
- Empowerment
- Relationships and communication
- Flexibility
- Optimal performance
- Recognition and appreciation
- Morale

The leader can be seen as a team facilitator, serving to help the team maximize success by providing the basic structure and tools that the team needs to function at a high level. The tools will vary depending on the make-up of the team. Blanchard et al. state, "Effective team leaders adjust their style to provide what the group can't provide for itself" (Blanchard et al., 1990, p. 74).

Managing a team consisting of members with diverse backgrounds, personality styles, work ethics, and interests presents a challenge for any leader. The midwifery leader who can bring the team together under a common vision, mission, and values is one who can flex into the appropriate leadership style dictated by the current situation. Maintaining the principles of emotional intelligence enhances the quality of team interactions and serves to provide a foundation for trusting relationships within and outside of the team.

Coaching: The New Leadership Skill

In decades past, it was thought that the role of the leader was to direct or to dictate to others in order to get the job done. Today, leaders are thought to be more effective if they assume the role of coach to support their staff and empower them to do the job they were hired to do. The concept of coaching can be applied to day-to-day interactions, mentoring, and development, as well addressing performance issues. Many *Fortune* 500 companies have invested in an executive coach or a business coach for key leaders to improve in certain areas of their job. The International Coach Federation is one of the leaders in the executive coaching arena. Seek out information on coaching and the role of the coach on their Web site at http://www.coachfederation.org.

A leadership style that integrates coaching leads to increased trust between a leader and members of the group. A philosophy of coaching as a foundation for communication between staff members provides an opportunity for staff to learn from each other in a manner that honors the expertise and experience of each team member. The skill of coaching is not necessarily intuitive for many leaders. It, like many other leadership skills, is a learned behavior that takes time, effort, practice, and patience to achieve.

Consider the following myths about coaching for midwifery leaders:

- *Coaching is something a midwife does, not something she needs.* Wrong! In fact, individuals at all levels of an organization benefit from coaching to help them process and organize their thoughts, integrate new ideas, and modify their approach to an issue or challenge.
- *Coaching is only warranted when dealing with negative performance or performance that needs improvement.* Wrong! Coaching can be useful in dealing with a variety of topics from clinical situations to interpersonal conflict and even career development. The role of the coach is to listen, provide support and insight into an issue, and encourage expansive thought and alternative solutions from the individual. In fact, a regular "coaching session" can serve to develop a foundation of trust in the leader/ employee relationship and to build self-esteem in the individual being coached.
- *Coaching is more about being nice to employees than being constructive.* Wrong! Coaching certainly isn't about being mean to your staff, but it is important for a coach to communicate honestly and directly. Staff appreciates positive feedback and kind gestures, but they also value your integrity, and that includes learning about the pluses and minuses of their performance.
- *Coaching leads to an environment where your employees do most of your work.* Wrong! Coaching takes you and your team to a higher level of productivity and accountability. In this new environment, the role of the coach has even more importance in keeping the team members focused on the vision, mission, and values and constantly seeking out new opportunities to raise the bar.

In summary, coaching is a leadership skill that is useful in many situations faced by today's midwifery leader. It is a tool that facilitates growth and resiliency in our staff and helps us maintain focus on the issue at hand and the positive attributes of the employee. A leader who effectively integrates the skill of coaching appropriately can communicate with employees about a variety of issues yet retain an environment of trust and respect. Teaching staff how to integrate the concept of coaching into daily team interactions can help a team survive challenging situations and move them forward to a higher level of effectiveness and success.

The Leader and Change

Although the concept of change as has been explored in depth in the literature, the following quote by James Rowland Angell provides timeless insight, "Change is no modern invention. It is as old as time and as unlikely to disappear. It has always to be counted on as of the essence of human experience". For midwifery leaders, this couldn't be truer. Changes in the clinical arena impact midwifery practice every day, influencing our practice models, profitability, and success. We are also faced with profound changes in the health care system, our society, and our world, which in turn impact our patients, our practice, and our profession. A strong midwifery leader not only faces change with courage and manages change successfully, but also anticipates and embraces change as an ally. A successful midwifery practice is positioned to adapt quickly, whether it be a simple change in coding regulations or an in-depth performance-improvement project.

Knowing that change is inevitable, a midwifery leader should assess the ability of a candidate for employment to change as early as the first interview. Ask direct questions about how the individual manages change and request specific examples describing how she has managed change in the past. It's always a warning sign when a prospective staff member simply states, "I hate change." For existing members of your practice, consider offering a training on change that provides an assessment of the individual's change management skills and information about successful change in the workplace.

Heller (1998) describes a simple structure for addressing change in a small pocket-sized book called *Managing Change*. The first step described is to understand change, including the causes and sources of change and the types of change. The second step is to plan change, which begins with focusing on goals and identifying essential changes and stresses the importance of anticipating the effects of and possible resistance to change. The third step is to implement change, which requires clear communication about the change and engagement of team members to build commitment. The final step is to consolidate change including monitoring and evaluation and building on change to maximize the success of the organization.

The ability to cope with stress and change, both minor and major, is often referred to as "resiliency." Resilient individuals tend to achieve a healthy balance in their personal and professional lives. Some of the key characteristics of a positive, resilient mindset described by Brooks and Goldstein (2004) include feeling in control of one's life and learning from both success and failure. Orioli (Essi Systems, 2003) developed an assessment tool that offers a great deal of information about resiliency, the Resiliency Map. Orioli and her team at Essi Systems describe six major areas in which to explore resiliency:

- Environmental Demands
- Environmental Assets
- Resilient Beliefs and Values
- Personal Coping Skills
- Social Coping Skills
- Health and Functioning

In addition, Orioli outlines building blocks for change that include 1) Reflect, 2) Specify and Declare, and 3) Build Accountability and Support. Specific guidelines for successful change management are reviewed and individuals are encouraged to formally plan for change.

In summary, the successful midwifery leader must be a change agent both within and outside of the practice. Investment in learning strategies for change management will benefit the individual, the practice, and the organization.

Leadership and Power

We all have faced a situation where an individual in a leadership position uses the authority of the position to exert power and control over employees. In a healthy work environment, the leader does not need to use power to influence others, but instead strives to empower individuals so that they can achieve at a higher level. This concept is sometimes referred to as "participative leadership," and is a leadership skill that builds trust within an organization. Kouzes and Posner (2002) described four leadership essentials to strengthen others:

- Ensure self-leadership.
- Provide choice.
- Develop competence and confidence.
- Foster accountability.

This "paradox of power" is summarized in one simple statement: "We become most powerful when we give our own power away" (Kouzes & Posner, 2002, p. 284). Implementing this concept in a midwifery practice leads to more engaged practice partners and increases the effectiveness and success of each individual as well as the practice as a whole. Without the need to micromanage minor details, the practice leader can focus on external relationship building and business strategy. Empowered team members are more comfortable taking risk and are more likely to embrace change. Building a practice culture of empowerment also serves to develop leadership skills in individual practice members, which aids in succession planning.

Steps to Developing as a Leader

Look back to the beginning of this chapter and consider again the background of most midwives who are currently in a leadership role; a highly competent midwife is promoted into a leadership role because of her excellent clinical skills. This promotion does not automatically make the individual a leader. The journey to becoming a successful leader is one that is launched well before we accept a formal leadership role. And it is a journey that requires on-going self-discovery, reflection, growth, and learning. Leaders change and adapt to meet the needs of the organization. The leader you are today is very different than the leader you will be in the future. Purposeful planning for developing as a leader will ensure that you will be successful on your journey. The result will be greater success for you as an individual as well as for your practice and the profession of midwifery. Consider the following steps in your development as a leader:

Step 1. Learn more about yourself. Consider an investment of time and energy in one or more of the self-assessment tools that have been introduced in this chapter. Whether you select a simple paper and pencil test or seek out the services of a professional consultant or coach, learning about your personality style and your individual strengths and vulnerabilities is an exciting first step in developing as a leader. Once you have a solid grasp of who you are, you can begin the process of building on your strengths and learn to manage your vulnerabilities.

Step 2. Learn more about your team. Invest in the success of each individual in your practice and the organization as a whole by offering others the opportunity to learn about themselves. What are their dreams and goals? What talents do they have and how might they develop and grow? When you have a better understanding of what makes the members of your team tick, you can adapt your communication and leadership style to work more effectively with each individual and the whole team.

Step 3. Learn more about leadership. You don't have to obtain a master's degree in business to build your leadership skills. Read about leadership styles and skills and experiment with various approaches to determine what might work best for you in your current environment. Seek out learning opportunities through seminars or workshops that focus on leadership. The Midwifery Business Institute offered through the University of Michigan is one example of an excellent program that provides continuing education on business for midwives. Join the Service Director's Network to meet other midwifery leaders. Find a mentor or coach to support you on your leadership journey.

Step 4. Learn more about business. Many of the concrete and practical skills that work in the business world are applicable to midwifery practice. A better understanding of basic business concepts such as strategic planning and marketing can help you to bring your practice to a new and stronger level of success. Knowing the language used by those in a decision-making position in your organization helps you to more effectively communicate and will increase respect and acknowledgement of your leadership abilities. The Mini MBA: Strategies for Successful Midwifery Practice is a business-focused training that offers a broad spectrum of business content for all midwives.

Step 5. Develop relationships and partnerships. Look at the relationships within your practice and the community at-large that can influence your success as a leader. Determine which relationships need to be strengthened and identify new relationships that need to be developed and focus on building those relationships. Communicate in a purposeful manner, offer your talents in areas outside of your comfort zone, and get involved in activities and organizations that can enhance who you are as a leader. Your local or state perinatal organization and the March of Dimes are examples of strategic partnership opportunities.

Step 6. Enjoy the Journey. Have fun along the way and seek opportunities to celebrate the minor wins and the major victories. Maintain your sense of humor as you face challenges and find ways to build fun into your daily activities. Journal, archive photographs, and occasionally take a "time-out" to reflect on where you've been and where you are going. Enjoy the small pleasures that are part of the leadership journey and revel in the sunlight of those around you whom you have led and supported on their own individual journeys.

Summary

In closing, being a leader is one of the most fulfilling and rewarding roles a midwife can assume. Whether you hold a formal leadership position or are a key member of a team or committee, you have the wonderful opportunity to impact individuals, families, and organizations in a way that will forever leave your imprint. Our profession needs creative and powerful leaders to improve the health of women and babies as well as communities and organizations. Take the giant leap into leadership and remember to enjoy the journey.

Chapter Exercises

1. **Exploring Leadership Attributes**
   First, think about the leaders who have influenced your professional life. List the attributes that impacted you and made a difference in your

professional life and role as a leader. Next, think about the people you have influenced in your professional life including students, staff, and colleagues. List the attributes that you exhibit that have made a difference in their lives. Now, summarize the leadership attributes that you currently see as your strengths, and those that might present you with an opportunity for improvement. Finally, develop an action plan to help you develop the leadership attributes that will most impact your success as a leader.

2. **Vision, Mission, and Values**
   Refer to the beginning of this chapter and review the section on vision, mission, and values (pages 334 to 335). Now, craft your own personal leadership vision, mission, and values. Take some time with your peers and staff exploring these concepts and identify opportunities for you to more fully live your potential as a leader every day.

References

Bar-On, R., & Parker, J. D. A. (2000). *The handbook of emotional intelligence: Theory, development, assessment, and application at home, school, and in the workplace.* San Francisco: Jossey-Bass.

Blanchard, K., Carew, D., Parisi-Carew, E. (1990). *The one minute manager builds high performing teams.* New York: William.

Blanchard, K., & O'Connor, M. (2003). *Managing by values: How to put your values into action for extraordinary results.* San Francisco: Berrett-Koehler.

Blanchard, K., & Shula, D. (2001). *The little book of coaching: Motivating people to be winners.* New York: Blanchard Family Partnership and Shula Enterprises.

Brooks, R., & Goldstein, S. (2004). *The power of resilience: Achieving balance, confidence, and personal strength in your life.* Chicago: Contemporary Books.

Brounstein, M. (2000). *Coaching and mentoring for dummies.* Foster City, CA: IDG Books Worldwide.

Buckingham, M., & Coffman, C. (1999). *First, break all the rules: What the world's greatest managers do differently.* New York: Simon & Schuster.

Byham, W. C., & Cox, J. (1988). *Zapp! The lightning of empowerment.* New York: Ballantine Books.

Charan, R., & Tichy, N. M. (1998). *Every business is a growth business: How your company can prosper year after year.* New York: Random House.

Cloke, K., & Goldsmith, J. (2000). *Resolving conflicts at work: A complete guide for everyone on the job.* San Francisco: Jossey-Bass.

Cooper, R. K. (1997a, December). Applying emotional intelligence in the workplace; training and development. *Training and Development, 31–38*

Cooper, R. K. (1997b). *Leadership metrics and mechanisms: The executive EQ model; Q-Metrics.* San Francisco: Advance Excellence Systems.

Cooper, R. K. (2001). *The other 90%: How to unlock your vast untapped potential for leadership & life.* New York: Crown Business.

Cooper, R. K. (2002). *Excelerating: Speeding through challenges with calm effectiveness in leadership and life.* San Francisco: Advanced Excellence Systems.

Cooper, R. K. & Sawaf, A. (1996). *Executive EQ: Emotional intelligence in leadership and organizations.* New York: Grosset/Putnam.

Covey, S. R. (1989). *The 7 habits of highly effective people.* New York: Simon & Schuster.

Covey, S. R. (2004). *The 8th habit: From effectiveness to greatness.* New York: Free Press

Developmental Dimensions International. (1996). *Retaining talent: The leader's role.* Pittsburgh, PA: Author.

Essi Systems. (1997). *The EQ map: An integrated EQ assessment and individual profile: Q-Metrics.* San Francisco: Author.

Essi Systems. (2003). *The resiliency map.* San Francisco: Author.

George, B. (2003). *Authentic leadership: Rediscovering the secrets for creating lasting value.* San Francisco: Jossey-Bass, Wiley.

Goleman, D. (1994). *Emotional intelligence: Why it can matter more than IQ.* New York: Bantam.

Goleman, D. (1998a, November–December). What makes a leader? *Harvard Business Review,* 91–102.

Goleman, D. (1998b). *Working with emotional intelligence.* New York: Bantam.

Goleman, D. (2000, March–April). Leadership that gets results. *Harvard Business Review,* 79–90.

Goleman, D. (2002). *Primal leadership: Realizing the power of emotional intelligence.* Boston: Harvard Business School Press.

Gordon, D. (2001). *Handling conflict.* Mason, OH: South-Western Educational Publishing.

Gorman, T. (1998). *The complete idiot's guide to MBA basics.* New York: Alpha Books.

Harvard Business Review on Change. (1998). Boston: Harvard Business School Press.

Harvard Business Review on Culture and Change. (2002). Boston: Harvard Business School Press.

Heller, R. (1998). *Managing change.* New York: DK Publishing.

Institute for Motivational Living. (2001). *Introduction to behavioral analysis.* New Castle, PA: IML DISC Insights.

Johnson, S. (1998). *Who moved my cheese?* New York: GP Putnam's Sons.

Kouzes, J. M., & Posner, Z. (2002). *The leadership challenge.* San Francisco: Jossey-Bass.

Lencioni, P. (2000). *The four obsessions of an extraordinary executive.* San Francisco: Jossey-Bass.

Lundin, S., Christensen, J., & Paul, H. (2000). *FISH! for life.* New York: Hyperion.

Lundin, S., Christensen, J., Paul, H., & Strand, P. (2002). *FISH! tales: Real-life stories to help you transform your workplace and your life.* New York: Hyperion.

Lundin, S., Christensen, J., & Paul, H. (2003). *FISH! sticks: A remarkable way to adapt to changing times and keep your work fresh.* New York: Hyperion.

Lundin, S., Paul, H., & Christensen, J. (2000). *FISH! A remarkable way to boost morale and improve results.* New York: Hyperion.

Lynn, A. B. (2002). *The emotional intelligence activity book: 50 activities for promoting EQ at work.* New York: American Management Association.

Maxwell, J. C. (2002). *Leadership 101: What every leader needs to know.* Nashville, TN: Thomas Nelson.

McClure, L. (2000). *Anger and conflict in the workplace: Spot the signs, avoid the trauma.* Manassas Park, VA: Impact Publications.

Nigro, N. (2003). *The everything coaching and mentoring book: How to increase productivity, foster talent, and encourage success.* Avon, MA: Adams Media Corporation.

Pachter, B. (2000). *The power of positive confrontation: The skills you need to know to handle conflicts at work, at home, and in life.* New York: Marlowe & Company.

Ryback, D. (1998). *Putting emotional intelligence to work: Successful leadership is more than IQ.* Boston: Butterworth-Heinemann.

Scott, S. (2002). *Fierce conversations: Achieving success at work and in life, one conversation at a time.* New York: Penguin Putnam.

Senge, P., Kleiner, A., Roberts, C., Ross, R., Roth, G., & Smith, B. (1999). *The dance of change: The challenges to sustaining momentum in learning organizations.* New York: Doubleday.

Thomas, J., & Thomas, T. (1998). *The Thomas concept.* Austin, TX: Inpsyte.

Varney, H., Kriebs, J., & Gegor, C. (2004). *Varney's midwifery* (4th ed.). Sudbury, MA: Jones and Bartlett.

Wheatley, M. J. (1999). *Leadership and the new science: Discovering order in a chaotic world.* San Francisco: Berrit-Koehler.

Zemke, R., Raines, C., & Filipczak, B. (2000). *Generations at work: Managing the clash of veterans, boomers, Xers, and nexters in your workplace.* New York: American Management Association.

Index